EVA SCRIVO
ON BEAUTY

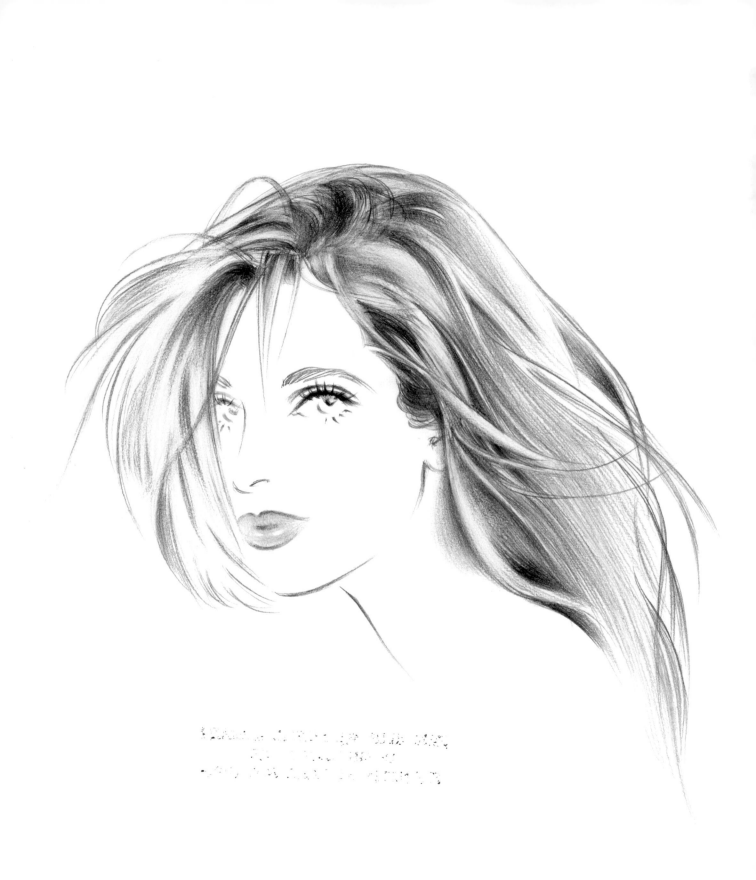

EVA SCRIVO
ON BEAUTY

THE TOOLS, TECHNIQUES, AND
INSIDER KNOWLEDGE EVERY WOMAN
NEEDS TO BE HER MOST BEAUTIFUL,
CONFIDENT SELF

EVA SCRIVO

WITH GINA WAY AND ARIK EFROS

ATRIA BOOKS
NEW YORK   LONDON   TORONTO   SYDNEY

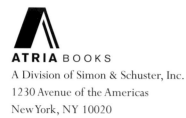

ATRIA BOOKS

A Division of Simon & Schuster, Inc.
1230 Avenue of the Americas
New York, NY 10020

First Atria Books hardcover edition April 2011

ATRIA BOOKS and colophon are trademarks of Simon & Schuster, Inc.

For information about special discounts for bulk purchases,
please contact Simon & Schuster Special Sales at
1-866-506-1949 or business@simonandschuster.com.

The Simon & Schuster Speakers Bureau can bring authors
to your live event. For more information or to book an event,
contact the Simon & Schuster Speakers Bureau at
1-866-248-3049 or visit our website at www.simonspeakers.com.

All haircuts, color, styling, and makeup by Eva Scrivo

Designed by Deborah DeStaffan

Photography by Marcqui Akins
Contributing photographer: Rebecca Greenfield
Illustrations by Jennie Yip

Manufactured in the United States of America

10   9   8   7   6   5   4   3   2   1

Library of Congress Cataloging-in-Publication Data

Scrivo, Eva.
Eva Scrivo on beauty : the tools, techniques, and insider knowledge every woman needs to be her most beautiful, confident self / by Eva Scrivo.
p.   cm.
1. Beauty, Personal. I. Title.
RA778.S37   2010
646.7'042—dc22   2010039581

ISBN 978-1-4391-6471-6
ISBN 978-1-4391-6486-0 (ebook)

To you, Dad

CONTENTS

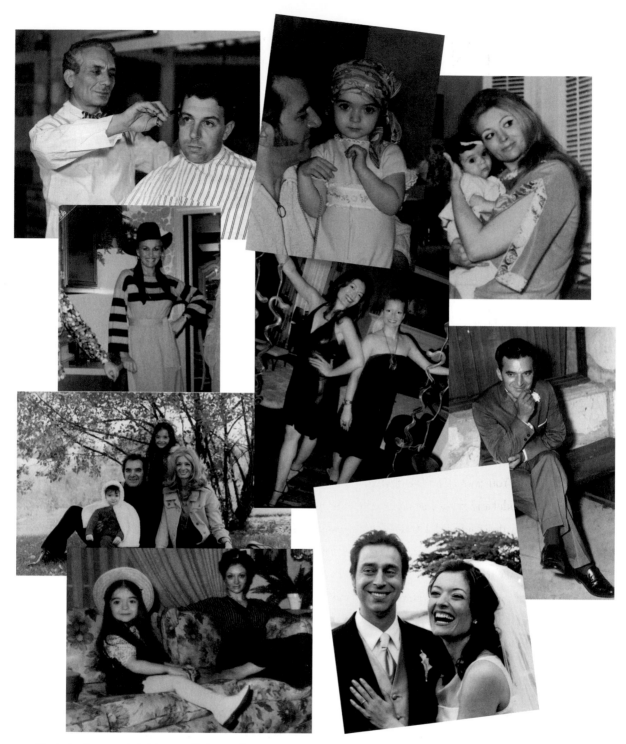

Clockwise from top left: My grandfather, Raffaele Scrivo, cutting hair in his barbershop, circa 1952. Mimicking my mom with her head scarf, with my dad, Vincenzo. My favorite photo—me with my mother, Saundra. My father, Vincenzo, on his wedding day, 1959. Me and my husband, Arik, on our wedding day. I've always loved to accessorize! Family portrait. Aunt Jan wearing her famous knit dress. With my best friend, Lynn.

INTRODUCTION

MY LIFE IN BEAUTY

I was born with a full head of hair. Not the wisps that come with most newborns, but actual two-inch-long, baby-soft black hair. My grandmother neatly tied a pink ribbon that she had removed from a soap set from the hospital gift shop (the only thing she could find with a ribbon) into a bow at the front of my head. Thus, I wore a hair accessory before ever wearing a piece of clothing. Perhaps it was a sign of things to come. I have been consumed by beauty and fashion for as long as I can remember.

You could even say that it is in my DNA. My mother was a professional model and my father, an interior designer by trade, was also a frustrated fashion designer and a trained hairdresser (his father was a barber). Even as a small child, I innately understood the rejuvenating power of beauty. While other three-year-old girls played with dolls, my favorite toys were hair curlers, which I loved to put in everyone's hair. I was fascinated with playing beautician. My aunt Jan, who had chronic back problems, loves to tell the story of how, at around that age, I would insist, "Why don't you let me curl your hair? It will make you feel better!" The relationship between how one looks and how one feels made perfect sense to me even then.

By the age of nine, I was studying drawing, painting, and sewing, and attending theater school. While my background in the dramatic arts has certainly come in handy for running a salon and managing creative personalities, learning to paint helped hone my eye as a hair colorist and makeup artist, and sewing taught me how to cut a straight line. I began to utilize these skills sooner than I'd expected. When I was about eleven, my father handed me my grandfather's shears and gave step-by-step instructions on how to cut his hair while he held a hand mirror to see what I was doing. At around the same time, my mother bestowed on me a hair-color brush and a mixing bowl and showed me how to touch up her ever-budding roots. (I remember her telling me that a famous colorist had given her the formula twenty years earlier, and since then she had mixed it herself every three weeks. A great professional is never forgotten.)

My parents' plan to raise a personal hairdresser had become perfectly clear, and word traveled fast among our huge Italian family! Soon I was being asked by my aunts, uncles, and cousins to bring my scissors to family functions. You can only imagine how exhausting holidays were for me! I still remember the horror of cutting my Grandma Scrivo's hair for the first time. She had always worn it pinned up, and on the day of her first appointment with me I found her sitting at the kitchen table with a garbage bag wrapped around her and her thin gray hair hanging down to her waist! She looked like a ghost of herself. With meatballs and "gravy" simmering, I snipped away while she made me promise not to take off too much length. This served as a poignant lesson that no matter who or how old, everyone wants to look good. Beauty is a part of all our lives, and this was the beginning of my personal journey.

By the time I entered cosmetology school at age seventeen, I had already been doing hair nearly half my life. With such powerful and supportive influences, my career in beauty seemed destined and came about very naturally. I never agonized about what I wanted to do with my life, as this profession quickly evolved into a true passion. I have had the good fortune to perform a craft that I love while being creative and making people happy on a daily basis.

After graduating from beauty school, I left my hometown in Michigan to live and work abroad. During those few years, I worked with some very talented hairdressers and fashion photographers in London and Milan. It was an amazing personal and professional growth experience that laid the groundwork for my eventual move to New York City. As is true for most of those brave enough to move to Manhattan on their own and in their early twenties, the first couple of years were about survival. I had no money and hardly knew anyone. I rented a one-bedroom apartment on the fourth floor of a walk-up building in the East Village, which at that time was still rather dangerous but also interesting and eclectic. Many artists lived there, and it was inspirational and exciting for me to be among them. I started doing hair and makeup on small jobs with equally small budgets. Some of the people I met there would ask me to cut their hair, so I invited them to my apartment. As I got busier, I decided to set up a makeshift salon in my living room and even installed a professional sink in my kitchen. New clients would often say to me, "You must be good, for people to walk up four flights of stairs!"

For the clients, going to a young, talented, but unknown hairdresser in an obscure apartment building felt like an experience in itself. For me, it was an amazing opportunity to connect with many intelligent and interesting women in an intimate setting. My clients came from all walks of life, and nearly every one of them enriched me far more than monetarily. Some have even made a profound impact on my life. I am proud to say that many of these clients still come to me today.

When people ask me how I built my business, they are always surprised that I did it strictly through word of mouth and out of a fourth-floor walk-up apartment. It wasn't until a few years later that I opened a small salon. I worked with my sister, Vinnetta, who did everything from making appointments to helping me blow-dry hair and shape eyebrows. We got busier and busier and soon had a waiting list of new clients. Although we were bursting at the seams, the thought of getting a bigger space felt overwhelming. Until one night I met a handsome man while hanging out in the Village, and my life changed.

His name was Arik. I remember the first day I invited him in for a haircut. He looked around my tiny but bustling salon in amazement and pointed out that I could have a much larger business. Arik held an MBA from a prestigious business school and was just as sensitive and creative as he was intelligent. Having spent several years in the corporate world, he had recently moved to New York and was working as a professor of marketing at a local university. In addition, he was an avid writer with an entrepreneurial spirit. As our personal relationship evolved, he also became more curious about my business. He helped me realize that women looked to me in ways that went beyond my role of a hairstylist. To many of them I was also a trusted beauty resource. My new boyfriend/consultant/mentor started teaching me about ways I could expand my small business. Our romance budded into a personal and business partnership that led to a proposal (of marriage!). Arik and I got married in

2004, about one and a half years after opening our first salon together (we often joke that it was like having a child out of wedlock). Most successes result from great partnerships in which both parties share the same dreams. I could not have done it without him.

At first, my passion for beauty was expressed through my hands, and people took notice. What started in my apartment led to a small salon that grew into a larger one, and then into a real company. When the media began to take notice and ask for interviews, I realized how much I loved talking about my craft. It gave me the opportunity to connect with people beyond my chair, while the beauty editors truly valued my insights. I understood how many misconceptions there are about beauty and the confusion created by the myriad of products advertised to women. In all the messages we are bombarded with, the missing element was honest education, and I was in a unique position to provide just that. Magazine articles and profiles paved the way to more television appearances, and in 2005 a radio talk show on beauty was born. Ultimately, it led to this book.

Having worked with thousands of women, while helping them with questions on everything imaginable relating to beauty, wellness, and fashion (and even relationships!), I consider teaching one of the most gratifying aspects of what I do. It is just as important as the physical transformations I create. I believe that the job of a beauty professional does not stop at the chair but should extend into a client's daily life and incorporate all elements of beauty. In addition to talent, skill, and hard work, this desire to continually hone my expertise, expand my knowledge, and share it with others has been instrumental in building my beauty business. I have always loved to connect with people and to freely share my insights, whether with clients, magazine readers, radio-show listeners and website subscribers, or my staff.

I am excited for this opportunity to establish a similar connection with you, to make professional techniques easy to understand, to empower you with newfound knowledge and skills, and ultimately help to improve the quality of your life. I hope that the information in the following pages will help encourage and inspire you to believe in your beauty and in yourself. By giving you an insider's view into the beauty business and the work of the professional, my objective is not to teach you to become a hairdresser or a makeup artist, but to simplify the technical information, translate industry terms, and make you a more knowledgeable consumer. Learning some of the methods and tools we use in the salon will better enable you to effectively communicate with your hairstylist to get the results you want and to work with your own hair at home. It will also give you a deeper understanding of and respect for the craft.

Realizing that you have more control than you ever thought over how you look and feel, and the energy that you exude, is inspirational and can be nothing short of life-changing. Beauty comes from a balance between your body and mind. It's an equation comprised of your hair, skin, makeup, lifestyle, physical and emotional health, and sense of style. You rarely need to change everything about yourself in order to look or feel better. Subtle shifts make a big impact—whether it's an adjustment to your hair or makeup, diet, or even attitude. Every day I see and speak with women who are unhappy with some aspects of their appearance. Most of the time, they find it hard to put their finger on what exactly is not working. It might be their hair, boredom with their overall look, or fear that they look older. Usually these women are missing just one or more pieces of the beauty pie, and it throws off the whole picture. The solution can be simple. For example, a slight deepening of the hair color can enliven the entire face, and the right hair length and layers can make one look ten years younger.

We all want to feel good about the way we look. This desire is not superficial, self-absorbed, or vain. On the contrary, it is natural, liberating, transformative, and, most important, within your reach. My father used to say, "A less beautiful woman who knows how to take care of herself can be far more attractive than one who is more physically perfect." Every woman can learn to be her most beautiful. It involves a set of skills that anyone can develop with the right instruction, and does not have to be confusing, intimidating, or difficult.

My own learning process on beauty continues each and every day. The beauty lessons have turned into life lessons, all of which I am honored and eager to share with you. I want to welcome you into my chair, and not just for an hour but for as long as you choose to stay in order to attain the tools and the knowledge you need. Now that you know a bit about my journey, let's get started with yours!

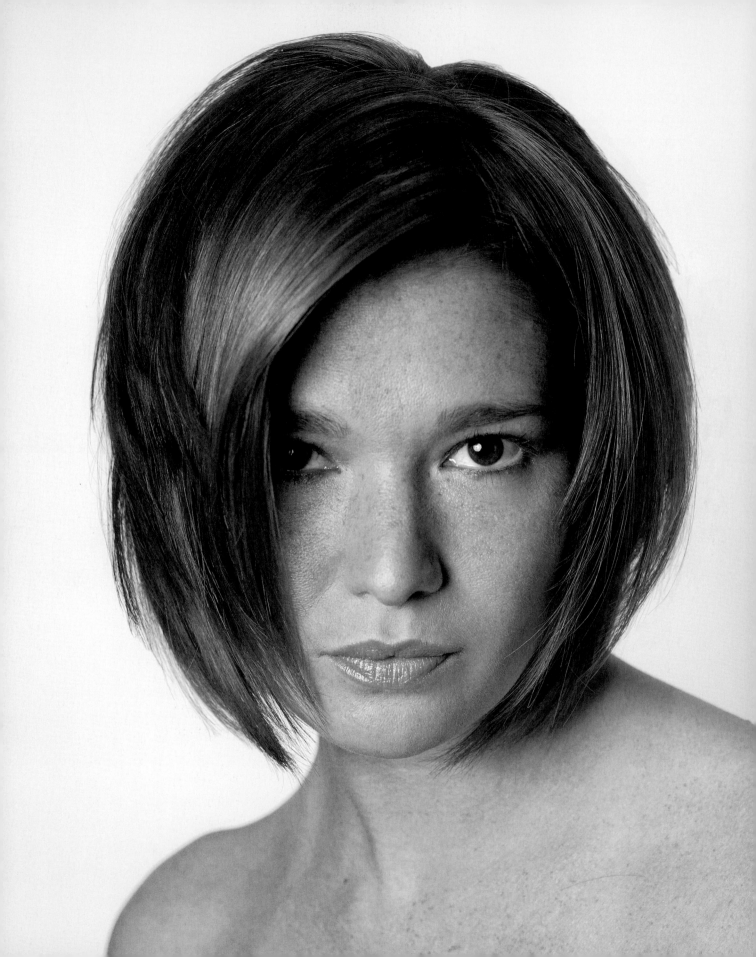

1

THE HAIRCUT ARCHITECTURE OF HAIR

I notice a woman's face when she walks into my salon for the first time, even before she sits in my chair to have me cut or color her hair. Her expression is one of eagerness and anticipation—as if she is wondering, "Will this haircut be 'the one'?"

Often a new client discovers me by word of mouth. She lives in New York and just loved what I did with her friend's hair. Other times, a first-time client has made a special trip to see me, perhaps from another part of the country. She may have saved up for this appointment, and this could be the first time she has decided to invest in herself and her appearance. Her expectations are high and rightfully so. She regards this as not just a haircut but a potentially life-changing experience, so I have a lot to live up to. I find these types of situations the most rewarding and gratifying.

Once we meet, I ask her what she likes about her hair and what she does not. I learn how she usually styles it and how she would ideally want it to look. Then I explain my vision for her hair and begin to work. I am confident that I will create the look she desires, but what is even more exciting is that I know this will actually change how she sees herself.

I witness this all the time in my clients, and I experience it myself when I get my hair cut, colored, and blown out. Suddenly, I feel twenty years old again, empowered and glowing from the experience. Many times, this physical transformation will also lead someone to modify other aspects of her life, such as making healthy dietary changes or starting a fitness program. It ignites a spark! This feeling that anything is possible produces a profound domino effect. More important, it does not have to wear off the day after the salon experience.

After cutting a new client's hair, I teach her how to re-create and maintain the new look at home by guiding her to the right styling products and showing her how to blow out her hair or dry it naturally so that the curl is brought out. After all, if she looks great only for that day, I have not accomplished my goal of giving her a cut she can work and live with. I am always happy to give away my "secrets" to empower the woman in my chair. This is what building a loyal, trusting relationship with a client is all about. These pages are filled with the same professional techniques and beauty education that I share in my salon, to put you in control of your looks.

HAIR AND YOUR IDENTITY

Your hair is often the first thing people notice about you. It represents who you are—your personality, sensuality, and sense of style. The relationship we have with our hair has a tremendous impact on our self-image and is so tied to our identity (for women and men) that it carries great psychological weight. It's no wonder that a woman will walk out of a salon very differently from when she walked in. Her hair—how it looks and how she feels about it—affects her energy and how she moves through the world.

The significance of hair is more than just personal. It is inextricably linked to our ideas about beauty and femininity. There is also a history and memory to how we think about it. When you look back on specific hairstyles you had in the past, they make you reminisce about those times in your life. You probably have mental images of how your mother wore her hair or how a friend wore hers that conjure up wonderful (and sometimes hilarious) memories. While our conception of hair is very personal, it is also iconic and universal. Consider the signature hairstyles of certain movie stars, such as Louise Brooks's bob, Audrey Hepburn's pixie cut, Brigitte Bardot's sexy bangs, and Jane Fonda's famous shag. These definitive representations of beauty and fashion have become an enduring part of our culture, and influence our perception of beauty.

Not surprisingly, how our hair looks engenders strong emotional reactions. A grown woman will cry when her hair is cut badly or damaged by a negligent color job. Some women don't want to go anywhere when their hair looks terrible. On a more poignant note, one of the most traumatic side effects of cancer treatment is hair loss. Many women have told me that they bravely managed to deal with everything else, but when they lost their hair, it all hit home. That is when they broke down.

Very often, hair is the first thing a woman wants to alter radically in a time of major transition. At the end of a relationship or before embarking on something new, there is a desire to shed this emotional weight and the memory that is bound in our hair. When you cut it off, or change the shape or color, a great sense of freedom and release often comes with it. This metamorphosis is not just physical but emotional, and actually makes you feel better and somehow lighter as the weight of your hair (and your past) is shorn. You become a new woman.

THE COMPOSITION OF HAIR
What It Is and Why It Behaves the Way It Does

Despite the enormous feeling we attach to it, hair has no nerve endings and no actual life at all. The strands that have sprouted from the follicles on your scalp are dead fibers composed primarily of keratin, the same hard protein that makes up your nails. Therefore, if hair is truly damaged, it should be cut off, because there is no way to "bring it back to life." Everyone's hair has essentially the same chemical composition. What makes your hair strands different from someone else's is their density (the amount of hair), weight (how thick or fine the strands are), and texture (straight, wavy, curly, or kinky).

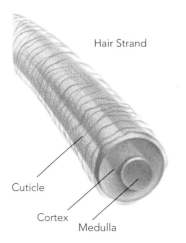

Hair Strand

Cuticle

Cortex

Medulla

The cuticle is the outer layer that encases the hair strand like the scales of a fish. If these scales are raised, the hair will feel coarse and look frizzy. If they are flattened, the hair looks and feels smooth. It is also shinier, since a flat surface better reflects light. A lifted cuticle allows light to scatter and makes the hair appear dull. The cuticle can be influenced and controlled by many factors: humid or dry air, heat from blow-dryers or irons, products that coat or manipulate the scales by smoothing or elevating them, chemicals in hair color, and the tools used to cut and shape the hair. Even though hair is not a living part of your body, you can affect its texture and how the outer layer feels and looks. If you understand on a fundamental level the basic composition of hair and how it reacts to cutting, coloring, styling, products, and the environment, you will find it easier to realize why yours behaves the way it does and how you can work with it more effectively. Many women mistakenly believe it is just their bad luck to have unruly, frizzy, or limp hair. However, a great haircut and color, the right hair care, and the right products, as well as adept styling, can transform it completely.

THE VALUE OF GREAT HAIR

When you buy something cheap, you lower the value of your own life.

—Noriko Hama, influential Japanese economist, on the deflationary price wars in Japan

Opposite: Cameron's hair has square layers cut with scissors and a razor. The color is a copper-based red.

Hair is like fine fabric. It can be tailored, colored, heated, molded, and styled. Like any delicate material, it must be expertly cut and properly cared for in order to feel and look its best. An exceptional cut and color is similar to a classic, made-to-measure garment—only it is something you live with and showcase each and every day. Designer clothing is more expensive not just because of the famous label, but because of the integrity and beauty of the fabric and the way that fabric is cut, draped, and sewn. The workmanship necessary to create a designer piece takes more time and money, but the finished product is more beautiful, longer lasting, and higher in quality.

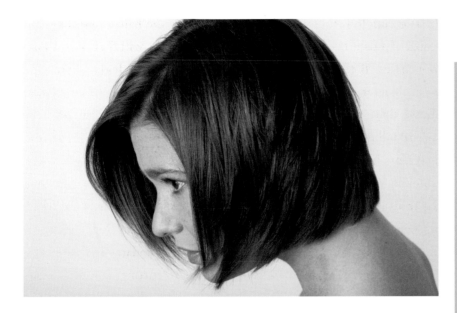

The same holds true for a great haircut. It is a permanent accessory that complements your every step and makes you feel confident, sexy, and beautiful. Yet this is where many people decide to scale back. Women spend a lot of money on expensive shoes or handbags. A night out on the town (with dinner, movie, babysitter, etc.) could easily run over $200. However, many will question spending that same amount on a service that actually makes them look and feel better, makes their life easier, and has a longer-lasting payoff. We tend not to prioritize things that make us better, healthier people and bring us happiness on a daily basis—such as a gym membership, a hair appointment, or a facial. Many consider these unnecessary, frivolous luxuries, or even vain indulgences. On the contrary, caring for yourself makes good common sense. You are certainly worth the investment!

Three things primarily measure the success of a haircut: how well it complements your face, how long it takes you to style, and how well it grows out. If your hair enhances your bone structure, strengthens your features, and makes you feel sexier and prettier, you have a great haircut. If it takes more than twenty minutes to pull and tug your hair into a style that still does not look right, then it is certainly not worth the money you spent on it—whether the cut was $20 or $200. This frustrating struggle

BEAUTY SECRET

A chef behind every chair

When a great chef prepares a meal, his or her goal is not to fill your stomach but to create an amazing experience for your taste buds. Many steps and a painstaking attention to detail are required to make a beautiful and memorable meal. You will likely never know what took place in the kitchen or the time and training required to reach this level of proficiency. Likewise, when a good stylist cuts your hair, the objective is not to make it shorter but to create a design around your face. The best in the business cut hair in several stages that include sectioning, cutting in thin sections, polishing the hair with a blow-dryer, and dry-cutting to refine the shape, all the while designing the cut based on your facial structure and head shape.

has a negative value or an opportunity cost associated with it. Dissatisfaction with the way your hair looks and behaves is distracting. Women tend to obsess over it—constantly thinking about their hair, hating it, battling with it, and feeling bad about themselves because of it. This is not surprising, since a bad haircut or color actually takes away from your beauty. On top of that, consider what you have spent on different styling products in an attempt to mask the shortcomings of a bad cut. It all adds up to time, money, and energy you could use for something much more fulfilling, fun, or lucrative.

A well-executed cut also grows out better and lasts two to three times longer than a less-competent one because of the structure that has been cut into it, thereby actually saving you time and money in the long run. It must be not just artistic, but architecturally sound. If the hair is cut with precision and balance, it will keep its shape as it grows out, fall attractively into place, and behave for you. On the other hand, while an uneven and sloppy cut may initially be masked with deft styling, it soon starts to show a lack of shape and attention to detail as the hair grows out. A good cut also gives the styling flexibility of air drying or blowing it out straight (or with a diffuser). Since your hair naturally falls into place due to its strong foundation, you are able to wear it with minimal effort and styling products. Everything you want is built into the cut: the right length, height, shape, and movement. An impeccable haircut has a life force of its own—it is the foundation and the first step toward great hair.

COMMON MISTAKE

Underestimating what it takes to become a good hairstylist

Cutting hair is both extraordinarily technical and artistic, yet there is a great misconception about hairdressing. People often think that great hairdressers are just born with a "gift," which might be true if you factor in good taste and an eye for scrutinizing your own work. But when it comes to actually cutting and coloring the hair, it is very much a craft, and like any other, it requires years of education and practice. It is only after a high level of proficiency has been achieved that a hairstylist has the ability to create a transformative experience around your face.

The bottom line: If something does not work or does not look good, or if you simply don't like it, it carries a cost that is usually far greater than what you would have spent on a higher-quality service or product. It's like purchasing an item of clothing that does not fit you, just because it's on sale. Real value is a haircut that makes you feel good about yourself, makes your life easier, and has longevity. Quality can be incorporated into most budgets. The only question is your priorities.

THE IMPORTANCE OF A GOOD HAIRCUT FOR A MAN

Women are always trying to change men, but it is wise to remember that one of the few things you actually *can* change is his hair. This is where most men are only too happy to take guidance from their wives or girlfriends. While women have an arsenal of personal beautification items at their disposal, from makeup to jewelry, all the accessories that men really have are their watches, shoes, and haircut. Yet so many men still have the same cut they had as boys, which does not complement their face shape or compensate for any changes in hair texture or density. They think nothing of spending $50 to $100 on a round of drinks or tickets to a sporting event but would not even consider investing that much in a good haircut.

I have found that most often this stems from simply not understanding the difference that a quality cut can make in a man's appearance. I also witness, time and time again, the amazement of a man who gets what may be the first great haircut of his life. It not only strengthens his facial structure, but actually makes thinning hair look thicker by building volume on top. This is also why a man who finally gets the right cut typically becomes the most loyal client. Understandably, some men do not feel comfortable going to the same salon as women (although about 20 percent of my salon's clientele is actually male). Therefore, seeing a good, old-fashioned barber is perfectly fine. I say "old-fashioned" because the majority of today's barbershops that cater to men do not use traditional barbering techniques like scissor-over-comb and thinning shears (real barbering scissors have longer blades than those generally used by stylists). Instead, they cut hair with electric clippers, in wide panels rather than thin sections. This makes it very difficult to tailor the cut to the shape of the head and causes the hair to grow out badly.

My grandfather Raffaele Scrivo was one of those old-fashioned barbers who took great pride in his work. I learned early in my career that there is a big difference between using proper shears and taking a buzzer to someone's head. Spending time with my grandfather and my dad gave me the opportunity to learn many of the old-world European cutting techniques, for which I am so grateful. I still have the shears that my grandfather used every day in his barbershop. They are framed and hang on the wall of my salon.

THE CUTTING GUIDE
Designing Your Perfect Cut

The architecture of a good haircut comes down to simple geometry: an understanding of how different shapes, lines, and angles work together and fit into one another. Cutting hair involves constructing an initial shape and length, then customizing that shape to a client's face, body, and hair texture.

The *perimeter* of the haircut consists of its length and its overall outline. *Layering* is done within that perimeter, in much the same way as a sculptor chisels detail into a mold or an artist adds shading and dimension to a sketch. The length, lines, and layers can soften, strengthen, camouflage, or emphasize specific facial features. Since your hair quite literally frames your face, the right cut has the power to improve and enhance it, or even modify its structure to a certain extent.

The *lines* in the haircut include the layers cut within it, the bangs, or a section that ends at a specific point around the face. If I want to bring attention to a certain feature, I will put a line there (for example, at the cheekbones). To soften or downplay a facial feature, such as a wide jaw, I make the pieces a little bit longer in that area so the eye is directed downward and away from it. It never ceases to amaze me how a few strategically positioned layers around a woman's face can enhance her look.

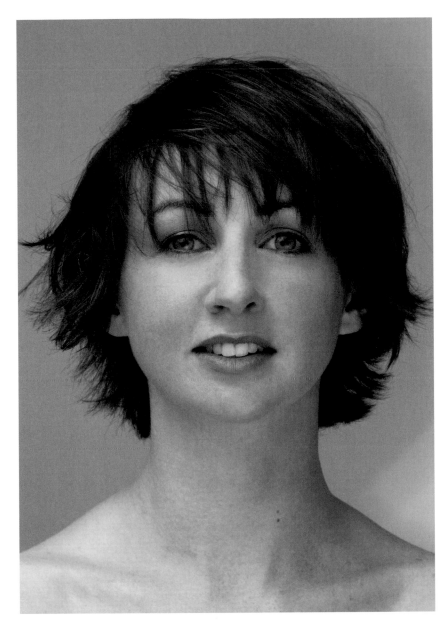

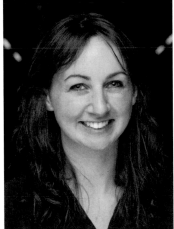

Joanna does not like to fuss much with her hair, but her long, one-length style with bangs was overwhelming and dragging down her small features. Her new short haircut was designed to complement her face shape. I cut layers with a razor so the haircut maintains its shape when air-dried. I also lightened her base color by one shade and added subtle highlights to create more dimension and enhance the shape of the cut.

Women always ask me, "How long do you think my hair should be?" "Should I grow my hair out?" "Would it look good short?" You may actually already know the answers. After growing out bad haircuts and learning from past mistakes, I bet you have a pretty good idea of what works for you and what does not. While you may not know exactly the look you should have, most women are pretty clear, even if intuitively, about what they do *not* want. It is important to listen to your own voice and trust your instincts, as well as to convey those ideas to the person who is about to cut your hair. Often women say, "I'm afraid to speak up." Don't be! By communicating your desires you are providing the hairdresser with essential information. We want you to be happy with the haircut. After all, you are the one who has to live with it.

WHAT LENGTH AND SHAPE ARE RIGHT FOR YOU?

There are six important factors that come into play when I am deciding how to cut a client's hair:

1. **WISH LIST:** Her personal preferences and desires about how she wants her face and hairstyle to look.
2. **HAIR TEXTURE:** The density of her hair and how curly or straight it is naturally.
3. **BEAUTY LIFESTYLE:** How she prefers to style her hair and how much time and effort she wants to put into it.
4. **PERSONALITY:** Her sense of style, her confidence, and how she presents herself to the world.
5. **FACE AND NECK:** Her facial features as well as the length and skin condition of her neck.
6. **BODY:** Her height, weight, and silhouette.

Your Wish List

For me, the most important guides to establishing the length and shape of a client's haircut are her personal preferences, or her wish list. Some of the first things I ask are: "How do you feel about your hair? Is there anything you would like to change?" and "What might you want to improve or modify about your features and which attributes would you like to bring into focus?" She may tell me that she does not like it when her curly hair looks flat on top and too poofy on the sides of her face. Maybe she is self-conscious about the condition of her neck and wants to bring attention to her eyes and cheekbones, or would like to make her face appear slimmer.

Perhaps she wants to look taller or thinner. The architecture of a well-designed haircut should support all these desires.

A good hairstylist is a problem solver. When I meet a client for the first time, I begin to envision how the geometric lines of a hair shape can strengthen, balance, or soften certain areas of her face. These lines perform a number of flattering optical illusions, accentuating your best features and minimizing the ones you are not crazy about. In short, the perfect haircut can make your wish list come true.

Your Hair Texture

Hair texture and density influence the choice of length and shape enormously, since they affect how the hair falls and moves. Is it curly, frizzy, or coarse? Straight, fine, or perhaps a combination of textures? After years of working with all types of hair, a skilled professional can predict how a particular texture will behave with certain cutting tools and techniques and will adjust the cut accordingly. For instance, curly hair tends to behave better and lie a little flatter if it is longer, because length creates weight. The same principle dictates that fine hair that is too long gets weighed down and can look flat or lifeless.

Your Beauty Lifestyle

Before I begin the cut, I always ask a client how she usually styles her hair and how she would ideally like it to look. (These questions often produce two very different answers.) Then I ask practical, detailed questions like, "Do you blow it out straight or do you let it air dry?" and "Do you like to pull it into a ponytail when you work out, or on the weekends?" (If so, she will obviously need enough length to pull back.) "How much time do you have in the morning to style your hair?" and "Do you know how to use a round brush?" All these questions and their answers provide the feedback I need to create a haircut that not only complements the client physically but is one she can work with easily at home.

A well-shaped haircut should provide styling versatility and look good whether it is worn wavy or blown out straight. Nevertheless, how a woman works with her hair daily will also help to determine how I will

My sister, Vinnetta, has triangular layers cut with a razor, which adds fullness to her fine hair. Her natural soft black color was enhanced with a dark glaze.

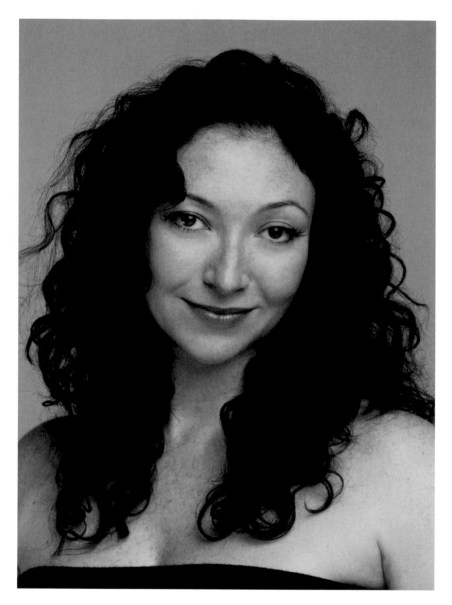

cut it. For someone who air dries her curly hair, the layers need to be left a little longer on top of the head, since curls (by virtue of their S shape) will shrink up as they dry. If I were to cut this woman's hair and blow it out straight in the salon without first asking how she usually wears it, she may find that it looks too short later when it dries naturally.

When a client tells me that she styles her hair with a blow-dryer, I want her to show me exactly how she uses it. Most women are not pro-

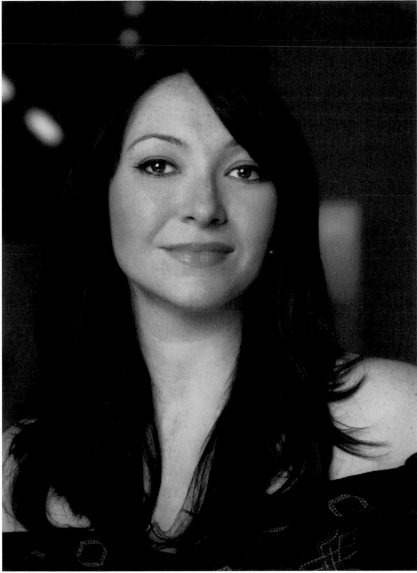

Vinnetta with the same haircut blown out straight. A round brush was used to create a smooth finish.

ficient at using a round brush and dryer together, so blow-drying may mean literally just blowing the hair around haphazardly. If she is not able to style it perfectly smooth herself, I will leave the length a bit longer because her hair will probably not be stretched to its longest when she styles it at home. If I know how someone works with her hair, I can better understand how it is going to look every day and I can compensate for that with the cut.

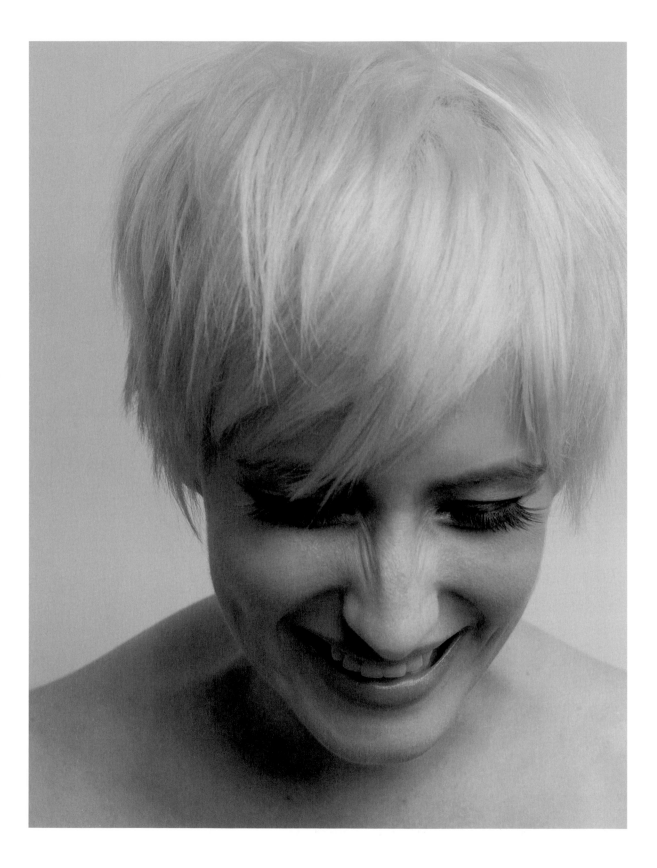

14   EVA SCRIVO ON BEAUTY

Your Personality

The power of your personality and your individual style is what makes you special and allows you to carry off a length, style, or hair color that might go against the general rules. Going for a supershort haircut, keeping the length long, or adding layers can be appropriate at any age and can work for almost anyone if the style suits the personality. In chapter 8, "Ageless Makeovers," you will see this "Why Can't You?" attitude in action. A hairstyle looks best when it is tailored to the woman who wears it, because it complements her physical features as well as her unique character. If you love to wear your hair very long (and you have the free-spirited and bohemian sensibility to go along with it), then why not embrace it? There is a way to make that length work for you. Or, if you are attracted to the classic style of a blunt-cut bob and horizontal bangs, it can be executed without looking too severe or retro. It is all about bending the rules and skillfully modifying the layers, the color, and the lines of the hair. Breaking away from the societal conventions means trusting your instincts, staying true to yourself, and communicating your desires effectively, in which case a talented hairstylist can make your signature look work beautifully for you.

Your Face and Neck

As I consult with a client, I take stock of all the visual cues available to me in order to assess her facial features and gauge what kind of hair shape would balance her facial structure. I look at a woman face-to-face, in the mirror, and I evaluate her profile (often I will give the client a hand mirror, so she can see her side view as well). Most of the time we look at ourselves head-on, but that is not how the world sees us. By looking at someone from all angles, I can clearly see the true shape of her face and neck, and understand where the lines of her haircut should hit to create the necessary optical illusion.

Opposite: Gwynne's razor cut was created with short, graduated layers.

MAKING A LONG OR NARROW FACE APPEAR FULLER: Diamond-shaped layers with the widest points at either side of the head help to broaden the face by creating the impression of width. For this face shape, I especially like using The UnCut™ (my signature layered cut), since the technique makes it easy to create a slightly fuller look at the cheekbones.

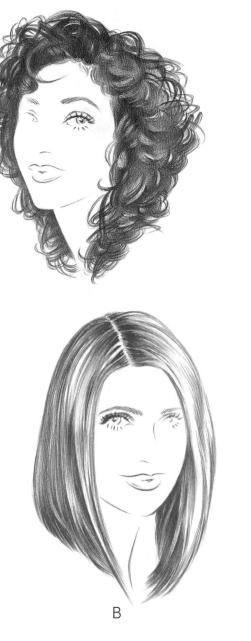

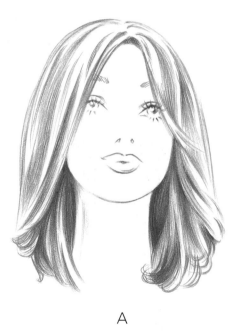

A

B

SLIMMING A ROUND FACE: Longer layers that fall on either side of the face (like curtains, in effect) will elongate a full face. The lines of the haircut should not end in the middle of the face, as this would add even more width there (A).

If you prefer a shorter alternative, an A-line bob, which is shorter in the back and longer in the front, with a side part, also works for this face shape (B).

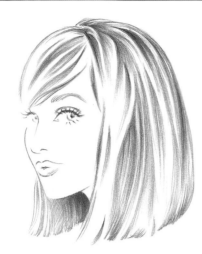

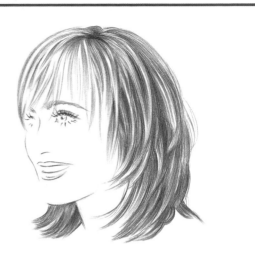

BALANCING A LONG NECK: Cutting a perimeter line that ends just below the middle of the neck will add more width there and make a long neck appear a bit shorter.

LENGTHENING A SHORT NECK: Instead of covering that area, I would subtly open it up by layering the hair between the jawline and the clavicle bone to remove some of the heaviness and help elongate the neck. A haircut ending at the clavicle or just below it is the perfect length to maintain.

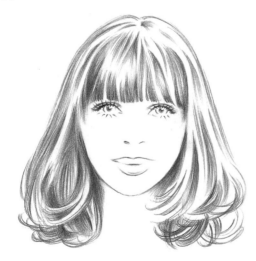

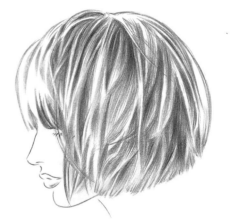

BALANCING A HEART-SHAPED FACE: A haircut that is fuller at the bottom creates an illusion of width at the jaw to balance the broader cheekbones. Shoulder-length hair also adds lateral depth to balance the strong cheekbones and a pointy chin.

STRENGTHENING THE JAWLINE AND OVERALL BONE STRUCTURE: A chin-length bob line not only helps to define the jaw but frames the entire face for a strong yet feminine look, which is accentuated by the exposed neck.

SOFTENING A STRONG JAW AND A SQUARE FACE:
Longer-length hair with soft layers helps to
soften strong facial features. Adding an asymmetrical line with a side-swept bang further
softens hard angles of the face. For a shorter
alternative, a longer bob (hitting one to two
inches above the clavicle bone, rather than at
the chin) creates a more vertical line, directing the
eye downward and softening the jawline. (Refer to
Balancing a Long Neck illustration on page 17.)

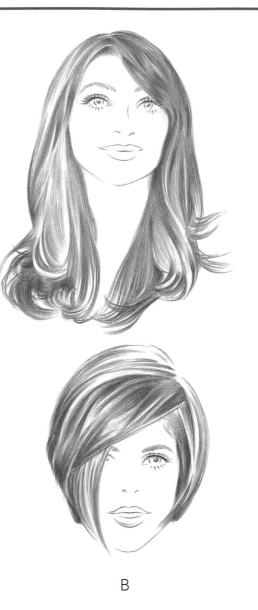

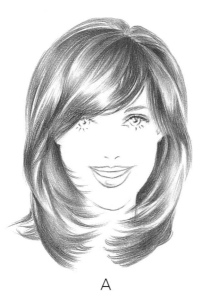

A   B

CAMOUFLAGING PROBLEMATIC JOWLS AND NECK: This situation can be dealt with in one of two
ways. Hair that ends at the jawline is not the way to go, since it brings attention right to the point
of distress. One option is more length (three inches below the jaw or longer with layers), cutting
longer pieces that can be styled inward to slightly obscure and soften the lines of a sagging neck.
Longer layers provide a diffusing effect and make for a wonderful method of camouflage (A).

   The second option is a much shorter length that hits just above the jaw and has height at the crown.
A longer side-swept bang can lift the focus upward to your eyes and detract from the jowl area (B).

Your Body

Considerations for choosing the right cut should not stop at your neck. The length and shape of your hair have to work in proportion to your entire body. When a woman comes to me for a haircut, I consider her height and silhouette. I know, for example, that someone with a larger frame could benefit from growing out her hair to her clavicle or longer, in order to slim and elongate not only her face but also her body shape. Yes, the right length and lines in your hair can actually make you appear thinner and taller. Creating a more vertical shape in a haircut, adding height at the crown, and cutting internal layers around the sides (to make the hair narrower at the cheeks and jaw) will extend the lines of the hair, face, and body from top to bottom. Hence, an illusion that you have lost a few pounds and gained a couple of inches in height is created. Remember that all good design comes back to "the line." Designers, decorators, and architects all speak of the line your eye follows when looking at a shape. It must have a flow and a continuum to feel and look right.

Usually a petite woman who wears her hair very long can seem even smaller in stature because the scale of the hair is not proportionate to her figure. The length tends to overwhelm a small body. If the hair were shorter, however, the focus would move up toward the face and visually lift up a petite frame. Despite that useful guideline, there are always exceptions to the rules, and plenty of petite women with bombshell-long hair look fantastic. This is because a woman's personality and style often manage to trump conventional laws of proportion.

HOW TO WEAR BANGS, AND WHICH STYLE IS RIGHT FOR YOU

Bangs or Botox? —Eva Scrivo

Bangs are a versatile, simple, and transformative way to customize most cuts. There is a world of different bangs out there. There are blunt, straight-across bangs; textured, softer bangs; side-swept and grown-out "rocker" bangs—all of which the British refer to as a "fringe."

Not only do bangs help to conceal fine lines and cover a short or a high forehead, they are youthful and fun. Bangs can make a woman look younger because they soften her face and provide a line in the haircut that can play up the eyes, lift the cheekbones, and produce a multitude of other subtle visual effects. For instance, if you want to put the focus on your eyes, then cutting bangs just above the brows will place the emphasis right there. A longer bang that hits below the brows will bring attention

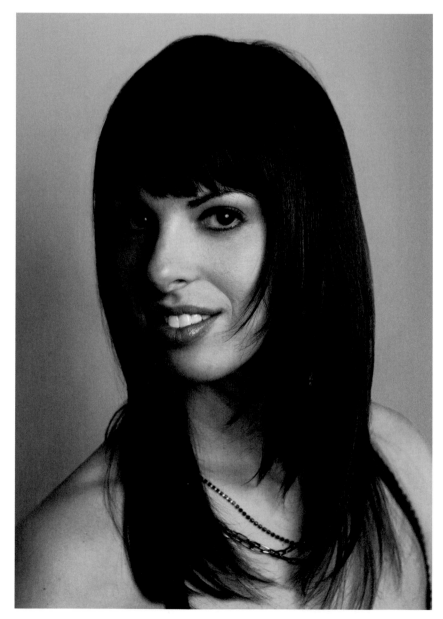

Christine has triangular layers cut with scissors. Her bangs end above her brows, bringing attention to her eyes. The hair color was enriched with a clear glaze, and a midnight-blue clip-in extension was added for a pop of color.

to your lips. Meanwhile, an asymmetrical fringe can help to minimize a broad nose or slim a round face by basically drawing a diagonal line across it, thus breaking up the width.

Bangs can be the perfect answer when a woman is seeking a change in her look but does not want to cut off the length of her hair. What she actually wants is more shape around her face, and a fringe creates that frame. This is why bangs are so frequently requested, are such a common

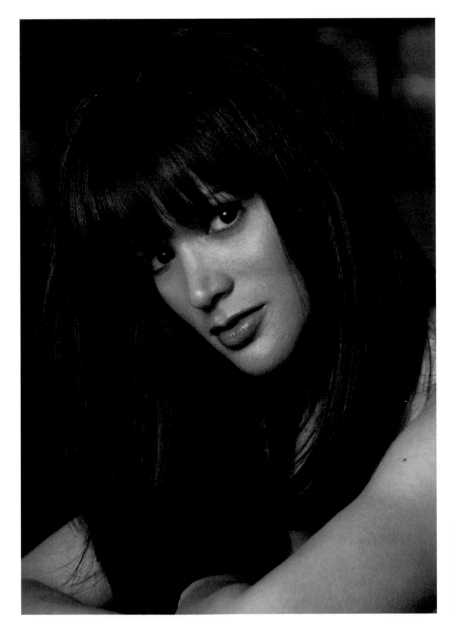

Marisel has concave layers cut with scissors and longer bangs that hit below her eyebrows, bringing attention to her mouth. A cool-tone espresso shade was added with demi-permanent color.

impulse decision, and why the question of whether or not to cut bangs is worth discussing with your hairdresser. Granted, you may not be chopping off all your hair, but cutting bangs is still a gamble that you don't want to end up regretting. After all, it can take up to a year to grow out that fringe. I have learned that most women have some kind of personal trauma associated with cutting bangs. A memory of a bad haircut often seems to include a bad bang experience. Many people associate bangs with the horizontal style they may have been forced to wear as a child, which looked like it was lopped off in one big snip. A well-executed bang does not look as if your grandma placed a bowl on your head and cut around it.

Not every texture has it easy when it comes to wearing a fringe. Bangs and curly hair are two elements that are not easily combined, but it is possible. You may not be able to wear a straight-across bang, but you can have slightly shorter pieces that tendril around your face. Someone with curly hair who wants a full-fledged bang has to accept that she cannot blow out just that section every day. The rest of her hair will have to be integrated with the smoothness of the bangs; otherwise, she will be sporting what is known as a "mall bang." This is not a look you want. (There is also the option of having the bangs chemically straightened. But this can be tricky,

OPTICAL ILLUSIONS

How slight variations in bangs can balance your facial features

- If a blunt bang is kept a bit longer at the temples, the look is more blended, softer, and slimming, since it directs the eye downward.
- Cutting those edges shorter at the temples makes a thin face look wider.
- Keeping the midpoint of the bang (in between the brows) a tiny bit longer can direct the eye inward and make wide-set eyes look not so far apart.
- For someone with close-set eyes, cutting that center part slightly shorter and texturizing it to remove a bit of weight will create the illusion of more space in the center of the face and of larger, wider-set eyes.

since the chemical process has to be very light to avoid ending up with two different textures, i.e., a permanent mall bang.)

GETTING YOUR HAIR CUT
The Process

Usually, once seated in the salon chair, most women zone out, having very little comprehension of what is happening on top of their heads. That is perfectly fine if you have been going to the same hairdresser for a while. (In fact, most of my clients think of their hair appointment as time for themselves and a welcome opportunity to relax.) But, especially at the initial visit, it is a good idea to be reasonably aware. This is not to say that you should become a backseat driver during your haircut. On the contrary, it is not advisable during the cut itself to chat too much with your stylist, who needs to concentrate on your hair. However, it is important to talk with him or her before the cut begins about how your hair will be shaped and how you want it to look. After reading this section, you will better understand what your hairdresser is doing and why.

CUTTING TOOLS

Hairstylists primarily use three types of tools to cut hair: scissors, razors, and thinning shears. Each creates a very different effect and is used in conjunction with numerous cutting techniques. Your hair texture and density help to determine why a hairstylist chooses a particular cutting tool or technique to either play up your natural hair texture or compensate for the way your hair tends to fall or behave.

Scissors

Scissors create a straight line, which is why they are typically used to cut the length and create a strong initial shape. A simple pair of scissors is an extraordinarily versatile implement that lends itself to different cutting techniques. In addition to cutting a precise line, they are used to create layers and build a specific shape, and to further texturize and soften the overall haircut when dry.

Ena has square layers that were cut with a razor. Subtle red highlights were added to bring warmth to her skin tone.

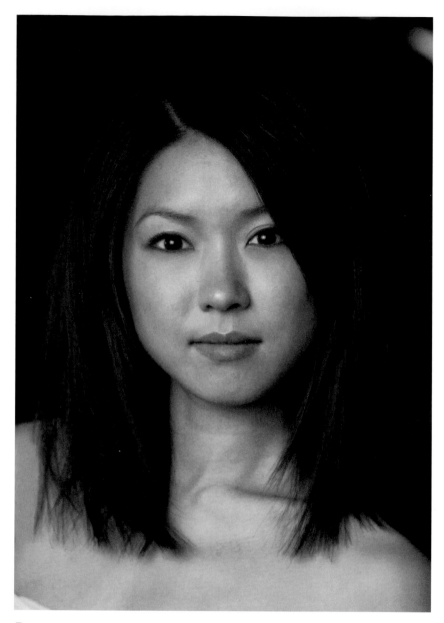

Razors

The straight blade of a razor, when combined with the slightly angled up-and-down motion of the wrist while making the cut, creates a broken but even line (rather than the solid one produced by scissors). Think of a zigzag stitch compared with a solid stitch done on a sewing machine. This is not a jagged, messy, or uneven line. (Consider that a straight blade is what surgeons use to make an extremely precise cut.) When employed correctly on the hair, this tool removes bulk and creates movement and

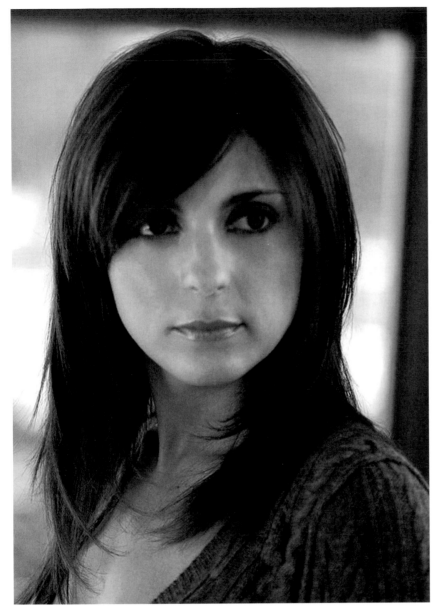

Leila has triangular layers cut with a razor. Her hair is colored a rich auburn that complements her complexion.

separation. It also allows curls and waves to spring up, since they are not dragged down with weight on the ends.

Because most stylists don't have proper training in razor cutting, unless yours has truly honed this skill, do not trust him or her to use a razor on your hair. However, a stylist with razor-cutting expertise gained through extensive training and experience can yield magnificent results. A razor is a truly amazing tool when used correctly.

THE RULE

Never cut curly hair with a razor, because it creates frizz.

THE RULE BREAKER: A straight blade is a misunderstood and

underappreciated cutting tool. In the hands of a skilled technician it does not cause frizz at all. In fact, I have seen many women with so-so curls walk out of my salon with glorious, defined curls after having their hair cut with a razor. I have also witnessed the razor phobia on a client's face when I suggest cutting her curly hair with one. Many women are understandably apprehensive, especially if they have had a terrible razor cut in the past. The razor's bad rap has less to do with the tool itself than with the way it is wielded by the hairstylist. In the wrong hands, a good pair of scissors can also create a disaster. Used the right way, a razor reduces heaviness with its zigzag line by individualizing, defining, and lifting each curl. With a razor, I am able to texturize and cut the ends simultaneously, making the perimeter line a little softer.

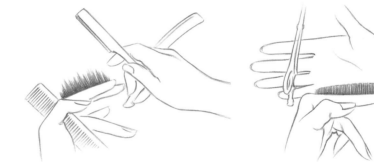

A line cut with a razor.   A line cut with scissors.

Thinning Shears

Thinning shears remove weight from the interior of the hair without affecting the exterior outline. They should be used sparingly on dry hair as a method of fine-tuning the weight distribution, which influences the shape. Instead of smooth, straight blades, these texturizing scissors have serrated teeth that notch into the hair and cut only the pieces in between those teeth. This literally thins out sections that are too dense, either in the middle of the hair shaft or closer to the ends. I may use thinning shears near the edges of a solid bob line, for example, if it feels heavy. This way, I retain the shape and length, while getting more movement and lightness at the ends.

COMMON MISTAKES

Using a razor *with* a guard

Destructive results can occur when using a straight blade with a safety guard. A guard protects stylists from cutting themselves but also makes the blade not as sharp. Consequently, more pressure must be applied to cut the hair, scraping the serrated guard over it. This friction burns the hair, shreds the ends, and even pulls keratin out of the hair shaft, which is what causes frizz (you can actually see that white keratin protein on the ends). The added tension on your hair can also be painful, and if your haircut hurts, it's all wrong! A razor with a guard should never be used to cut hair. Then why is it used? Just as a proper razor in inexperienced hands can wreak havoc on your hair, it can also wreak havoc on the stylist's inexperienced hands! The extremely sharp blade's downward motion is directed at the index and middle fingers. When used properly, it stops within an eighth of an inch of the skin. I have certainly seen my share of razor accidents, from deep cuts that required stitches, and even the tip of a finger being sliced clean off, to the smaller cuts that are simply a part of life at every salon. In addition, a razor is almost always used on wet hair, since it is imperative that the blade can glide through slick strands. Using a razor on clean, dry hair (without an oily or waxy product to provide some slip) will cause the blade to drag on the hair and create damage and frizz.

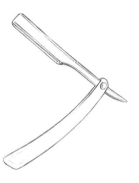

Razor without a guard.

Scraping the hair with scissors

The razor and thinning shears are not the only tools that can damage hair if used improperly. The most frequent damage actually happens from scissors. It can be caused by overtexturizing (removing too much hair to the point where it feels thin) or by dragging the scissors over the hair and pulling on it so that it actually hurts. This shreds the ends of the hair and pulls the keratin out of it in the same way as when a razor with a guard is used, resulting in frizz.

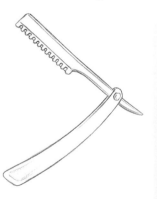

Razor with a guard.
(If you see this, run!)

Haphazardly using thinning shears

Like a razor, thinning shears are often misused or overused, resulting in a wispy, overly thinned texture or a haircut that is unbalanced. Used correctly, this tool should not make hair frizzy or fuzzy. Some stylists cut too deeply into the hair and end up cutting too much off, while others thin out the hair unevenly throughout the haircut. Weight must be removed equally unless the hair naturally grows in heavier on one side. Cutting into the hair with thinning shears haphazardly creates an unbalanced shape that is especially noticeable on straight hair.

CUTTING TECHNIQUES

It's not the tool but the skill with which it is used that sets great hairstylists apart. The combination of tool and technique is what creates a particular effect, feeling, or movement in the haircut. There are many methods of cutting and layering the hair, and it is helpful to know a few of the basic techniques and the terminology. Understanding what the stylist intends to do should not only make you feel more comfortable but give you the opportunity to intercept a miscommunication before it manifests itself in your haircut.

BUILDING THE STRUCTURE WITH LAYERS

It may seem as if a hairstylist cuts hair aimlessly in a passionate, artistic flurry. Nothing is farther from the truth. While there is certainly an intuitive aesthetic sensibility and creativity at work, the craft itself is technical and methodical. Haircutting follows a precise formula of connecting one section of hair to another, using each one that is cut as a guide for the length of the next. In the industry, this is called your "guideline." It makes every section even and in line with the others. The stylist always has a small piece of the previous section (her guideline) in her hand as she continues to build the shape. As the haircut progresses, all sections start to match up and connect in a very systematic way.

Most haircuts begin with the stylist dividing the hair, then cutting one section that will act as his or her guideline for the entire cut. She is basically connecting the dots in order to create a completely balanced, even form, so that every section eventually can be traced back to that first one. This precision cutting ensures continuity throughout the haircut for a sound structure. The bangs (typically shorter in length than the rest of the hair but can also be left longer) are the area most commonly disconnected from the rest of the cut. There are also advanced cutting techniques that are referred to as "disconnected," where, for example, the top may be longer than the sides and back, but the overall cut still feels balanced if properly executed.

Opposite: Kendra has round layers cut with scissors. Her highlights were created using the balayage technique.

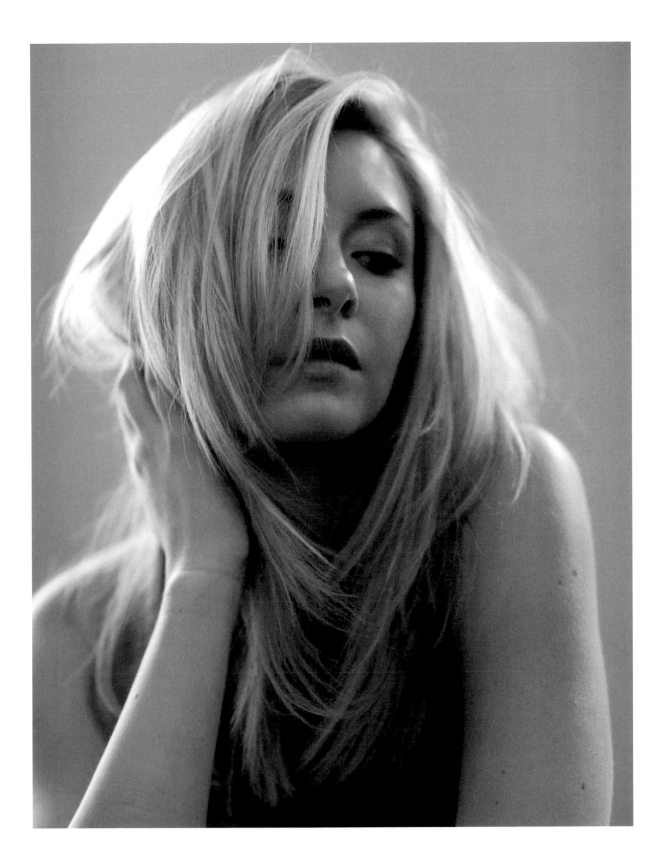

Great shapes are built from the bottom up, and a skilled hairstylist thinks like an architect: if a bottom floor of a building is off-kilter, the entire structure is not sound. Just as one would not begin constructing a building from the top floor, I have found that the haircuts that last the longest and grow out best are cut from the bottom up. Although many hairstylists do the opposite, they frequently cut the top shorter to get height and compensate for the lack of support within the structure, which is also not as long-lasting. For example, if you feel that your hair starts to collapse and becomes flat within two to three weeks of being cut, this may be the reason.

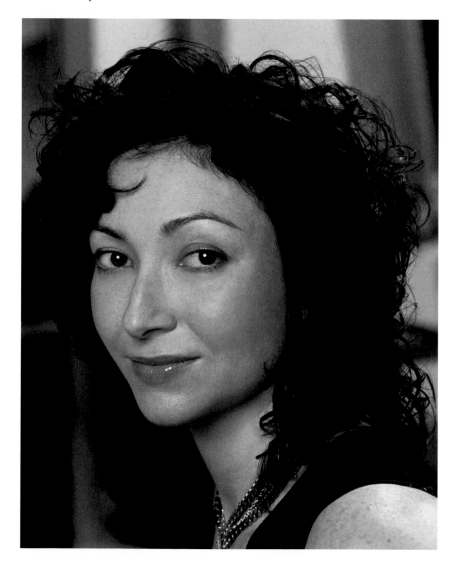

Vinnetta with my signature "The UnCut," done with a razor.

Layering is a pattern of cutting the hair to build a specific shape and add height at the top of the head. It refers to how the hair is elevated and held between the fingers while being cut. Various elevations create different types of layers, which in turn produce different overall shapes in the haircut. Layers also act as flexible girders that move from side to side, giving the hair movement.

Many women believe that one-length hair is easier to style, but that misconception usually comes from badly or overly layered haircuts. It comes down to choosing the right amount and type of layering for your hair. One-length hair is a specific look that some women like, which is fine if that is your preference. However, it does not give the framework, fullness, height, and movement that come with some gentle layering. Even the most geometric shapes, like a bob, look more modern with some movement to them. You can still maintain that one-length feel with gently cut round layers that will also give some height at the top of the head.

On pages 32 and 33 are five basic layering techniques that build different structure and movement into the hair. One of them will most likely be the way a stylist cuts your hair shape.

PROFESSIONAL TECHNIQUE

The UnCut™

At my salon, stylists perform my trademarked The UnCut, a method of razor cutting layers to create the initial lines and length and remove bulk, then using scissors to dry cut and refine the shape. I named it The UnCut because the evenly cut, zigzag line produced by the razor always looks natural and slightly grown out. Although based on the principle of triangular layering, the cut is more diamond-shaped. It produces soft layers that fall into place without the aid of a dryer or much styling. The UnCut is the solution for a common hair dilemma. Women with curly, wavy, or thick hair complain that they hate to wear it natural because the hair expands at the bottom as it dries and ends up looking like a tepee. But it is not necessarily the curl, wave, length, or texture that they don't like; it's the width around the bottom. I also use this technique on straight hair, and on both long and short lengths. This concept of cutting can be modified by using a razor with other layering patterns.

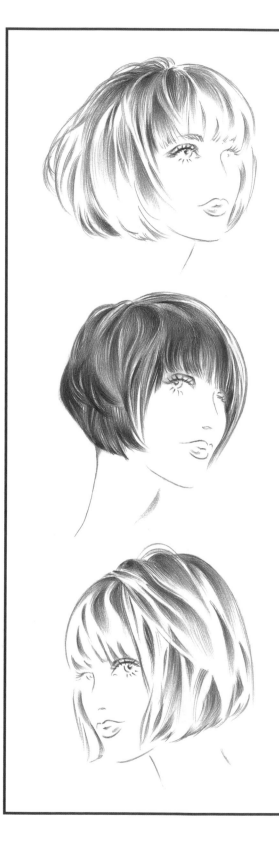

ROUND LAYERS: Round layers give the softest shape and are created by cutting the elevated sections of hair to the same length and in a circular pattern. If the hair was held out from all points of the head, it would actually form the shape of a circle. Round layers can be used on all hair lengths and textures and remove the least amount of length and weight. This technique is best for adding light layering without compromising the hair's natural thickness.

GRADUATED LAYERS: These are horizontally layered sections that build weight by stacking slightly shorter pieces underneath longer ones. They graduate from short to long, starting at the nape of the neck and getting longer as the haircut progresses toward the top of the head. Many shorter haircuts are beveled like this in the back so the hair at the nape can build support and height at the crown.

SQUARE LAYERS: Unlike round layers, square layers build a strong, geometric shape into a haircut with more solid lines. If all of the hair was pulled straight up at the top of the head, out at the sides, and back at the back of the head, it would literally form a square. This technique removes more weight around the face and adds volume at the top of the head. It is ideal for creating defined and modern shapes and also lends itself to more alternative, edgier haircuts.

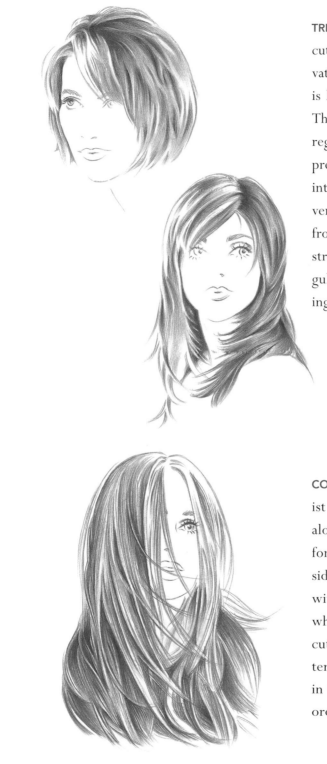

TRIANGULAR LAYERS: Triangular layers are cut straight across the top as the hair is elevated, and angled downward when the hair is held straight out at the sides and back. They form an upside-down pyramid shape regardless of the hair length. This actually prevents curly or thick hair from turning into a dreaded pyramid by creating the reverse effect and removing bulk and width from just above the ears down. On longer straight hair, which tends to go flat, triangular layering lifts the hair while maintaining the length.

CONCAVE LAYERS: With this method, a stylist layers the hair, allowing the thickness along the bottom to remain. It essentially forms a shape of a pyramid that is rightside-up; the opposite of the form created with triangular layers. It is perfect for those who want shape and definition in the haircut while maintaining a more solid perimeter line. The cut retains most of the density in the hair but still has some choppiness in order not to look one length.

TEXTURIZING

Texturizing is a method of weight removal that creates a more airy texture on the ends, adding movement to the haircut. This can be done on wet or dry hair: on the ends with a point-cutting or razor-cutting technique, or by cutting more deeply into the hair from the midshaft to the ends to remove bulk.

When hairdressers talk about "weight" and "bulk," we are (thankfully) referring to your hair density and texture—two elements that have an enormous effect on the shape and movement of the hair. Weight, or

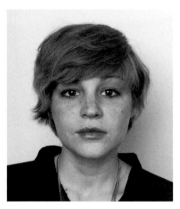

Before.

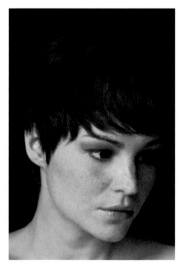

Olivia has square layers cut with a razor and colored a rich, fiery, violet-based ruby red.

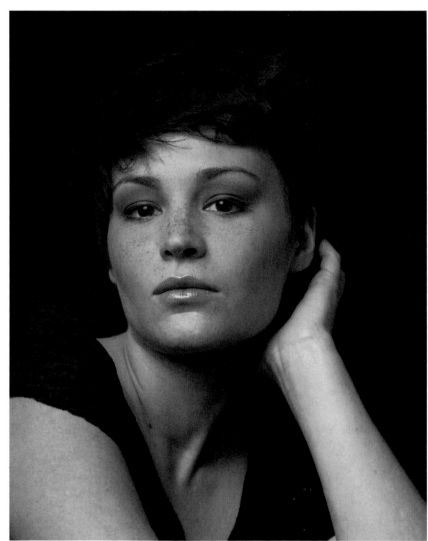

density within the hair, feels like heaviness and is not the same thing as length. It can be concentrated in one specific area of the hair or throughout the entire head. It is the combination of the right length and even distribution of weight that creates a proportionate haircut. Weight can also work to your advantage by weighing down frizzy or flyaway hair, for example. Or it can be something you want to remove if it makes the hair look too bulky and detracts from the shape of the haircut.

If your hair tends to flatten at the top, removing excess weight around the bottom by softly layering the last three to four inches can reduce the heaviness and lift the shape. Women with wavy or curly hair often complain that it is too puffy and round, in which case I may cut into the ends, with either a razor or scissors, to create some airiness and separation. This individualizes each curl and prevents the overall hair shape from looking like a solid mass. I may also layer the hair to remove excess bulk and make it lie closer to the head. It is not unusual to have different textures in one head of hair. Many women have ringlets underneath, while the top layer is wavy and fluffy. To balance that, I reduce the bulk on top, perhaps by using a razor to remove some of the heaviness and bring out more natural curl in that area. On the other hand, if a woman with pin-straight, fine hair tells me that she is frustrated with how flat and thin it

COMMON MISTAKE

Getting a bouncy, voluminous blowout right after a cut

After a haircut, you may desire to have your hair blown out with some wave and lots of lift, and I don't blame you. A luxurious, bouncy blowout softens the face and can last for days. Unfortunately, it also masks imperfections in a haircut and should not be done until the cut is completely checked dry. The volume and wave created by the blowout alter the lines of the hair, which is precisely why it is a bad idea before your stylist dry cuts it. Many hairdressers make this error and are unable to clearly see mistakes or imbalances in the haircut. Following the initial wet cut, your hair should be dried straight and smooth so that your stylist is able to go over his or her work with more clarity. After the dry cut is completed, you can ask your stylist to go over the blowout and add body and lift with a round brush or Velcro rollers. This helps to ensure that your haircut is perfectly balanced and that you are able to style your hair easily at home.

looks, I would cut a crisp, solid line at the bottom so that her hair does not seem so wispy. I would then create more volume by adding round layers, and *not* texturize her hair, in order to maintain its natural weight.

Point Cutting

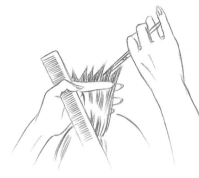

Point cutting technique.

This texturizing technique involves cutting into the ends of the hair to remove weight and give it more movement. The scissors are held at a higher angle and their tips are used to cut a tiny V shape into the ends with each snip. This is a way to soften the lines of a haircut on straight hair so that everything feels more blended, or to create separation by individualizing curls in wavy or curly textures.

Your hair should not be point cut if it tends to become thin on the ends and feels as though it never grows past a certain length. In such instances, it is best to keep crisp, solid lines.

PROFESSIONAL TECHNIQUES

Adjusting a haircut for the climate

I always ask new clients where they live because the climate affects how the hair behaves. For someone who lives in a more humid environment, it may be better not to cut into the ends of the hair, allowing the strands to remain heavier to help weigh down frizz and flyaways. Since removing weight in the ends gives the hair more body and lift, it is just what you do not want in humidity, but do want in a dry, arid place that is not conducive to creating body in the hair.

Adjusting a haircut for the shape of the head

An often overlooked factor in how the hair should be layered is the shape of the head, which along with texture determines how the hair lies. A good hairdresser needs to know how to work with that variable (I feel up all my clients before I cut their hair—to gauge the shape of their skulls, of course). By building weight or removing density, or by creating height where the hair tends to be flat, I can rebalance the face and head shape with the right lines and layers cut into the hair. For example, if the head is slightly flatter on top, cutting layers and adding more shape at the back of the head creates volume at the crown. A slightly cone-shaped skull causes the hair to hang flatter, and proper layers can fill out the sides. If the skull seems more flat on one side (or if a woman prefers to wear a deep side part in her hair), I will texturize the heavier side and cut a few shorter layers on the other. It is all about balance and compensation.

THE RULE

Regular trims will help your hair grow faster.

THE RULE BREAKER: Since hair grows from the roots, not the

ends, that logic is false. I advise my clients who are growing out their hair to go as long as they can without cutting it. If you are trying to grow your hair longer, trimming the ends too often will get you nowhere, but not trimming them at all will lead to long hair that is unhealthy and unattractive. In addition, if your ends are split, you will ultimately have to cut off the damage, or those damaged ends could end up simply snapping off. Either way, you will lose length.

Try to wait at least eight to ten weeks between micro-trims to keep the ends healthy. A wonderful way to freshen up a haircut without altering too much of its length is to have your haircutter blow it out smooth and straight and then just dust the edges with scissors when it is dry. Because wet hair stretches, it is easy to cut off too much length when trimming the ends. If you are growing out a shorter, layered cut, have the layers just around your face trimmed every six to eight weeks without touching the bottom length. This creates more shape around the face and gives you an instant feeling of lift, making the growing-out process more palatable—and prettier.

Thinning

Thinning is used to remove weight and bulk from the interior of the hair without altering the length or perimeter lines of the cut. It can be accomplished with thinning shears, razor, or scissors. When it comes to thinning the hair, moderation and good judgment are important. This technique has received a bad rap because stylists frequently overdo it by cutting too deeply into the hair, creating too many shorter pieces to support the long ones (ironically, this can create the appearance of more volume). Whether on short or long hair, it is best to use thinning shears only on the ends (approximately on the last one to two inches on short hair and three inches on longer lengths).

Dry Cutting

Although the technical groundwork—constructing the shape and length—is usually done when the hair is wet, it is easier to see the lines of the haircut when it is dry. This is why dry cutting is used to fine-tune the hair shape after the initial wet cut. Cutting a head of hair without dry cutting at the end is like chiseling a shape into a sculpture without sanding and polishing it. This essential final step is the finishing work. After the hair has been dried and styled, I am able to see how it falls and where it may be out of balance.

Since hair stretches to a longer length when wet, checking the cut again once it is dry provides an accurate, realistic look at the length and shape. Additionally, since it is impossible during the initial cut to pull each section of hair with the same amount of tension and to precisely the same length as the last section, it is important to recheck those measurements. Curly hair, in particular, tends to be unpredictable, and it is hard to tell exactly where the ends are going to hit or what the shape will be until the hair is completely dry. At that point, I look at the exterior shape as if it were a topiary, making final tweaks and adjustments to create more overall balance and better definition in the individual curls.

THE BOB: *A Classic*

Shake it, love! —Vidal Sassoon

Of all the haircuts, the bob stands out as the most noteworthy. Since its inception around the 1920s, this cut has served as an inspiration for hairstylists around the world and has laid the groundwork for many other haircuts. A classic bob has a solid, straight line at the bottom and is even in length on all sides, like a box (it is sometimes called a "box bob" for this reason). The strong square shape traditionally falls just below the ear. While it can be left longer, the finite length must rest on its own, above the shoulder. This is what makes it a bob: it does not bend or break by hitting the shoulders, but rests at the neck. The benefit of the bob line, and one of the reasons why it has been so enduringly popular in all its incarnations, is that the defined structural lines add strength to the shape of the face.

When it came into fashion, the bob was a shocking sign of the times. It originated just as women were joining the workforce during World War I and no longer had the time or the endurance to wear their hair in the ornate Victorian upsweeps of the preceding era. Cropped hair became a

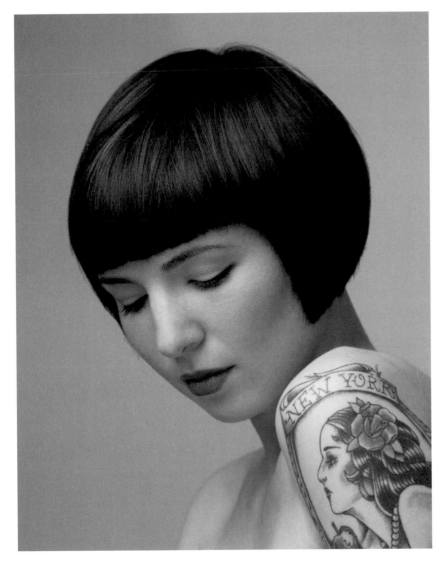

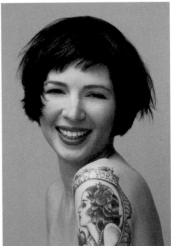

Mara has a short bob that was cut with scissors. Graduated layers were added with a razor, and the shape was enhanced with golden highlights.

badge of freedom, rebellion, and independence for working women who had also just gained the right to vote. Their short hair was very much a political statement, just as long hair made a very different political statement for both men and women in the 1960s.

The bob set off the flapper era of the 1920s as the freethinking female population, now emancipated from their long tresses and old-fashioned hairdos, broke free of other constraints and started wearing short dresses and lipstick. Bobs transitioned to longer hairstyles in the 1940s and 1950s but were brought back into fashion by legendary hairstylist Vidal Sassoon

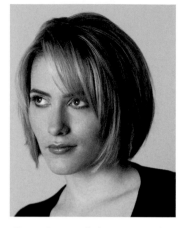

Above: Donna's bob was cut with triangular layers, using a razor. Her strawberry blond was created with the balayage technique.

Right: This classic bob with lightly graduated layers was cut with scissors. A combination of foils and subtle balayage was used for the pale blond highlights.

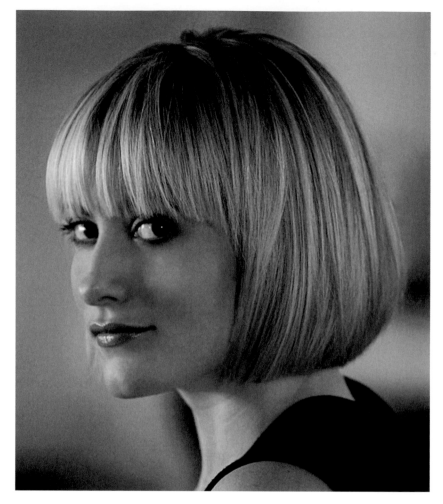

in the 1960s. (It was Sassoon who also cut Mia Farrow's famous pixie crop in the 1960s.) Sassoon's geometric interpretation of the bob was angular and modern as well as sculptural. It is not surprising that Sassoon said his geometric cuts were inspired by modern Bauhaus architecture even more than by fashion. The look had lift, movement, and swing. (He was famous for telling his models, "Shake it, love!" after he had cut and styled their hair.)

The bob is still an amazingly versatile and adaptable style, since the lines can be modified to flatter any face shape. Within the parameters of the bob style come a variety of forms and lengths. Bobs can be curly, wavy, or stick straight. They can be one solid length or layered. They can have bangs or not. The bob is the incarnation of modern haircutting.

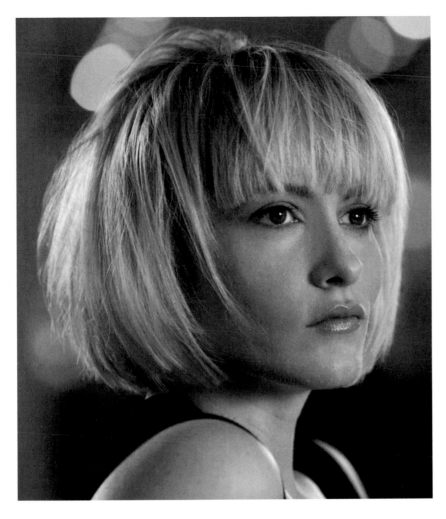

Same haircut as in the larger photo on the opposite page, styled with more movement by adding a drop of pomade to loosen and "open up" the cut.

PROFESSIONAL TECHNIQUE

Adjusting a bob for curly or fine hair

Curly hair, once bobbed, can instantly turn into a triangle. To prevent this pyramid from forming, the hair can be layered to reduce the width and texturized slightly at the ends while maintaining a solid perimeter line. To make a fine texture look much fuller, a graduated bob would be the best choice (refer to Graduated Layers illustration on page 32).

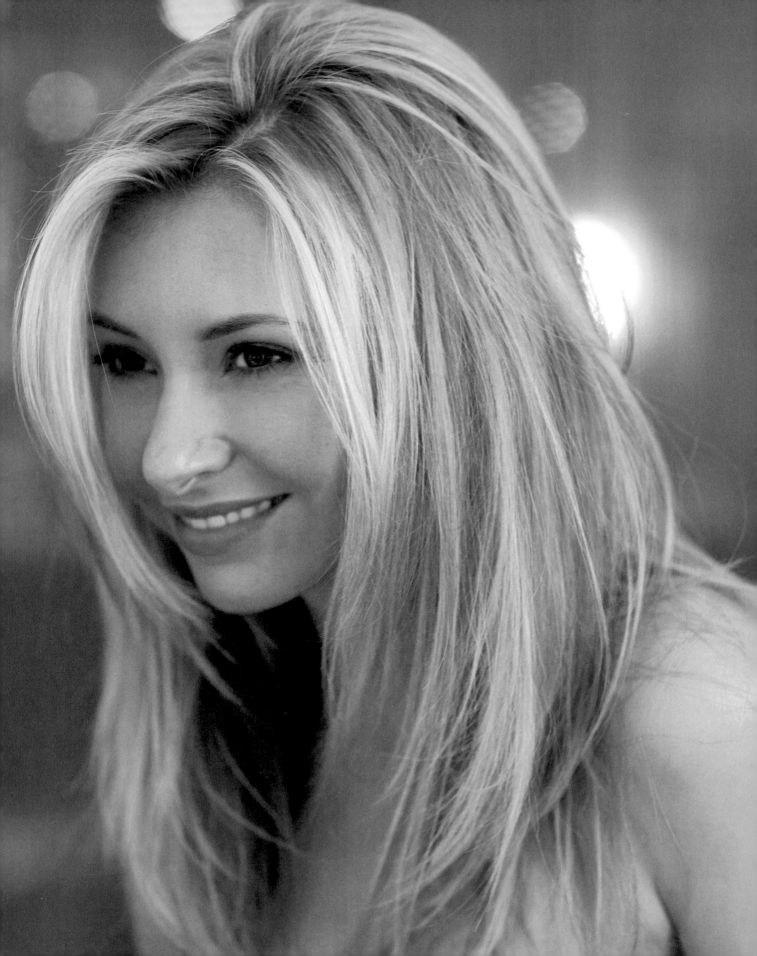

2

HAIR COLOR FROM ARCHITECTS TO PAINTERS

Cutting hair is like creating a sketch or an outline, while color adds depth and fullness to that shape. Artfully applied hair color is a remarkable yet understated makeover tool. Color, in general, has a profound effect on one's mood and frame of mind. When you paint the walls in your home a different color or reupholster a piece of furniture, it changes the entire feel of a room. Consider the positive reactions from others when you wear clothing in flattering hues. Hair color has an even more powerful and personal impact. It works with the cut to help enhance facial features and to emphasize the movement and texture of the hair. The right hair color can give you a more radiant-looking complexion, making you appear refreshed and rested. It can make your eyes look brighter and even give the impression of a slimmer face or thicker hair. However, like a bad haircut, the wrong color detracts from your appearance and can make you look pale or tired. In addition, it can simply look fake, which may not be your goal. Unless you are going for a completely new look, hair color changes can be so subtle and natural that people cannot pinpoint exactly what is different or improved about your appearance: "Did you go on vacation?" "Have you lost weight?" "Have you had something done?"

"Are you in love?" Beautiful hair color that complements your skin is something that everybody notices, even if indirectly. People may not say, "I love your hair color," but they will mention how much they love your hair or comment on how great you look.

Altering your hair color even slightly is the quickest way to feel a sense of change, especially if you don't love your haircut. If you do not want to shorten the length or cut bangs, adding a few highlights or deepening or lightening the base color can provide a satisfying sense of transformation. Color enhances a hair shape that might look flat or boring on its own.

Hair color is just as important as the cut. They play off each other and both should be customized to a woman's hair texture, lifestyle, and personality. When you are adding dimension to your hair with highlights or lowlights, the color should complement the haircut. It is like a three-dimensional canvas. A colorist can see which areas to lighten or darken to bring out the movement and lines in the hair, literally coloring them in and bringing them to life.

While cutting the hair involves building a structure, coloring is a combination of painting and science. A colorist must understand the chemistry of mixing pigments and how these formulations process on different types of hair. Because there is so much complexity and subtlety to color, the best colorists are also true artists. It has taken me years of practice to become proficient. I am not simply taking one color and putting it all over someone's hair. A unique formula is customized for every client, often using up to three or four different colors to get just the right shade and tone—and this is just for the base color (the color in the root area, which affects the overall tone). In addition to a client's current hair color, I also consider her natural hair color, skin tone, and eye color; the shape and lines of her haircut; and the health of her hair.[1]

There is such a wide range of hair colors and there are so many types of red, blond, brunette, and even gray, that it is actually rare for two women to get the exact same shade. Color can be individualized by several methods: creating shading and dimension with highlights or lowlights, adjusting the tone with a glaze, or separately formulating for different areas of the hair for an even, balanced, and beautiful result. A great colorist knows how to work with many variables to create the client's perfect hair color, such as the movement of the haircut, the environment that the hair is exposed to, the color that has been previously applied, and the condition of the hair. Often, subtle adjustments will give the color one has always wanted. If a dark brunette tells me that she dreams of being a blonde, I can fulfill this wish without damaging her hair or making the color look fake. I may lighten her base color one shade and weave in a few brighter highlights just around her face to create an overall sense of lightness and a realistic version of blond hair that suits her natural coloring. (See Lori, below.)

In the hands of a talented and skilled colorist, the possibilities of hair color open up to you. There are so many amazing tools available to a professional, and learning about these options will help you to have a

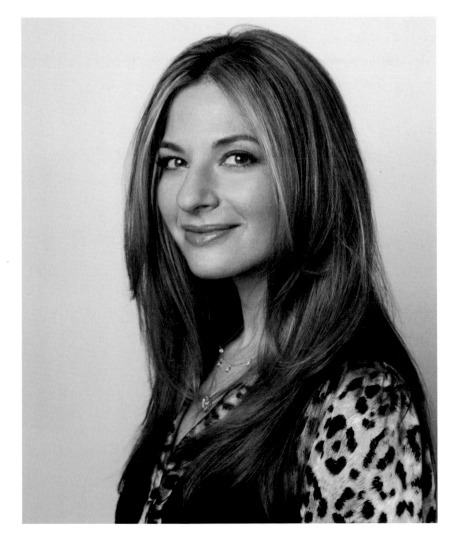

Lori naturally has medium ash-brown hair. Her highlights and lowlights were painted using the balayage technique. Her triangular layers were cut with scissors.

THE RULE

Hair color is damaging to the hair.

THE RULE BREAKER: Hair can absolutely be damaged by color or

bleach. In fact, such damage occurs every day in salons around the world (and especially at home). However, as I will explain in this chapter, the most common cause is professional error—the wrong type of formulation for one's hair, as well as improper and sloppy application and processing. As long as you are in the hands of a skilled, experienced, and conscientious colorist, your hair will not become damaged. On the contrary, I have seen many cases of already damaged hair that looks smoother, shinier, brighter, and healthier *after* the coloring process.

When professional hair color was in a state of technological infancy and used to contain high levels of ammonia, it was difficult even for a skilled professional to use. A great deal of advancement has since been made. Not only do modern permanent-color formulas contain minute levels of ammonia, if any; they also contain more conditioning ingredients. All of this makes color much gentler and safer on the hair and scalp. Additionally, ammonia-free permanent hair color that delivers professional results has been recently introduced and other technological advancements are continually being made.

much more gratifying salon experience. In addition, it is a good idea to have at least a basic understanding of the chemicals that are applied to your hair and scalp. This will lead to a more honest and informed consultation with your colorist and ultimately to more beautiful hair color and healthier hair.

More than 70 percent of women in the United States color their hair, whether at a salon or at home. Most of them have very little knowledge of the formulation being used or how it affects their hair. The professional coloring process might seem even more mystifying than haircutting: a colorist mixes some kind of concoction (usually in a back room of the salon) and puts it on your hair, and you magically walk out with a different hair color.

Colorists also speak in code such as "levels," chemical formulas, and "tonal values." While it is not necessary to know all the technical intricacies of hair-color formulation (and you probably don't want to), lifting the veil on the process gives you a better understanding of and appreciation for the expertise that goes into the service. This basic knowledge results in a stronger element of trust between the client and colorist and enables you to understand what type of coloring service is right for you.

HOW DOES HAIR COLOR WORK?

Hair color falls into four main categories: temporary, semi-permanent, demi-permanent, and permanent. The main difference among them is in their chemical compositions, which determine how deeply each type of color permeates the hair strand: resting on top of it, sneaking inside it to a certain extent, or completely penetrating the cuticle to deposit or lift away pigment inside the cortex of the hair shaft. In addition to the actual colorant, the agents that facilitate the hair-coloring process are hydrogen peroxide, monoethanolamine (or MEA), and ammonia. These agents are also the determinants for how long the color will last.

Hydrogen peroxide is the oxidant (also referred to as "developer"), which serves as the catalyst for the hair-coloring process with demi-permanent and permanent color formulations (the same hydrogen peroxide used to clean cuts and scrapes, or to whiten teeth). When colorists talk about the "volume of peroxide," they are referring to the strength of peroxide used with hair color or bleach. Higher volume means stronger peroxide and therefore greater lightening capability.

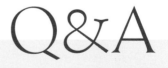

Q: *I'm trying to lead a healthier lifestyle and would like to use fewer chemicals on my hair. Is natural hair color used in salons, and is it as effective?*

A: Some salons offer vegetable-based hair dyes. These have many limitations but can be a decent alternative for those who are allergic to traditional hair color and have little to choose from. At my salon, we often use ammonia-free color for clients who have sensitivity to it or just prefer to not have it on their scalps. Whether demi-permanent or permanent formulations, ammonia-free hair color gives beautiful results if correctly formulated and applied.

MEA is an alkaline agent that helps to open the cuticle of the hair strand. It is found in demi-permanent color as well as in some permanent formulations. Ammonia is the strongest alkaline agent that is found in most permanent color and bleach. It lifts the cuticle wide open to let color be deposited inside the cortex of the hair shaft, or to allow bleach inside to break down, lighten, and remove the natural pigment molecules.

Temporary Hair Color

Temporary color is made to wash out after one shampoo. Examples are coloring sticks or mascara-like tints to mask emerging gray hair around the hairline, spray-on color, and color-depositing shampoos. These formulations alter or enhance existing color by temporarily depositing pigment on the hair until it is shampooed out.

THE RULE
Henna is a natural, healthier alternative to chemical hair color.

THE RULE BREAKER: Henna pigment, a powder ground from the
dried leaves of the henna plant, is undoubtedly natural. But is it a healthier alternative to synthetic color? Absolutely not! In fact, henna can permanently stain the hair and over time can even destroy it. The henna pigment builds up on the hair with repeated applications and eventually becomes impossible to remove, preventing conditioning agents from penetrating into the hair shaft. Therefore, treatments, conditioners, and even natural oils from your scalp are not able to get through that heavy layer of gunk covering the cuticle. With consistent use, the hair can become so dehydrated and brittle that it begins to break.

Unlike professional hair color, natural henna cannot be controlled and the results are often unpredictable. Hair colorists hate henna because it is so difficult to remove from the hair. (We have all attempted to fix quite a few at-home henna coloring mistakes.) Because henna forms a hard coating on the hair, it can be next to impossible for any other dye to penetrate it. Consequently, any new color is likely to result in a two-tone look, since it will take only in the root area (on the healthy regrowth).

Henna was traditionally used when nothing else was available. (It also became popular because it has a cooling effect on the scalp and lowers the body temperature in a hot climate.) Times have changed, thank goodness. Even in India, where henna had been the most popular, many women prefer not to use it on their hair. For people who want to live a more natural and holistic lifestyle, there are far better alternatives for hair coloring than henna. My best advice: stay away from it.

Semi-permanent Hair Color

Semi-permanent formulas do not contain peroxide or alkaline agents. Instead, they are made of slightly stronger colorants than those in temporary formulas, which deposit pigment and coat the cuticle with color. An example is a color rinse that removes yellow from the hair or provides subtle tonal changes. The color gradually washes off over eight to ten shampoos.

Demi-permanent Hair Color

A demi-permanent formula is mixed with peroxide to initiate the chemical process. It is ammonia-free with MEA as its alkaline agent. It can darken the hair to any desired shade, or lighten it by one shade. If the client has only a few grays, I use demi-permanent to cover gray hair. Since it cannot penetrate the hair shaft as completely as a permanent formula, the color fades after about twenty-four shampoos and does not leave an obvious demarcation line as the hair grows out. Depending on their level of expertise, colorists can use demi-permanent in a variety of ways. It is my go-to product whenever possible: for refreshing previously colored hair, deepening the color, lightening it a shade, or altering the tone.

Permanent Hair Color

Permanent color does not wash out or fade away—it grows out. As a result, a line of demarcation emerges near the roots as the new hair grows

Q&A

Q: *Why does my hair feel so good after having been colored?*

A: Today, color can actually improve the texture of the hair and enhance its condition. Besides imparting pigment, hair color coats the strands and smoothes the cuticle, which then reflects more light and looks shinier. It also fills in any tiny holes in the cuticle. On a damaged hair strand, this outer layer is like a rocky road filled with potholes, and hair color basically repaves it by filling in the dips with color molecules. Thus, hair becomes softer, smoother, and less frizzy. This additional layer on the hair can also add volume and density to strands, making them look and feel thicker. Highlights similarly affect volume, since bleach raises and expands the cuticle.

in. A permanent formula is used to darken or lighten the base color to any desired shade and to give 100 percent gray coverage. It gives the widest range of color possibilities. Historically, all permanent color has contained ammonia, which over time was reduced from more than 20 percent in the 1960s to less than 1.5 percent today. More recently, innovations in permanent color have enabled the complete replacement of ammonia with the alkaline agent MEA.

Bleach

Bleach primarily comes in the form of powder, cream, or paste. When combined with peroxide, it breaks down the color molecules in the cortex, causing color loss (thus lightening the hair). Bleach gives permanent results but is not considered a color, because it does not contain direct dye molecules. It is used to lift hair color by removing color molecules from the hair shaft to create highlights (strategically placed streaks of lighter hair). Some women get highlights only and may not use any permanent hair color at all. Most bleach contains ammonia, but there are ammonia-free bleach formulations available to salons. If this is a concern, ask if your salon carries them.

WHICH TYPE OF FORMULATION IS RIGHT FOR YOU?

If you were coming to see me for a new hair color, I would consider five factors to determine the right type(s) of color for your hair.

1. HOW MUCH GRAY DO YOU HAVE?

Covering gray is the most common reason why women color their hair. If your hair is more than 50 percent gray and/or you want complete coverage, I would choose a permanent hair color. Gray hair is resistant and needs a more potent formula to open up the cuticle and get the pigment into the cortex. However, if your hair is less than 50 percent gray, it is possible to get effective coverage with a demi-permanent formula that is processed with heat. (See "Gray Hair," page 71.)

2. WHAT IS THE COLOR YOU WISH TO ACHIEVE?

The desire for change is another common reason why women get their hair colored. If the color you want is two or more shades lighter than your present hair color (whether natural or dyed), you will get better results from permanent color and/or highlights. For more subtle changes a demi-permanent may suffice.

3. IS YOUR HAIR ALREADY COLOR TREATED?

If you have virgin hair, a semi-permanent can enhance your natural color and the pigment will wash out gradually. If your hair has been colored previously, you can also deepen that color with a demi-permanent. If you wish to lighten your hair, you may have to prelighten it first with bleach to remove the dark pigment before applying your desired lighter formula, especially on the ends, where color builds up over time and becomes more difficult to remove.

4. WHAT IS YOUR PREFERRED COLOR-MAINTENANCE PLAN?

A permanent color that is no more than one to two shades lighter or darker than your natural base color will allow the hair to grow in without a strong line of demarcation. A demi-permanent color will fade over time (and over many shampoos), also making the regrowth less noticeable. Generally, semi- and demi-permanents require the least amount of maintenance and the fewest salon visits. Highlighting can also be low maintenance if the highlights are incorporated in moderation.

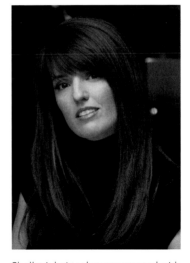

Shelley's hair color was created with a permanent formulation in the root area and demi-permanent on the ends, both in a copper-based red. The haircut has square layers cut with a razor to make her long, thick hair more manageable.

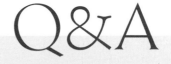

Q: *Is it safe to color my hair when I'm pregnant?*
A: Ultimately that decision is up to you and your doctor. Some expectant mothers are advised not to use hair color during their first trimester, but it is generally fine to use ammonia-free color. It is also considered safe to highlight the hair because when highlighting is done correctly, the bleach does not touch the scalp and therefore poses no risk of any chemical absorption into the bloodstream.

5. HOW DAMAGED, DRY, OR POROUS IS YOUR HAIR?

The dryness of the hair drastically affects the way color is absorbed. Depending on the level of porosity, even a temporary color can stain dry areas, like the ends. This must especially be taken into account when using demi-permanent and permanent color, so the hair does not turn out darker than expected.

FORMULATING THE COLOR
The Level of Porosity and Color Balancing

The porosity of the hair determines how much moisture (or color) it can absorb. Hair is typically the healthiest near the scalp and gets dryer toward the ends. Depending on the amount of wear and tear, environmental damage, chemical processing, and heat styling, these more porous ends are usually where hair grabs the most color. This is why they can so easily become darker than the rest of the hair, especially in the hands of an at-home colorist.

Women who color their hair may have experienced roots that are brighter than the rest of the hair (referred to as "hot roots" in the industry), ends that are too dark, or even "bands" of color down the hair shaft from bouncing between colorists (literally a different shade from each salon). Such color needs to be balanced to look even throughout. Color balancing also refers to getting the color right: finding the complementary tone for a woman's complexion and having everything work harmoniously together.

A conscientious colorist adjusts the formulation of color and the length of processing time based on porosity throughout the hair. Prior to the introduction of ammonia-free permanent color, I used a demi-permanent throughout the hair to the ends, even if applying a permanent color at the roots to cover gray. This was absolutely crucial for the health of previously colored hair, since overlapping permanent color that contains ammonia while doing a root touch-up can cause damage. (When two different formulas need to be mixed, a colorist would most likely charge you a bit extra, because a single process is truly just covering the regrowth. This is for the health of your hair; your colorist is not trying to overcharge you.) Another method to refresh the previously colored ends is the classic "soap cap" technique. After the permanent formula has processed for about thirty minutes at the roots, I work some water and a drop of shampoo through the rest of the hair and apply the remainder of the permanent color onto the wet hair. This dilutes the chemical formula so that it can safely be used throughout the hair.

DETERMINING YOUR PERFECT HAIR COLOR
Hair Color and Skin Complexion

Often, the hair color we are born with can be a bit drab for our complexions. It is not until we warm the shade and deepen it to make it richer, or lighten it, that it feels "natural." The key is to enhance what nature gave us. So how can you tell if you need a new hair color, a lighter or darker version of your natural color, or just a change in tone to a warmer or cooler shade? The best way to assess your hair color is by the way it works with your skin tone. Since it frames your face, the tone and color of your hair can dramatically affect how your skin looks, which influences how you feel about your overall appearance. If you are not happy with the color of your complexion, there is a good chance that the real problem is your hair color. The right color can make you look healthier, younger, and fresher. It can brighten the skin or neutralize a tone that has too much red or pink. The wrong shade or tone will do the opposite, by pulling color from the face.

If you feel that you look tired, sallow, or pale, or notice that your skin looks blotchy or too ruddy, it is a good indication that your hair color is not right. Hair that is too warm or brassy will exacerbate redness in the skin, while hair that is too light or dark can make you look washed out, which is likely to be the case if you need to wear more makeup in order not to feel pale. Presenting your colorist with such a problem to solve can start the creative process of determining your perfect hair color. As with haircutting, coloring should not necessarily entail a big overhaul. One or two subtle adjustments, such as adding a few highlights, going half a shade lighter or darker with your base color, or altering the overall tone of your hair, can make a profound impact. When we tend to look tired, changing our hair color is not usually the first thing that comes to mind, but it often ends up being the solution.

THE TONE AND LEVEL OF HAIR COLOR

To find your perfect hair color, a colorist must first establish two things: the tone and the level of color that will be right for you. When colorists talk about *tone* or *tonal value*, we are referring to the warmth or coolness of the color. It can be a golden or an ash blond, a warm chestnut versus a cool brown. Adjusting the tone does not affect the level, but it does affect your overall color. *Levels* of hair color refer to the lightness or darkness of a color. Levels go from one to ten; ten is the lightest blond, one is black, and medium brown is five or six. Most women have the wrong tone, not the wrong color, for their skin. You may have a nice medium-brown level, which can be too red or golden for you, or flat and ashy. A slight adjustment in the tonal value will be enough to dramatically improve your hair color and the appearance of your skin.

The Tone—Getting It Right

The guidelines of color tones (warm, cool, or neutral) are actually quite simple. Most people are confused about the undertones of their skin, which are really not that complicated to understand. According to basic color theory, red is a warm color and green is cool. Yellow and olive are close to green and fall in the cool category. Most people think of darker skin with yellow or olive undertones as "warm," but it is actually those with pink or red in their skin who have warm complexions. Ultimately, you want to be more neutral and balanced overall. Therefore, if you have red in your skin, go cooler with your hair color. A gold or red tone in the hair will only exacerbate the redness. Conversely, if your skin has

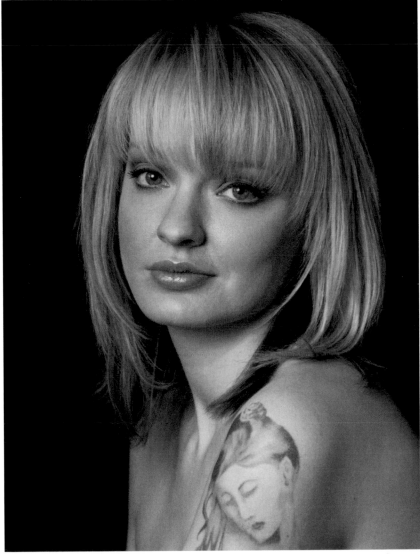

Kerstin has a neutral skin tone—a balance of warm and cool undertones that gives her the widest range of colors to choose from. She prefers a light golden blond, created here with a combination of foils and balayage highlights that frame her face. Her triangular layered cut was done with scissors.

yellow or green undertones, tends to tan easily, or looks sallow when you have not been in the sun, it will be complemented by a warmer hair color. For example, because I have fair yellow skin, the red in my auburn hair adds warmth to my complexion. Some find that their skin falls somewhere in the middle—a neutral tone with an equal balance of yellow and pink. These women have a wider range of hair colors that complement their complexions and can usually base color choices on personal preference.

My fair yellow complexion is balanced by the warmth in my hair color, which is created using ammonia-free permanent color in the base with face-framing balayage highlights. My concave layers are cut with scissors.

For an example of a warm complexion that is balanced with cool-toned hair color, see Marisel on page 21.

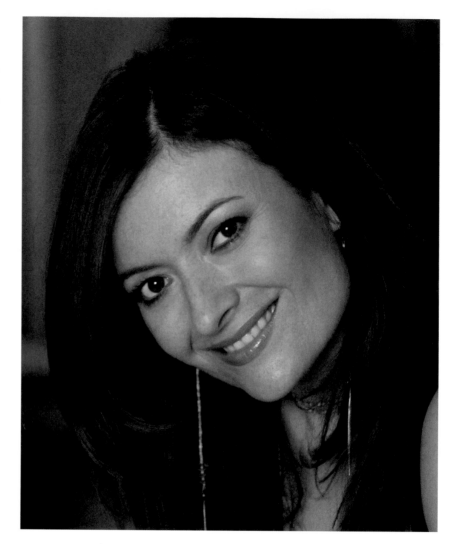

BEAUTY SECRET

How to tell if you need a darker hair color

If you fear that your hair has become too light or overhighlighted, you can do a simple test at home. Hair becomes two to three shades darker when wet. Wet your hair, put on your daytime makeup, and comb the hair next to your face. You will instantly see if your complexion looks brighter. Then, reevaluate your complexion once the hair is dry. If you prefer the way you look with wet hair, this is a good indication that it will probably look better darker. I frequently do this easy test at my salon, especially on blondes, to show how much better a client's skin looks with a little more contrast between her complexion and hair color.

The Right Level

When you have the correct tone and shade of hair color, your skin automatically looks more radiant. With the right amount of contrast between hair color and skin tone, the hair will not fade into or clash with the complexion. Choosing the right level of brunette, blond, or red should be based on your natural hair color. Usually, a good range for your base color is within one to two levels of your natural shade, whether lighter or darker, which will also look the most natural as it grows out. (Your highlights can be lighter than that.)

THE COLOR CONSULTATION
Pictures Speak a Thousand Words

A good colorist, like a good haircutter, is a problem solver. Therefore, during the color consultation you should address any issues you want resolved, such as gray coverage or the tendency for your hair to go brassy. Even though many of these concerns will be apparent to the colorist when she sees you, some are more subtle, so it is important to convey what is bothering you. For example, if you hate the red undertone in your brown hair, you need to communicate that detail; otherwise, the colorist may use a warm color, thinking that is your preference.

During the initial consultation, the colorist usually has to do some decoding. Often a woman knows that she wants something different but is not sure what it may be or how to clearly describe it, and words often just don't cut it. People can have a different concept of "blond" or "natural brown." My idea of "sun-kissed," "golden," or "caramel" highlights may be very different from yours.

Even though after reading this chapter you will have a better working knowledge of hair color, I have one important piece of advice when it comes to conveying what you want: bring color photographs to your appointment. They allow your colorist to understand more clearly what type of color you are attracted to and help establish a precise direction in which to go: how blond you want to be, how many highlights you want and where you want them placed, the amount of red in your natural brunette that you feel comfortable with, or how much gold you like in your hair. Nothing beats a photograph for narrowing the communication gap between client and colorist. You can rip out pictures from magazines or bring photos of yourself with different hair colors or even a childhood photograph of your natural color. Sometimes it is important for a colorist to see what nature gave you and it can help him or her to formulate the color more effectively.

Another worthy topic to discuss during the consultation is your budget and lifestyle. How can your hair color and cut fit comfortably into both? Don't be shy about telling your colorist how often you prefer to come for color maintenance and how much you want to spend on your hair annually. If you need a low-maintenance hair color, you may have to reconsider the idea of lightening your brown hair to an all-over blond or becoming a fiery redhead. Your colorist should be happy to devise a hair-color strategy that will work for your budget and time constraints. That could mean touching up the highlights two or three times a year instead of every time you do your base color or applying a glaze at the roots in between touch-ups to lift the base slightly and revitalize the brightness of the highlights. Talk to her about ways that you can stretch out salon visits for your single process from every four to every six weeks.

THE ART OF LAYERING COLOR

The most beautiful hair color has numerous subtle shades within it. This is how nature intended our hair to be. Look at a child's hair for inspiration: it has multiple variations of the same tone and different shades of blond, gold, or brown beautifully blended together. That combination of light and dark is what looks the most natural and appealing. Putting just one shade of color all over the hair will rarely maximize the lines and movement of the cut or the texture of the hair. Layering hair color is a concept similar to the shading in a charcoal drawing: it is not until depth is added and light and dark are in harmony that you see the true shape of the image. It becomes more three-dimensional and is brought to life. Adding various levels of color into the picture makes even a very simple haircut look more alluring and feminine.

Highlights

The word *highlight* is defined as "an area of illumination," which is in fact what highlighting does for the hair. A few strategically placed pieces that are two to three levels lighter than the base color can add just the right amount of contrast to define the layers and shape of the cut. The placement and painting of highlights (and lowlights) are where the artistry of hair coloring becomes truly profound. Before adding highlights, I consider how they can illuminate the face, bring out the lines of the haircut, and enhance the texture of the client's hair. How I customize the color depends

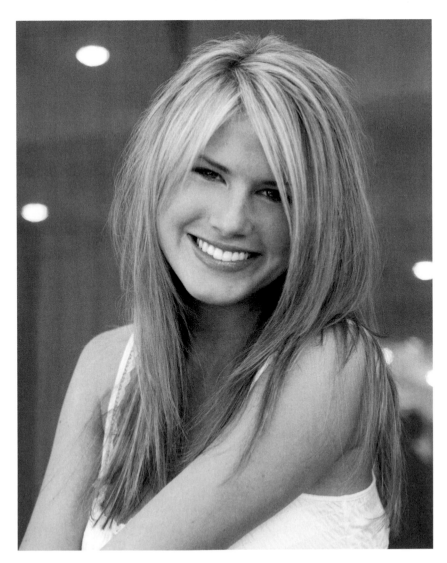

Anne Marie has foiled highlights and a golden glaze. Her square layers were cut using scissors.

Kirsten's highlights and lowlights were created with the balayage technique. Her haircut with concave layers was designed using a combination of scissors and a razor.

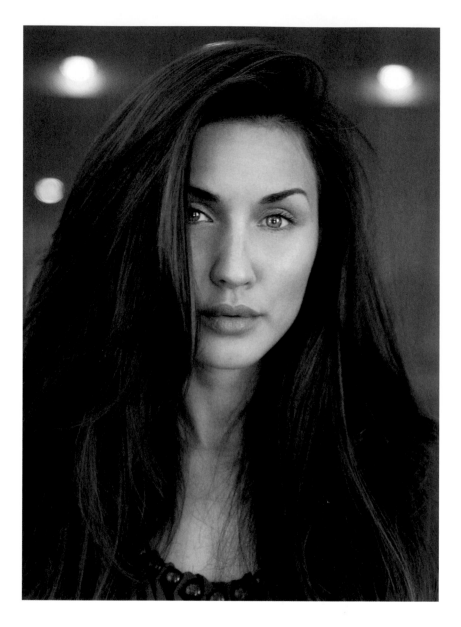

on the individual in my chair. I might paint finer highlights around the face or the bang area to brighten the eyes and complexion. Thicker highlights may be flattering on one woman, while on another, the same wider panels can look too chunky. You can use highlights to become an overall blonde or place just a few of them around your hairline to enhance your natural color. Whether the base color is your natural shade or one that your colorist has formulated for you, adding highlights will brighten your complexion, reflect light, and bring out dimension within any haircut.

Often a woman will start with a few highlights, then add more with each successive appointment. Gradually, her hair becomes too light. Whether the hair starts to feel overprocessed or the color begins to look flat and one-dimensional, she may have ended up with too much of a good thing. A simple way to avoid this is to touch up only the regrowth from the previous highlights, rather than add blond to new sections of hair. Additionally, to prevent your hair from becoming too light, highlights should not be placed too close together. Some lowlights can always be added if you have gone overboard. If your hair has become dry or damaged, give it a rest by having only a few highlights added around your face.

If a client wants to be an overall blonde and her hair is in good condition, highlights should be woven closer together in finer, thinner sections. Such placement will create the "wow factor" that she is looking for. I would also consider using a single process to lighten her base color and remove the shadow in the root area.

Hair Damage Can Start in the Salon

Most hair damage occurs from applying color (especially that contains ammonia) or bleach to hair that has been previously colored. Highlights should be placed only on the new growth, yet when a section of hair is cov-

BEAUTY SECRET

Have a decent shape to your hair for your first color appointment

Many think that since they are going to a salon, they should not bother doing their hair beforehand. This seems to make sense, since you are going to have your hair done by a professional. However, it is difficult for the hairdresser to see how your hair moves if it is dirty or pulled back into a ponytail. Hair also looks a shade or two darker when it needs to be washed, making it harder to accurately assess the color. When your hair is not styled in the way you typically wear it, your colorist is operating with limited information. By no means does it have to be perfect, but when a client comes in with her basic hair shape in place, I can see clearly what needs to be done. It is also easier for me to find the inspiration to create something different for her that day. This is especially good to keep in mind for first-time clients, but it remains important if your regular colorist is making any changes to your hair. Your colorist needs to see the texture and density of your hair, as well as how it moves, where it parts, and the amount of wave or curl it has when you style it yourself, for the proper placement of highlights.

ered with bleach, placed between aluminum foil, and heated, the bleach begins to expand and migrates beyond where it was initially applied. This is why so many blondes experience breakage. When using foils, it is critical that the colorist allow room for the bleach to expand by not overly saturating each section of hair and actually stopping about a quarter of an inch short of the previously highlighted area. This type of breakage is so common that in the industry it is sometimes referred to as a "chemical cut." It can inadvertently create unwanted layers or even bangs, in addition to more extreme damage. Most often it is caused by neglect or inexperience. One of the reasons I am so partial to the balayage method of highlighting, which does not require aluminum foil, is that it enables the colorist to see exactly where the bleach stops. Also, since the lightener is typically mixed a bit thicker than for foils, it is more likely to stay put.

It pays to be aware and to speak up if you start to notice breakage in you hair. You can say something like, "I know how careful you always are, but I just want to remind you that I am experiencing breakage. Please be extra careful about applying lightener only on my regrowth." A gentle reminder like this can prevent a great deal of heartache, avoid potential damage, and save your relationship with your colorist. A true professional will appreciate the input and that instead of going to someone else, you are giving him or her an opportunity to pay closer attention.

Highlighting Techniques: Balayage or Foils?

When it comes to choosing the right highlighting method for you, a few factors should be considered. Foiling the hair is the most traditional and common. No matter where you are in the world, the majority of salons use this simple and easy technique. With foils, you can effectively lighten the hair in a multitude of shades and a variety of tones. Foils allow the colorist to stay organized in the application.

The balayage technique is the one I am truly in love with, and the beautiful effect it produces is completely different from that of foils. The word *balayage* is French for "sweeping" or "to sweep." It is a true art form, since the colorist literally hand paints the hair, using a brush and palette. She applies the lightener to specific sections of the hair with short, sweeping strokes. Mastering balayage has been inspirational for me as an artist

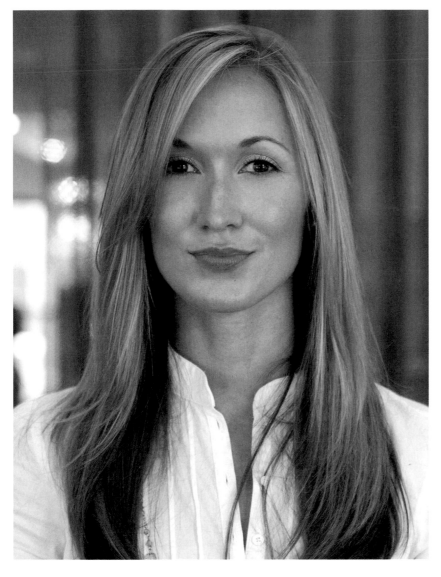

Ashley's highlights were done using balayage.

and has allowed me to take my color work to a whole new level. All of the colorists to whom I have taught this highlighting method have also fallen in love with it. To professionals, it feels like we are learning hair color all over again in a fresh, new way. Balayage gives me the freedom of placing color exactly where I want it, as opposed to following the more rigid placement that foils require. The color looks more natural, with subtle dimensions and variations, and it grows out beautifully. By hand painting, I can create a more profound impact with fewer highlights; this is why I also believe that it is healthier for the hair.

So why use foils at all? The highlighting technique I use depends on how dark your hair is and what tone of highlights you desire. Foil is an excellent conductor of heat and gives a colorist the ability to lighten the hair all the way from a naturally dark shade to a pale blond. If my goal is to get cool-toned highlights from dark hair that has a tendency to go red, I would use foils. But to create light beige to warm-golden highlights, I would prefer to balayage the hair.

Most people associate highlights with blond hair, but on dark brown or black hair they can create beautiful definition and dimension. Since dark hair tends to absorb light, it can appear flat in its natural (or manufactured) state. Weaving in a few highlights adds more light to the hair and brings out the shape of the haircut. However, correctly highlighting brunette hair is not without its challenges. Because the underlying pigment in dark hair is red, when the brown is lifted with bleach, the red colors emerge. Some women do not mind the warmth that highlights give, while others hate it. Bleach is tough to control (you know this if you have ever accidentally gotten some on your clothing while doing laundry). If it is left on the hair for too long or not long enough, the highlights can end up orange or yellow, which is why many brunettes shy away from them. Despite that, you should know that an experienced and skilled colorist understands how to work with the underlying red pigment in dark hair to create the effect you want.

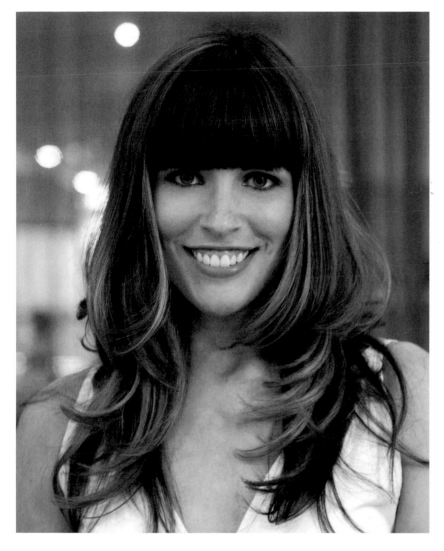

Kristen's highlights and lowlights were done using balayage.

Lowlights

Lowlights are usually about two shades darker than the highlights and are woven throughout for added depth and contrast, which makes the hair color look more authentic and multidimensional (the way nature intended). To choose the most appropriate shade, use your natural color as a guideline. Extending this slightly darker hue will also make the re-growth less noticeable, allowing for more time between salon visits. If your natural color is too dark, choose a level that is between the base color and your highlights.

If your hair has *not* been overly highlighted, your actual base color may act as the perfect lowlight and provide the necessary contrast and depth to complement blond highlights. I also like to add lowlights to medium brown and auburn hair to create more movement and richness, making a color that can otherwise look solid and one-dimensional more interesting.

Glaze

A glaze is a translucent demi-permanent color that is used to alter or reinvigorate the tone of the hair and to increase shine. It is the most effective way to blend away the "stripiness" after highlighting. A glaze, also known as a "gloss," does not have to change the level of the hair color, but it can make the tone cooler or warmer. An icy-toned glaze adds a cool tonal value, while a golden glaze will warm up the color. A cool-toned glaze also neutralizes warmth in all hair color and can defuse the brassiness of highlights or take down the yellow tint in gray hair.

A clear glaze or gloss coats the hair like a clear topcoat of polish on your nails, adding a smooth sheen to it. It does not mask your hair color but enhances it. Think of a glazed doughnut—you can still see the doughnut beneath the shiny glaze and it is still the same color; it just looks more enticing.

Natural hair color begins to fade in our thirties or forties and becomes much less vibrant. A typical example is a natural-born blonde who over time turns into a light brunette. Another is a redhead whose hints of sparkling copper and gold gradually fade. As a result, many women are unhappy with their hair color but are also afraid that having it professionally colored will look unnatural. They do not want to completely transform their hair color—they just want to enliven it! I have had so many clients convey their fear of never getting back their true color and going from their current drab shade to a fake-looking dye job. They also worry about the trap of starting to color their hair and having to contend with roots.

The good news is that the possibilities have really expanded for women who love their natural color but need just a little boost. A low-maintenance glaze can re-create their once-beautiful shade with nuances of red, copper, or gold, returning the hair to its natural beauty without completely altering the hue. It is a very subtle way of coloring hair that can make a dramatic difference.

Bear in mind, however, that these are demi-permanent formulations and it is wise to exercise some caution. Although they make the hair look healthier, having this done too frequently can dehydrate it. Even a clear gloss contains peroxide and can be drying to the hair over time. If your hair is healthy, you can have a glaze applied every time you visit the salon for color. However, if it is damaged, this should be done less often, or kept only in the root area. Women often overuse at-home glazing products thinking that the longer they leave them on, the shinier their hair will become. Be sure to read the label to see if the product contains hydrogen peroxide and follow the instructions carefully. If the glaze is peroxide-free, it can be used more frequently.

With blond hair, especially if it is particularly porous and dry, you can still use a glaze and reap its benefits; the key is to leave it on for less time. This way, it will not mask the brightness of your highlights or make your hair appear darker from over absorption. Stick to using clear or very pale colors and process for just one to three minutes. Ask your colorist to stay close and keep an eye on it. Every second matters when working with bleached hair. I typically stand at the sink with my assistant, waiting for the exact moment to rinse it off.

PROFESSIONAL TECHNIQUE

How to refresh your highlights

A glaze applied at the roots not only will refresh your hair color but will buy you another month before the next touch-up. (Highlights usually need to be touched up every eight to ten weeks, depending on how fast the hair grows.) If your hair is blond, I suggest a glaze four to five weeks after getting highlights. It will help blend the root area, minimizing that halo of darkness near the scalp to take the edge off the contrast between highlights and the natural base color. This quick, simple process makes the blond sparkle and brightens the entirety of the hair color. Another way to make your highlights look lighter and brighter is by adding a few lowlights underneath. The contrast makes the highlights stand out and almost look new again.

PROFESSIONAL TECHNIQUES

"Skinny hair" and other optical illusions

Hair color not only accentuates the haircut but can enhance your bone structure. For example, richer colors at the sides of the face provide shading, making the cheeks look a bit slimmer and more defined. So, for someone with a round face, I may lowlight the sides and keep highlights on top of the head. This shading creates depth around the frame of the haircut to minimize weight on either side of the face.

I call this technique "skinny hair." It entails strategically placed hair color on the sides of the head to narrow a full face. Conversely, lightening at the temples and sides of the head with highlights creates the impression of more width, which is perfect for someone with a long face.

Manipulation of light and dark shades in hair color can also make fine hair appear thicker. Expertly applied lowlights can add more visual depth to the hair. The trick is to weave in very fine, darker sections throughout the areas of the head that would benefit from looking thicker, such as underneath, above the ears, and lightly through the crown. Keep in mind, however, that lowlights that are too thick can make the hair look even thinner. The most natural and dimensional look is actually created by alternating fine with small-to-medium-size sections.

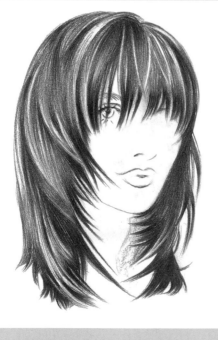

Making a round face appear slimmer.

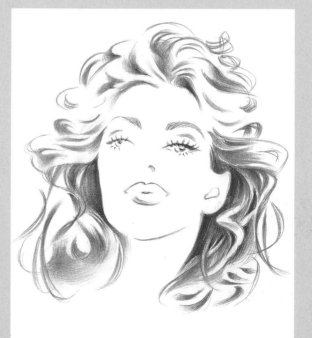

Making a narrow face appear broader.

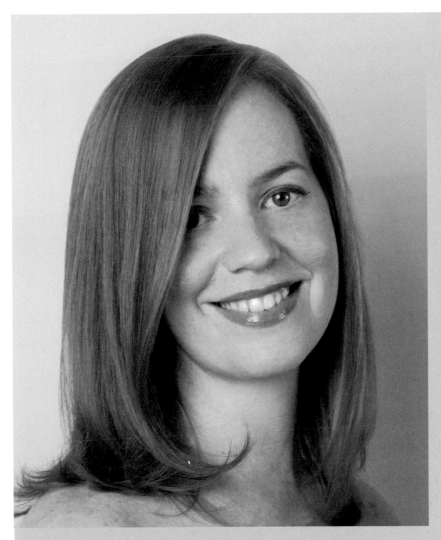

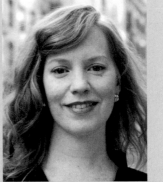

Before

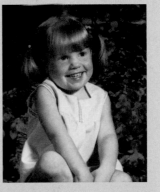

When I met Anny, she told me that her wish was to once again have her childhood hair color. She showed me this adorable photo, and I completely understood. I used a light copper demi-permanent color and a clear glaze. I cut her round layers with scissors. Her biggest fear was that the color would look fake. She never imagined that becoming a "natural redhead," once again, could be so easy.

Regaining your natural red hair

Red is one of the most gorgeous hair colors, but when it begins to fade, it is difficult to re-create that unique, natural shade. A perfect recipe for a beautiful natural-looking redhead begins with placing a few blond highlights around the face and lifting them only to a light golden color. The lightener should be left on for no more than ten minutes without heat. Then apply a golden red glaze that matches the hair's original shade all over for about ten to fifteen minutes. This will enrich the natural red and make the highlights a brighter, more beautiful strawberry color.

Personal Story

Communicating through pictures

Some pictures that clients bring are more helpful than others, and some are simply hilarious! I specify "color" pictures because a client once showed me a black-and-white photograph to demonstrate the blond she wanted. Although I could see the placement of the highlights, the color was a mystery. This, however, was not the most original visual expression of a dream hair color: another woman actually brought in a picture of her Irish setter and told me this was the type of red she wanted (that actually was helpful). And once, during a haircut consultation, a woman drew a stick figure with about seven hairs popping out of the head as an example of the hair shape she was going for. It looked like a Charlie Brown comic strip and was one of the only times I did not find a picture useful!

HAIRMARE

Obsessive-Compulsive Blonde Disorder

OCBD is a condition that may not yet have been clinically diagnosed, but it has long been identified and fretted over by hair colorists. This mental disorder occurs when a woman feels she is never light or blond enough, hopping from salon to salon and terrorizing colorists in her path. In her never-ending quest for that "perfect blond"—the holy grail of hair color, which does not exist—she is never satisfied and destroys her hair in the process. If you feel that you may suffer from OCBD, there is help, but you will not find it in a salon. On behalf of the industry, I urge you to switch from the salon chair to a therapist's couch, so that you can get to the "root" of the problem.

Common Mistake

Adding highlights because it's summertime

The notion of adding highlights for the summer is ingrained in so many women, but it actually should work in reverse. I prefer to weave in a few highlights in the wintertime when your hair color and skin tone can look dull. This brightens the hair and the complexion, giving you a boost in a gray, dark season. Adding highlights for the summer is often unnecessary, since hair naturally gets lighter from sun exposure. If you add more, by the end of summer the combination of bleach, sun, and salt water could make the hair too white, dry, or brassy. Especially if I know that a client is going to spend a lot of time outdoors, there is no need to give her a double whammy.

GRAY HAIR

Even if you have only a few gray hairs, you are likely to remember your reaction when you noticed the first one. Perhaps it was a combination of shock and panic: "How is this possible? I'm too young to go gray!" and "How do I get rid of it?" You probably plucked that offending hair out immediately. I did it myself when I found a gray hair—it was an impulsive reaction and I needed to get rid of the enemy. Thankfully, that myth about plucking one gray hair producing ten more in its place is just that. A gray-hair militia does not come in to save the tweezed strand. Although you cannot create more gray hairs by extricating one, the idea certainly taps into our worst fears: that they will proliferate like weeds. The truth is, once you notice one, you start to spot more and more because your eye is now tuned in to finding grays that may have been hiding from sight before. And of course, once hair begins to go gray, it does not stop with just one. It is not a bad thing to pluck a gray hair now and then, but it is not the solution.

Why Does Hair Turn Gray?

There are a number of theories about what causes gray hair, but two determining factors are clear: the aging process and genetics. If your mother or grandmother went gray at an early age, it is likely that you will, too. As we get older, melanin pigment decreases in the cortex of the hair shaft. Like all our cells, melanocytes (the body's pigment makers) slow down and ultimately retire for good. When melanin production stops, color in the hair does as well.

Scientific research about gray hair abounds in the hope that if an exact cause is found, it could lead to a discovery that prevents the phenomenon altogether. Recent studies have shown that hair turns gray as a result of hydrogen peroxide, trace amounts of which are naturally produced by hair cells. It acts as a pigment eraser, but is broken down and diffused by the enzyme *catalase,* which decreases as we age, eventually allowing hydrogen peroxide to build up and block the synthesis of melanin. This lightens the hair from the inside out, causing it to become gray or white.

Interestingly, this is the same chemical reaction as that which produces vitiligo, a genetic disease that causes loss of pigment in the skin.

A link between psychological stress and graying hair has not been scientifically proved, but there certainly seems to be a connection. Just look at every recent president of the United States; each one rapidly turns grayer with every passing year in office. Another theory is that a mineral deficiency in the body could cause hair to turn gray faster. It is noteworthy that Asian populations with a higher mineral content in their diets do not seem to go gray as early in life. This could be because edible marine seaweed, a staple in most Asian diets, has a higher mineral content than land plants. Increasing the intake of kelp and spirulina, whether through food or supplements, can maximize our levels of important minerals like sodium, magnesium, and iron, and perhaps slow the graying process.

Regardless of why it happens, women primarily want to know what they should do about it once it starts. It is important to realize that you have control, whether you want to camouflage or cover the grays or choose to embrace them.

Styling Away the Grays

It is frustrating that gray hairs show up right where they are most unwanted, at the part and around the hairline, as if they had some kind of evil plan. And they seem to pop up within just a few weeks of having your hair colored. New growth typically needs to be touched up every four weeks, but there are simple ways to extend your color by another week or two (as long as your roots do not exceed three-quarters of an inch).

Just moving your hair into a slightly different position, like changing your part to a spot where you have fewer grays, can do an effective smoke-and-mirrors job. Grays are also more apparent when they are flat against the head, so creating some volume at the root deflects the eye from them. Teasing your hair a bit at the crown adds height and makes the gray hair at the base less noticeable. In general, wearing the hair looser and fuller allows for more movement, which helps camouflage emerging gray roots. Do not style your hair in strict separations or parts and do not pull it completely off your face. Wearing the hair more forward on the face literally covers the grays at the hairline. In fact, if you feel that grays are especially prevalent around your face, consider talking to your hairstylist about cutting a longer, side-swept bang.

Covering Gray

The cuticle of a gray hair is less permeable and it takes more work for hydrogen peroxide and an alkaline agent to open it. It is like a door that is sealed shut. This is why most colorists use permanent hair color to cover gray. It gives perfect coverage and allows for more possibilities. However, when a client wants to blend her gray hair, instead of covering it completely, and to avoid a demarcation line, I often use a demi-permanent color.

Embracing Gray

There are a number of good reasons why a woman may decide to go gray, but ultimately the decision comes down to preference and personal choice. One motivation is certainly to eliminate the monthly touch-ups that gray coverage demands. It can be a relief to stop the continual upkeep of gray roots. Some would rather just accept their gray hair because they feel that coloring it is unnatural. Others are simply blessed with stunningly beautiful white hair, which is only one shade from platinum blond and can be very glamorous. For many, going gray can be a personal statement about self-acceptance—a way to embrace their age and who they are as women.

If you have been coloring your hair and have now decided to embrace your natural shade, you must begin by growing it out. This can require an uncomfortable six to twelve months. Gorgeous hair color does not come easily—even if you are going natural. Unless you do not mind a two-tone look as the gray roots grow in, you have to get rid of the previously colored hair. If your hair is already relatively short, say just below the ears, you might consider going with an even shorter, cropped style to eliminate most of the previously dyed hair. Wearing a little extra makeup and jewelry is my personal recommendation for feeling more feminine if your hair is temporarily shorter. During this growing-out period, a colorist may suggest applying a semi-permanent color over your hair to balance out the uneven tones and take the edge off. *Don't do it!* A semi-permanent formula will not fully cover the gray anyway and can stain your hair, especially if

BEAUTY SECRET

Using a brush to apply hair color

On hard-to-cover gray, a brush is the only application option because it physically drives the color into resistant strands. Applying color with the tip of a nozzle does not have the same force or friction. I gently jab at the roots with the tips of the hard bristles to create some agitation and help open up the cuticle layer for proper coverage.

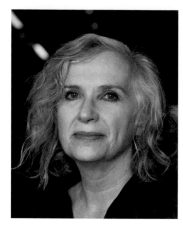

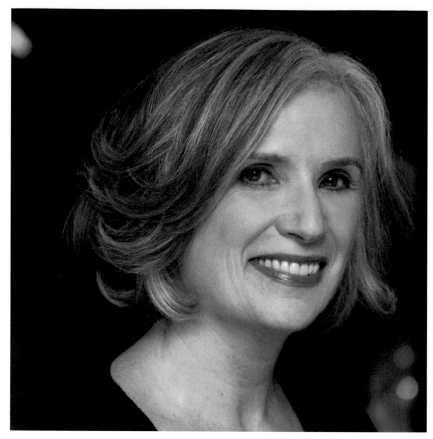

Before: Using a cool-toned permanent color, lowlights were painted onto Devin's naturally gray hair. Her solid bob line was cut with scissors, while round layers were added using a razor. Her eyebrows were colored one shade darker to help define their natural shape.

the ends are dry and porous. This only adds another layer of pigment to the hair and defeats the purpose of letting the artificial color grow out. Additionally, as a semi-permanent color fades, it can leave behind a yellow tint on gray or white hair. It is best to bite the bullet, cut off as much of the previously colored hair as possible, and start fresh.

Improving on Nature: Enhancing Gray

Very often, gray hair can benefit from some added dimension to prevent it from appearing dull or washing out the complexion. A few lowlights can make the growing-out process less painful by blending different levels of gray or silver throughout the hair. Lowlights, often the shade of your original pre-gray base color, can be woven in the underneath, back, and side sections of the hair. It is a great way to break up the overall lightness while still allowing the hair to look natural—essentially adding some pepper back to the salt. If you are mostly gray, think back to how your hair looked five to ten years ago. Lowlights return the depth your hair had before it went completely gray.

How Not to Look Washed Out with Gray Hair

Deciding to go gray is not necessarily about doing less; it is about doing something different. Gray, silver, and white hair do not impart any warmth to the skin, so makeup becomes imperative. Typically, gray hair tends to make a woman look older because the color palette is now a more drab tone, as opposed to the warmer browns, blonds, or reds. Therefore, it starts to wash out the skin tone. You will probably find that you need to compensate with makeup for this lack of color and contrast. You can go one shade darker with your foundation, wear a bit more blush, or warm the skin with a light dusting of bronzer. Lipstick also becomes much more important and is an easy way to enliven your face. I have found that a pale pink or peach eye shadow can be especially helpful to bring brightness to the eye area. A peach or brighter pink blush also works wonders.

Most women mistakenly overlook grooming their eyebrows, which can have an even greater impact when you have gray hair. Well-shaped eyebrows add sharpness to the facial features, which also helps to avoid looking washed out. They become a permanent type of makeup, bringing definition to the eyes. To bring them to life, I use a hair color that is similar to the base color the woman once had. It is important to choose a cool-toned color for the brows to blend with the gray shade above.

A few highlights can also be added around the face, especially if the hair is a darker gray there. It is important that the highlights and lowlights match the tonal value of the gray hair, which means that they need to be cool toned. Nothing looks worse than golden highlights next to gray hair. Highlights should be bleached to more of a white and lowlights should be a slate, pewter, cool black, or ash brown. Look at a piece of white marble for inspiration. These are the shades that blend perfectly. Because bleach tends to pull gold, I often prefer just to add lowlights and use the natural white hair as the highlight color.

BEAUTY SECRET

Why you should stay on schedule with root touch-ups

The reason why colorists tell you to come back every four to six weeks to have your roots done is not just to get you into the salon more often. It is actually for the sake of your hair. When hair color is applied at the scalp, your natural body heat helps to process it. This heat can radiate only one-half to three-quarters of an inch off the scalp, which is how much hair typically grows in four to six weeks. If your roots exceed that, the color is likely to darken or lighten the hair unevenly. This is evident when women have darker "bands" of color in their hair—perfect in the immediate area of the regrowth but a different shade beyond that. Trying to compensate for that body-heat disparity with artificial heat from a lamp will only make the color process faster all over and intensify the problem (since now you are dealing with both body heat and artificial heat). This is also how you end up with "hot roots." So stay on schedule if you want an even color.

Improving the Texture of Gray Hair

Okay, so now you are officially a silver fox! Don't think that because you are back to your natural color, there is no need to do anything with it. The wiry, coarse texture of most gray hair can look like a pulled guitar string and has to be appropriately cared for. This is why regular brushing is absolutely essential for gray-haired women. It greatly improves the shine by distributing the natural oil from the scalp down the hair shaft. After about six weeks of nightly brushing I promise that your hair will become smoother, softer, and glossier. Another easy way to bring luster and life to gray hair is by removing the residue (such as product buildup) that sits on the surface and dulls the hair. Once a week, wash your hair with a clarifying shampoo or mix some apple cider vinegar into your regular shampoo.

All my clients with gray hair get professional glossing treatments and they cannot believe the difference. This clear top coat gives the hair shine and the white appears more opulent. It coats the cuticle and makes the strands sleeker, blending the texture of grays with the rest of your hair. (Warning: If a glaze is left on too long, it can start to alter the color of your gray, turning it into a golden or light brown.) Because even gray hair still has a bit of natural pigment left in it, the small amount of peroxide in a glaze can pull warmth if left on too long. To keep your gray hair looking as healthy and shiny as possible, I suggest having a glossing treatment done at your salon every six to eight weeks.

Keeping Gray from Turning Yellow

The yellowing of gray hair is a common complaint. This is caused by external factors like exposure to the sun, chlorine, or even metal deposits from the water in your home. Gray hair often becomes discolored in the same way as a light fabric yellows in the sun or brunettes go brassy. To prevent this, protect your hair with a hat or a scarf. You can also buy a water filter for your shower that will help to eliminate mineral deposits.

The yellow tint can be corrected at a salon by applying a pastel glaze. This is a clear glaze with a violet-based pigment that helps to neutralize the yellow. It gives you a sparkling, brighter, and more beautiful gray, silver, or white shade. To get rid of the yellow at home, you might try using a violet-based shampoo once a week. These are available at most salons and beauty-supply stores. There are also temporary rinses that are formulated to remove the yellow. However, they can easily overdeposit color and create an unnatural cast over the hair. We have all seen older women with that odd blue, pink, or lavender hue to their hair, which occurs when a rinse is left on too long or repeated too frequently. A violet-based shampoo is much safer to use.

THE RULE
Never wash your hair before having it colored.

THE RULE BREAKER: Contrary to popular belief, it is a terrific idea
to wash your hair the morning of your color appointment, particularly if you have grays. The exception is when getting highlights, since the natural oils on the hair protect it from the drying effects of bleach. Because gray hair is already resistant to color, an additional layer of buildup from your natural oils, styling products, and pollution further inhibits absorption. If the hair is clean, you will achieve better coverage. Try using a clarifying shampoo the morning of your salon visit to more effectively remove residue.

DRASTIC MEASURES WHEN YOU NEED A MAJOR CHANGE

Extreme color transformations can mean deciding to go all gray, going back to your natural color after being blond for years, or becoming a blonde because it is what you have always wanted.

Nearly all women have fantasized at one time or another about having a totally different hair color. Brunettes wonder what it would be like to be a blonde or a redhead. And there are plenty of light-haired women who want to be dark, rich brunettes. Going to extremes is not necessarily a

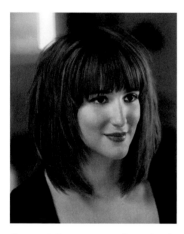

Gwynne's hair is copper-based red with round layers cut with scissors.

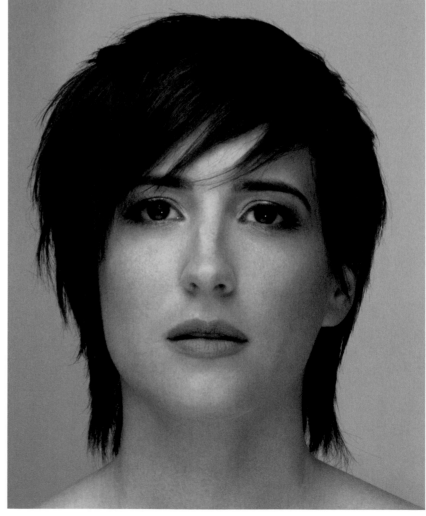

Her deep chocolate color was created with a demi-permanent formula. The square layers were cut with a razor.

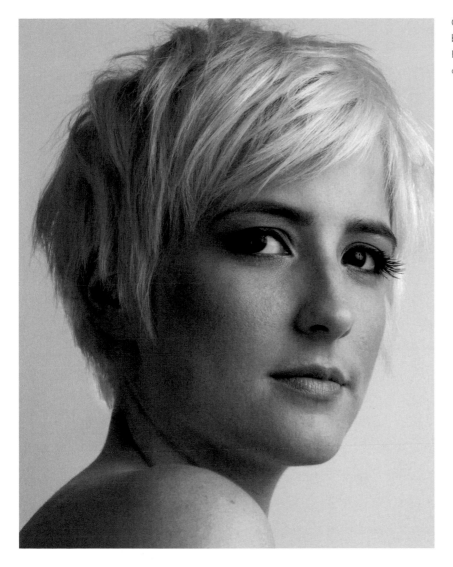

Gwynne was lightened to platinum blond and toned with a cool glaze. Her graduated short layers were done with a razor.

bad idea, but it is one to think about seriously. What kind of maintenance will it need? How damaging might the coloring be to your hair? And of course, will it be flattering for you? These are very important questions to talk over with your colorist beforehand. Often, when a woman needs some kind of change in her life, what she can control and make over immediately is her hair. (You can't always change your circumstances, but you can change your hair!) I have seen women make mistakes by taking their frustrations out on their hair and being too rash, impulsive, or eager for change. Take a moment to consider the consequences. That being said, there are times in one's life when I profoundly believe in personal change

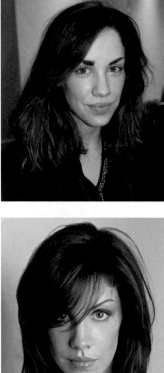

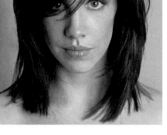

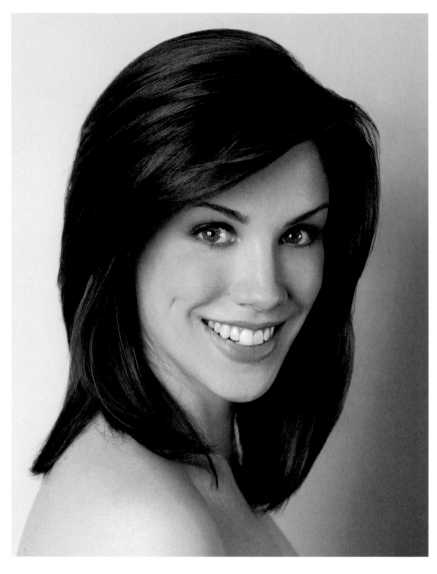

Heather's hair was first pre-lightened with balayage highlights. A rich red (violet and copper-based) demi-permanent color was then applied. Her triangular layers were cut with a razor. Her eyebrows were lightened and slightly warmed with permanent color.

and physical transformation. A makeover can be just what the doctor (or hairdresser) ordered.

Change is often best when done gradually. For example, if a dark brunette wants to go blond, I suggest that she start with some highlights around her face rather than bleach the entirety of the hair. Then, every eight to twelve weeks, I can integrate a few additional lighter pieces. Eventually I may lift her base color to pull all those highlights together and she will become a blonde. A slower transformation, in addition to being safer for the hair, is less shocking to you

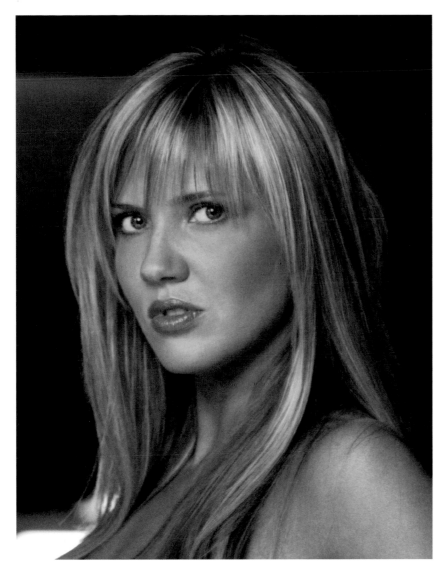

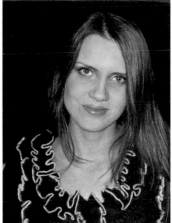

Before.

To create Alina's bombshell blond, her hair was highlighted to a pale shade using the balayage technique in combination with an icy, platinum glaze. Her triangular layers were cut with scissors and her bangs with a razor. This transformation was done over a few appointments.

and those around you. People will just comment on how great your hair looks.

Once you have made a significant change to your hair color, you should maintain it for a while. It is the constant back-and-forth of color extremes—going from blond to brunette and back to blond again—that stresses your hair, literally to the breaking point. There are trade-offs to consider. You cannot maintain long hair and frequently make drastic color changes, for example. With shorter hair you have much more freedom because you are regularly cutting off the ends, which typically experience the most damage.

CORRECTING AND REBALANCING YOUR COLOR

Women come to me all the time to have their hair color corrected (whether it's color they did themselves or from a salon). If your color has somehow gone wrong, it is definitely worth your while to look for a truly experienced and skilled colorist to fix it. The only way that a colorist becomes good at color correction is through years of tackling all kinds of nightmarish chemical circumstances. This person must have a combination of technical expertise and artistic sensibility to get your hair back on track.

Solutions to hair color mistakes can be quite challenging. The term *decolorizing* means removing the oversaturation of dye in the hair by using an array of professional products made specifically for this purpose. Perhaps the ends of the hair are much darker than the roots from an at-home color job or a temporary color has permanently stained blond hair.

COMMON MISTAKE

Judging your hair color in the wrong light

The reason why your hair color looks so gorgeous in the salon as opposed to how it sometimes appears elsewhere is a simple matter of lighting. The lighting in a salon has to be as accurate as possible. In the daytime, there is also an element of natural light diffused throughout the space. One day I glanced at my hair in the car mirror when the sunroof was open and thought, Oh my God, I'm a blazing redhead! Actually I'm a warm brunette, but the color looked much redder in the sunlight. Sometimes, when this scenario occurs, a woman comes back to the salon and requests to have her color corrected. However, what has changed is not the hair color but the environment in which she is viewing it.

The best way to gauge your true hair color is in a room that has a combination of natural light and eye-level incandescent (preferably halogen) light. It is well worth it to change the lighting in your bathroom to a warm incandescent bulb that mimics natural light and emits the softest, most flattering illumination. The addition of sconces on each side of your mirror will give you a much more accurate perspective of what your hair color really looks like (not to mention that you will look ten years younger). I will talk more about proper bathroom lighting in "Mastering Makeup," chapter 7.

It is important to remember that often a color problem cannot be fixed immediately, and it usually takes a lot more time and money to get out of a mess than it did to get into one. Extreme hair damage or color disasters could even take a few appointments and three to four haircuts so the bad color can be cut off. Going back to the analogy between hair and fabric, sometimes a stain cannot be taken out and the damage is irreparable.

Keep in mind, however, that color correction can mean fixing a drastic mistake or making a simple adjustment, like a color rebalancing when the hair needs a little more of one thing or less of another. It could even be simple enough to rebalance yourself. For example, if your hair color has ended up too bright or dark, washing it a few times with a clarifying shampoo can remove some of that pigment. If your hair is brassy, a violet-based shampoo will help tone it down. These shampoos have been around a long time and are usually recommended primarily for blond hair, but they can work just as well to get rid of brassiness in brunette hair.

GETTING BACK TO YOUR NATURAL COLOR

Rediscovering your natural color after years of dyeing or bleaching it is just as radical as going from a brunette to a blonde and the process should be just as gradual. You cannot just dump brown hair color on top of the bleached blond and expect your natural shade to emerge. Such a trans-

BEAUTY SECRET

Have the front of your hair dried first to make sure you like the color

Most professionals are experienced enough to assess tone and color when the hair is wet. But it is important that you approve of the color as well, and to see it clearly, the hair needs to be dry. Drying the entire head of hair and then checking the color is time-consuming. Many stylists automatically start drying the back, taking up to twenty minutes before they reach the front (the part you can see). Therefore, after having your color done, you should ask to have the bangs or the front of your hair blown dry first so you can immediately see if there are any adjustments to be made.

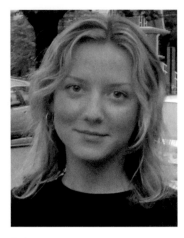

Before.

After years of highlighting her hair to a pale blond, Zhanna realized that this color washed her out. She wanted to become more of a "natural" dark blonde with just a few highlights. I deepened her overall color with a series of demi-permanent applications, then painted a few highlights around her hairline, to mimic what the sun would create. I then cut triangular layers with scissors. Darkening her eyebrows by two shades brought more definition to her eyes.

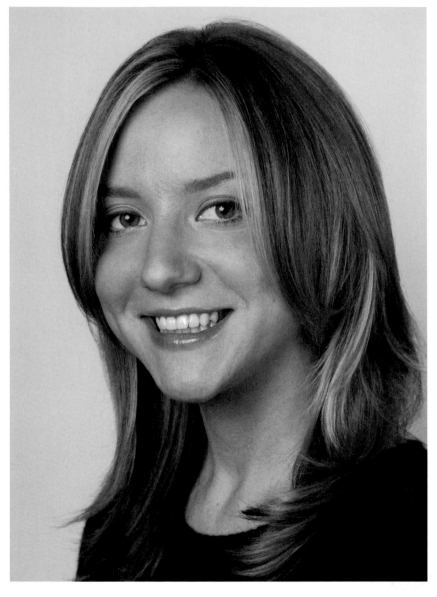

formation would require at least two steps. You literally have to replace the gold-red pigment that the bleach has stripped away and rebuild the cuticle of the hair with color.

As color is lifted from the hair with bleach, it moves through stages: brown, red, orange, yellow, and finally to pale blond. Now you must retrace your steps to find your way back home. Skipping a step could lead you to a different color altogether, which may be far from natural-looking. The first step is to apply a filler that is a gold-based demi-permanent

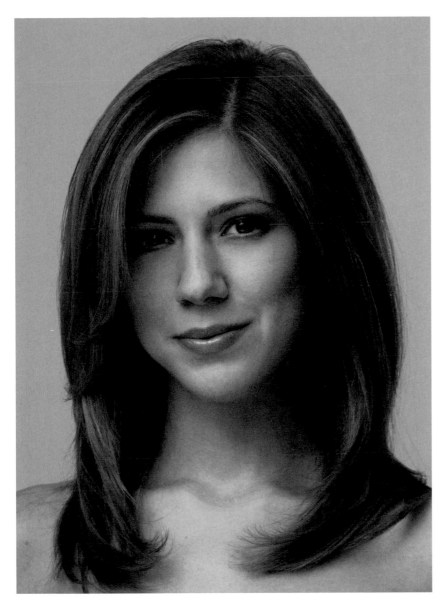

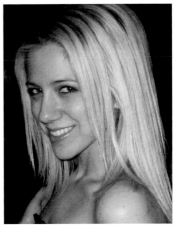

Before.

Having veered too far off course, Michelle wanted to return to her natural hair color, only a better version of it. After taking the appropriate steps to recapture her natural hair color, I painted (balayage) highlights around her face in order for her color to not look "flat." As a final step to this major color transformation, a golden honey glaze was used to add shine. The cut was done with concave layers, using scissors. This is a good example that sometimes nature knows best.

color that literally fills in the cortex with gold pigment. Without this filler to get the hair a few steps closer to the desired original shade, the darker dye would turn the hair green! Next, the colorist will choose the appropriate brown and apply it from roots to ends. At first, the new "natural" brunette color has a tendency to fade. Keep in mind that you are trying to rebuild the cuticle of the hair with synthetic hair color. In four to six weeks you will need to refresh your faded color with a demi-permanent formula or a glaze.

Kimmy has light blond highlights done with foils. Pale pink and lavender clip-on extensions were added for a fun splash of color.

BEAUTY SECRET

Try on wigs for a totally new color

This is a risk-free, fun way to experiment with a totally different look. You can see immediately if a certain color looks terrible on you, saving your hair in the process. I also like to add extensions for a commitment-free pop of color. If you want to be adventurous and experiment with different colors, you can just clip-in temporary pieces and have them cut to blend with your hair.

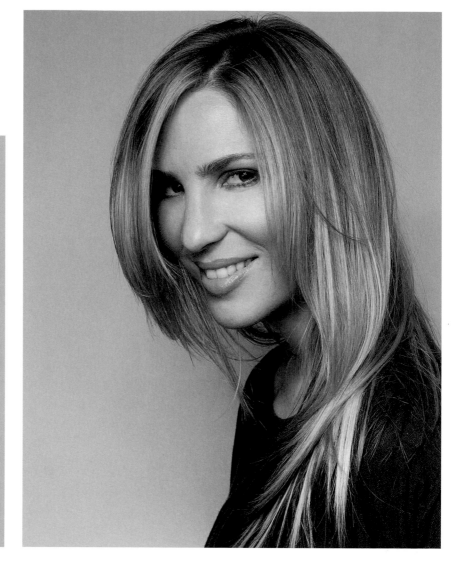

BEAUTY SECRET

Hollywood transformations

How do actors change their hair color so frequently and radically without completely frying their hair? First of all, they have a retinue of skilled hair pros at their disposal and the expense and maintenance are not an issue for them. Very frequently, however, the color changes you see are not real. Often, hair color is digitally enhanced in a photo or extensions are added. Wigs and extensions are frequently used in film and television to make it appear that an actress has a completely different hair color or length. Sometimes you just can't believe your own eyes.

COLORING YOUR EYEBROWS

Eyebrows are a central focal point on the face and yet, when it comes to color, they are almost always forgotten. Because I am also a makeup artist, I consider the brows a vital element of one's look. Coloring them can be transformative. Well-groomed brows bring definition to the face, like pemanent makeup. If the hair on your head affects your skin tone by resting next to it, imagine the importance of your eyebrow color. Brows that are a completely different color from the hair are also a glaring giveaway that the hair is tinted. I always consider lightening or darkening the brows when changing someone's hair color to make the overall color look more natural. Lightening the brows by one shade provides a subtle softening and lifting effect and can change the entire face by taking the edge off otherwise dark brows (see Heather on page 80). Actresses with brunette hair use this technique all the time. On the other hand, since eyebrows can fade and become sparser with age, darkening them slightly helps create more definition and makes the face look more vibrant and youthful (see Devin on page 74). Redheads need to warm their eyebrows to complement the warmth in their hair (see Anny on page 69).

Over time, I have perfected the art of eyebrow coloring, but keep in mind that most hairdressers are not eyebrow experts. You cannot use the same color as on your head. Many colorists make this mistake and end up turning the brows too dark, too red, or just all wrong. Because eyebrow hairs are finer than those on your head, they grab color more quickly and their typically ashier shade requires a different color formula.

AT-HOME HAIR COLOR
Know Your Limitations

Having learned about the intricacies of creating great hair color, you should understand why putting one shade of boxed color on your head at home will not give you the same results. I generally do not recommend that anyone do her own color. But if you do, you should know the constraints under which you are operating, manage your expectations, and be extra careful not to damage your hair. Hair coloring is such a complex and nuanced craft that even many professionals never become truly skilled at it. Without expertise or salon-quality products and tools, a do-it-yourself colorist is at a big disadvantage and is simply unable to produce the details and subtleties from the dumbed-down versions of color available for at-home use. At-home hair color is a big trade-off. Of course, there may be budgetary concerns, especially if you have to touch up gray roots every couple of weeks. Try talking to your colorist about ways that he or she can make your hair color more affordable. With some planning, good hair color can be factored into your lifestyle without breaking the bank.

Here are the five biggest limitations of at-home color:

1. BOXED HAIR COLOR IS NOT THE SAME QUALITY AS THE PROFESSIONAL COLOR USED IN SALONS.

Drugstore hair color is a different formulation from the kind used in salons. While the basic technology is similar, their chemical composition is different. Many people are under the misconception that all hair color is the same but you pay more for a colorist to apply it. Most professional color is made with finer and more expensive colorants and conditioning ingredients than mass-market brands, to make the hair shinier, keep it healthier, and achieve more beautiful results. In addition, salons are typically the first to gain access to the latest technological breakthroughs in color that usually do not reach the mass market for years, if ever.

2. ONLY ONE SHADE COMES IN A BOX.

A professional colorist mixes a specific recipe to create your formula— usually combining more than one pigment and adding a cool or warm tone to make your color more individualized and flattering. Colorists do not use a generic "light brown" to create beautiful light-brown hair. With boxed color, that one basic shade is all you have to work with. Even if you use a drugstore hair dye just to touch up the grays between coloring appointments, it can alter the base color completely, changing the palette and requiring your colorist to reformulate the color to even things out.

3. IT'S PHYSICALLY IMPOSSIBLE TO APPLY YOUR OWN COLOR ACCURATELY.

A professional applies color in a well-lit salon, looking down at your head as you sit in a chair that moves up and down. If you had that same viewpoint and lighting, you would have a better shot at applying your color correctly. Not being able to see what you are doing leads to mistakes.

4. YOU CAN CAUSE SERIOUS DAMAGE TO YOUR HAIR.

If your hair can be damaged by overlapping of color when a professional with a superior product and vantage point applies it, imagine how easily you can make this mistake at home. Now consider the disadvantage of working with a runny, liquid-based boxed color formula. Professional color has a thicker, creamy consistency that stays in place. We also use a brush to apply it. A liquid formulation is impossible to keep just in the root area, and will inevitably bleed into the rest of the hair. The at-home colorist can also create other problems, such as making the ends of her hair practically black or choosing the wrong tone and making the hair turn orange instead of the pretty golden brown shown on the front of the box. You can see why the combination of a nonprofessional product and lack of expertise forms a perfect storm that can easily create a hair-color disaster that you will then have to pay a professional dearly to fix.

5. THERE IS NO WAY AROUND IT: AT-HOME COLOR WILL LOOK FLAT.

Hair is rarely one solid shade, but a boxed color is exactly that, which is why it usually looks monochromatic. Colorists have numerous pigments to choose from in a salon dispensary to simulate the varying levels and dimensions that hair color should have naturally. A seasoned professional also knows how to work with different parts of the hair, formulating the color a little differently around the hairline and the more porous ends. You can be assured that the gorgeous hair color you see in at-home color commercials was created by a seasoned professional.

FOR THE AT-HOME-COLOR JUNKIES

Despite everything you have just learned about the complexities of hair coloring, I know that for you die-hard home colorists there is probably little hope for reform. You may have artistic tendencies or perhaps you just can't find a good colorist in your area. Since this is a beauty book, I feel it is my obligation to make the best of a bad situation. (Once I even received a panicked phone call during one of my radio shows from two teenage girls having a hair-color emergency while dyeing each other's hair!) Here are my five pro tips for at-home hair coloring:

1. Read the directions on the package (most people don't). Just because you have read the instructions on the box of color from one company does not mean that the same directions apply to all color.

2. Buy gloves that actually fit you. I have never figured out whom those gloves in the color package actually fit, but it's no woman. You will achieve more accurate application with the right tools.

3. See if you can coerce your significant other, best girlfriend, neighbor, or child to help apply the color to the back of your head. Not being able to see what you are doing is actually dangerous—not just for your hair but for rugs, wood floors, tile or marble, walls, doors, furniture, and drapes.

4. Set an actual timer. Many women leave the color on too long because they busy themselves around the house and forget to check their watch.

5. Get into the shower to wash out color. The faucet in the bathroom or kitchen does not have enough water pressure to successfully remove color. (The ones in your home are not like the sinks at a salon.) Proper removal of all chemicals is crucial for the health of the hair, since any remaining residue can cause damage.

EXTENDING THE LIFE OF YOUR COLOR

To make your color remain as vibrant and be as long-lasting as possible, you have to treat it with care. There are five simple ways to help ensure this.

1. WAIT SEVENTY-TWO HOURS TO SHAMPOO OR CONDITION YOUR HAIR.

This is no myth. It really is optimal not to shampoo or condition for at least two days, preferably three, after having your hair colored (if you absolutely have to, rinse with tepid water after twenty-four hours). This allows the cuticle to close and lock the color molecules into the hair shaft. When the cuticle is still slightly open, using a cream-based conditioner, a conditioning mask, or a hot-oil treatment could pull some of the color out. The professional shampoos and conditioners that are used at a salon after the coloring process are made with this in mind.

2. USE A SHAMPOO AND CONDITIONER FOR COLOR-TREATED HAIR.

This is not a case of big cosmetics firms trying to hoodwink you into buying something you do not need; these products actually make a difference. The coloring process takes some of the shine and moisture from the hair. Shampoos and conditioners specifically formulated for color-treated hair are more emollient and gentle. They are technologically designed to cleanse the dirt and oil from the hair without removing the color molecules.

3. PROTECT YOUR HAIR FROM THE SUN.

Just like fabric, hair fades and discolors from consistent exposure to the sun. There are hair products that contain sunscreen, but these will not completely block UV rays. The best sunblocks for skin and hair are physical. I recommend covering your hair with a hat or scarf to protect it in the sun. Ideally wear both, since many sun hats have tiny holes for ventilation and do not adequately protect the hair.

4. DO NOT RINSE YOUR HAIR WITH HOT WATER.

Heat lifts up the cuticle of the hair, allowing pigment to escape from the hair shaft. This concept is also why a conditioning treatment works more effectively when you apply heat or steam; it can penetrate better. Adjust the water in your shower to a warm or tepid temperature when rinsing or washing your hair. This tip is especially important for redheads, because red pigment tends to fade the fastest.

5. INSTALL A WATER FILTER ON YOUR SHOWERHEAD.

A water filter is a simple solution that removes chlorine and metal deposits which otherwise dry out your hair and fade hair color. Consider how chlorine in a swimming pool dehydrates the hair and can actually turn blond hair green. Chlorine, along with iron deposits, is a big reason why many brunettes go brassy. It is not just from sun exposure. Chlorine also dries out the skin. When I installed a charcoal filter in my shower, I noticed that my hair and skin felt softer.

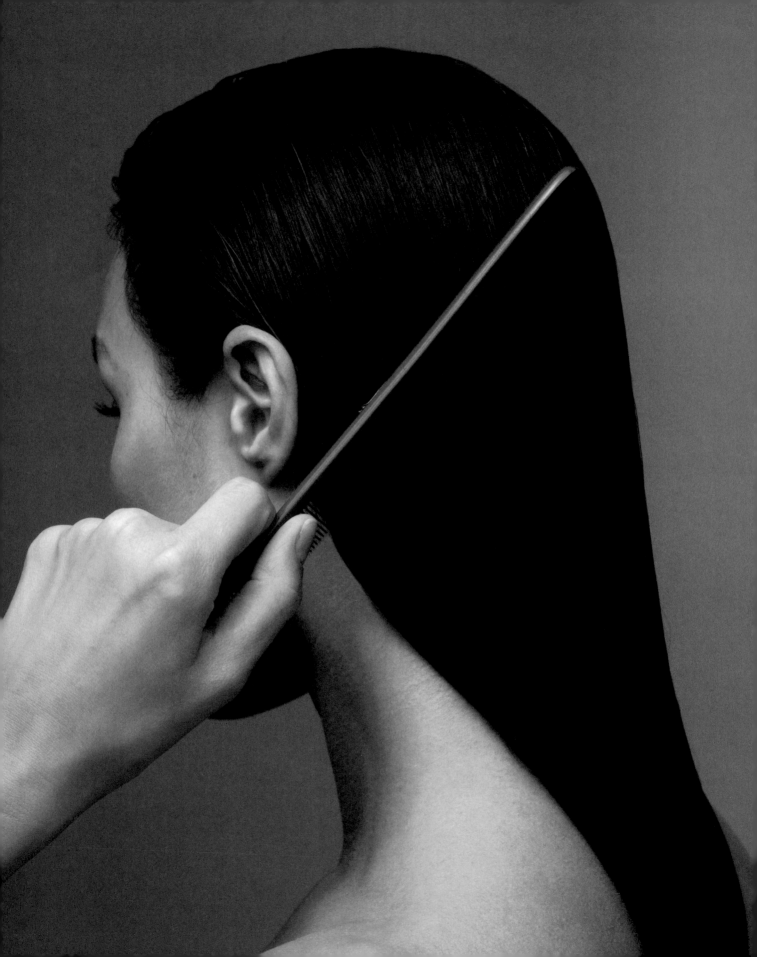

3

HAIR CARE

I never thought it was such a bad little tree. It's not bad at all, really. Maybe it just needs a little love.
——Linus, in *A Charlie Brown Christmas*

How we take care of our hair at home greatly affects its health and appearance. Nurturing and nourishing it supports a great haircut and gorgeous color and can prolong the time between salon appointments. Yet many women spend their time, money, and energy on having their hair cut, colored, and styled but neglect caring for it at home. This is like buying a designer dress and treating it like a T-shirt—throwing it into the washing machine with a harsh detergent and tossing it into a blazing-hot dryer. Often, women treat their delicate fabrics with more care than their own hair. Conscientious home care is the key to great texture, shine, and styling results. By not choosing the right shampoo or bothering to condition properly, not protecting your hair from the sun and hot styling tools, not brushing it regularly (if at all), you are doing yourself a disservice. The right products and care protect the investment you just made at the salon. Without them, you are not only wasting money on the wrong or inferior products but are adversely affecting the health of your hair and the look created for you.

No styling product can compensate for missing fundamental elements such as a great cut and color and, above all, healthy hair. Women tend to put so much hope and stock in such products, but styling actually starts in the shower. We have been brainwashed to believe that the secret to great hair lies in some miraculous styling products, but they only support—not create—healthy, well-cut, and beautifully colored hair. Proper care will actually allow you to use fewer styling products. For example, with a more gentle moisturizing shampoo and conditioner, you might not need to use as much styling cream or serum to make your hair feel softer or behave better. Too many people do not value the importance of shampoo and conditioner and most completely skip the one thing that is likely to make the biggest difference in the health of their hair: regular brushing.

STEP ONE: *Shampoo*

What you use to wash your hair is just as important as what you leave in as a styling aid. We protect our clothing by using the appropriate soap but try to save money when it comes to our hair, washing it with harsh detergents as opposed to something gentle and specific for our hair type. If you invest in a high-quality cleanser, you not only will feel a real difference in your hair but will need to use only a small amount each time you shampoo.

What Kind of Shampoo Should You Use?

Generally, hair care products should be geared to the type of hair you have and the look you are trying to achieve. If your primary objective is to smooth your hair or eliminate frizz, you can try a straightening shampoo that has been formulated to smooth the cuticle. Of course, these shampoos will not completely alter the texture of your hair. Naturally curly hair is not going to become straight—nor is straight hair going to become curly—just by being washed. However, a cleanser for curly hair will give it more bounce and moisture, while a straightening shampoo will help create a smoother texture. Volumizing shampoos remove some of the residue from the hair and deposit a fine layer of protein (sometimes from ingredients like wheat, rice, or soy extracts) to slightly strengthen and bulk up the strands. A shampoo formulated for color-treated hair is a mild cleansing option for all hair types, since it has more gentle detergents and a higher concentration of conditioning agents. Shampoo that is appropriate for your hair type will help to support the look you want, whether you blow dry or air dry your hair.

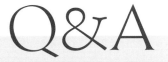

Q&A

Q: *I've heard that you should switch shampoos periodically because your hair gets used to one if used continually over time. Is this true?*

A: Different types of shampoo and conditioner really do affect the hair differently. You experience this when switching products and noticing a change in how your hair feels as a result. This is due to the different ingredients, not because your old shampoo and conditioner have stopped working. Your hair can also be more responsive to certain formulations depending on its health and the weather. Some shampoos are stronger than others and will make your hair feel a little cleaner and bouncier. If used regularly, however, that same shampoo may dehydrate your hair, and switching to a more emollient formulation will make it feel softer again. I like to change products depending on the climate or what my hair feels like on a given day. I will use a richer, moisturizing shampoo and conditioner in the winter and a straightening one in humid weather to tame the frizz. Occasionally, I use a clarifying shampoo to remove buildup. It helps to have some options to choose from.

When in doubt about what to buy, ask your hairstylist what he or she recommends. The person who works with your hair should know what will be best for you. Hair professionals are constantly being sent new products to try and go through the trial and error for you. It is wise to remember that much of what you read about products in magazine beauty articles is advertiser driven and may not be truly objective.

How Often Should You Shampoo?

How often you wash your hair depends on whether your hair and scalp are oily or dry, the density of your hair, your environment, and how much styling product you use. People with oily hair may need to shampoo every day. Those with curly or dry textures might find that shampooing once or twice a week helps to keep more natural oils in the hair and make it less frizzy. You may also need to wash your hair more frequently in the summertime, when it is hot and humid, or when traveling. Someone who works outdoors or around food preparation usually needs to shampoo more often than a person who works in an office. Keep in mind that you do not have to wash your hair every time you go to the gym and break a sweat. Perspiration is not dirt and your hair may not be unclean at all.

The amount of oil your scalp produces may even adjust, depending on how often you remove it by washing. Therefore, if you are used to shampooing daily and switch to every other day, your hair could initially feel oily on the second day, but it should soon adjust. The same holds true for oily skin, where more gentle care can calm overactive oil glands that contribute to acne. Try just rinsing and conditioning on the days when you skip the shampoo. Sometimes all the hair really needs is a warm rinse. You may be surprised at how your hair feels without the daily use of cleansing detergents. Generally, my recommendation is simple: wash your hair when it feels dirty or when your scalp feels itchy—listen to what your hair needs.

How to Shampoo

How much shampoo you need to use depends on the length of your hair: a nickel-size amount for short hair; for midlengths, a quarter-size; and for longer hair, about a half-dollar. You can also apply a small amount to the back of your head, add a bit more on the sides and end up at the top to ensure that it is evenly applied. Most people (especially men) put all the shampoo in the front of the head first and then have a hard time moving it through, inevitably needing to pile on more. This not only concentrates most of the cleanser in one place but makes it more difficult to rinse out. You need a fairly even distribution of lather from the scalp to the ends.

Q&A

Q: *Will a clarifying shampoo dry out my hair or strip some of my color?*
A: A clarifying shampoo typically contains citric acid to remove residue from the hair. It is generally safe to use on color-treated hair about once per month and can actually revive your color and make it look more vibrant by removing product buildup. To alleviate any concerns about your color fading, you can also use it just before going to the salon for a touch-up. You can even make your own natural clarifier by adding a tablespoon of apple cider vinegar to a quarter-size amount of shampoo in your palm. (Vinegar contains acetic acid, which removes deposits, even from your coffeemaker!) Massage this into your hair for about three minutes, rinse it out, and shampoo one more time to get rid of the vinegar smell. This recipe is also a gentler alternative for fine hair that is highlighted and may feel fragile.

STEP TWO: *Condition*

Many women and most men neglect to condition their hair properly, treating it as an optional step. Granted, although conditioning is important for everyone, it is usually more so for women because their hair is longer and often is chemically treated. Conditioner helps to smooth the hair follicle after it gets roughed up during the cleansing process, reestablishes the moisture balance, and helps strengthen and protect the outer layer of the hair. You can see and feel the difference when you use a great product. As with skin creams, emollient ingredients such as shea butter, jojoba oil, and ceramides work to hydrate and coat the surface layer of the hair, making it feel smoother and look healthier.

There are as many different types of conditioner as there are shampoos. One made for volume will not have heavy emollients and might contain wheat or rice protein to strengthen and stiffen the strands, making them look and feel thicker. A straightening conditioner may contain silicone, which will leave a sheath on the hair, helping to smooth the cuticle and make blow-drying easier. Conditioners for color-treated hair are made to hydrate and further protect you hair color from fading. Those for dry hair are richer in emollients, allowing a bit of moisture to remain on the hair shaft after rinsing. Formulations for damaged hair include protein to strengthen the hair and give it more support after cleansing.

Start with a dime-size amount; apply first to the ends and work your way up, applying more as you move to the top of the head. If you have oily hair, try skipping the root area, since it is naturally moisturized by the oils from your scalp. Those with damaged, bleached, or especially dry hair should use a deep conditioning treatment (instead of a regular conditioner) every time they wash.

Deep Conditioning Treatments

Deep conditioning treatments are concentrated, creamy conditioners that act like moisturizing masks for the hair. This step does not have to be time-consuming. Modern treatments are formulated to be left on only two to five minutes. First, wash your hair; squeeze most of the water out; apply the hair mask and gently comb through; then wash your body

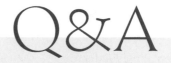

Q: *Is there a big difference between salon conditioning treatments and those you can do at home?*
A: Salon treatments, like most professional products and hair color, are formulated differently from those made for the general public. Many are liquid and penetrate the hair more easily. They typically have a higher concentration of botanicals, oils, and other moisturizing agents. Another benefit of salon treatments is that someone applies the product evenly through your hair while massaging your scalp, which improves circulation (and also feels wonderful).

and shave your legs while it conditions; finally, rinse the hair thoroughly. Because the emollient ingredients are so concentrated, you need to use only a small amount (start with a quarter-size).

Leave-in Conditioners

This conditioner is lightweight enough to be used in addition to the rinse-out conditioner applied in the shower. It is best for women with wavy or curly hair that needs extra moisture for better curl form with less frizz. It also doubles as a styling product, since it affects the overall look of the hair.

Hair Oils

Oil has been used to condition the hair and skin for centuries. Two oils that are especially beneficial are neem oil, extracted from the seeds of evergreen trees in India, and amla oil from the Indian gooseberry. They are moisturizing and nourishing for the hair, are healing to the scalp, and make for an easy and wonderful night treatment. Rub six to eight drops between your fingers and massage into the head and hair. Brush with your natural-bristle brush and shampoo out in the morning. Remember, these oils are concentrated and should be applied sparingly.

Salon Versus Drugstore Products

I work with professional products daily in my salon and I am constantly sent products to try, so that I may carry them in my salon or recommend them on my radio show. Having worked with and tested so many products over the course of my career, I can tell you that there is a distinct difference between the professional products and those sold at drugstores. Most professional hair care lines are superior because they contain more expensive and higher-quality ingredients. For example, there are different grades of alcohols and silicones. The finer formulations of these products also produce a more sophisticated consistency and scent, whereas many mass-market alternatives are heavily fragranced and smell synthetic. Professional products cost more because they are more expensive to make. Additionally, they are continually tested for efficacy by the most discerning and critical consumer—the hairdresser.

Lower-price shampoos also tend to have higher levels of detergent, which immediately results in a full, rich lather that strips the hair of its natural oils, not to mention the salon color in which you may have just invested. Although shampoo commercials have long romanticized lather, generally, lower-lather shampoos are healthier for the hair. Mass-market conditioners usually contain more silicone, which adds a slippery feeling to the hair and gives it a false sense of moisture. While silicone can be an effective ingredient that protects the hair from the environment and heat styling, it can build up a barrier on the hair that, ironically, prevents healthy conditioning ingredients from permeating it.

In addition, I have noticed that mass-market containers tend to have larger openings to dispense the product, so too much is dumped into your hand and ultimately wasted. Because the active conditioning ingredients in luxury products are more concentrated and higher in quality, they can be used in smaller amounts.

COMMON MISTAKE

Not rinsing out conditioner well enough

Rinsing out product from the hair is just as important as putting it in. Conditioners are formulated to leave just enough of the lubricating ingredients on the hair strands after rinsing. Women with dry, coarse, or curly hair often do not entirely rinse out the conditioner, assuming that what remains will act as a leave-in. In reality, it just sits on the hair, making it look flat and dull. A small amount of leave-in conditioner would be a wiser choice after fully rinsing the regular shampoo and conditioner from the hair.

There are exceptions, however. Within the realm of luxury and mass-market products there are also big differences in quality. Therefore, just because a product line is marketed and priced as "professional" does not necessarily make it good. (I have tested and worked with products in this category that I loved and others that I hated.) Similarly, not every mass-market brand is necessarily bad. In my experience, the best professional or luxury products are vastly superior to the best mass-market products, while the best mass-market products may very well be better than the subpar professional products.

Ultimately, I believe that either we pay now by purchasing a higher-quality product that lasts longer and performs better, or we pay later by having to buy multiple less-effective products while struggling with our hair. But it also is a matter of personal preference. If you love a less expensive brand of shampoo and conditioner, then by all means, keep using

BEAUTY SECRET

Do not be a victim of product diversion

After a hair service, people sometimes proudly declare that they have purchased well-known professional brand products in their neighborhood drugstore, thinking that they have managed to "beat the system" and save money. What they don't realize is that they were actually duped into wasting money—often spending 30 to 50 percent more than they would have paid for the very same products in a salon! Why? Because of an insidious industry problem called "diversion," which professional product companies have been trying to combat for years. It involves drugstores and other unauthorized retailers' purchasing products directly from salons (or from distributors who purchase them from salons) and reselling them to consumers at a higher price. This type of activity is also referred to as "gray market."

Because such products are typically sold only to qualifying salons and sometimes a few other select retailers, diversion is the only way for mass retailers to obtain them. The recourse that product manufacturers have (and frequently use) is to cut off the salons participating in this activity. You may think that this practice is limited to mom-and-pop drugstores, but it has involved some of this country's largest mass retailers. Meanwhile, consumers are so conditioned to believe that prices are always lower at drugstores or large discount retailers that they pay without question, thinking that they are saving money.

and enjoying it. The bottom line is that if a product works well for you, then it is a good value no matter the price. If it dries out your hair or strips your color, it has a negative value.

HAIR-APY SESSION
The State of Your Hair

Women are accustomed to relying on quick fixes to deal with their hair issues and keep up appearances, instead of getting to the root of the problem. Meanwhile, many abuse their hair on a daily basis. Rather than trying to mask problems with styling products, focus on the basics of hair care that are likely to eliminate them. Part of a hairstylist's job is to educate clients about proper hair care and styling beyond the chair.

Hair Brushing: A Miracle Treatment

If you learn just one thing from this chapter, I hope it is the miraculous benefits of hair brushing. Whether you are plagued by frizz, dryness, split ends, or even hair thinning, nightly brushing with a natural-bristle brush will help to alleviate if not completely cure the condition. A high-quality, natural-bristle brush is the one hair care tool you cannot do without. Today, the best natural bristles are generally made of boar hair, but other effective alternatives are being developed. A pure-bristle brush (without any other types of bristles added) is best for delicate or fine hair, while one mixed with nylon bristles is for medium to thick hair. The natural bristles distribute the oils from your scalp to the ends of your hair, whereas the nylon bristles allow the brush to get through thicker hair with more ease. Brushing is not just an old wives' tale or some archaic grooming ritual—I consider it a lost art and a holistic beauty secret. It is the best way to condition your hair because your natural oils are more compatible and effective than most synthetic conditioning ingredients. If you brush your hair for two minutes every night before bed, I promise you will see a change in your hair texture within about six weeks. I have experienced amazing results in my hair and have witnessed it in my clients' hair, which becomes smoother, more manageable, less frizzy, softer, and shinier—all from brushing. I also have received countless testimonials that brushing has changed the health of their hair and scalp, from women and men whom I have never met but who have followed my advice.

The scalp is an extension of our skin, with oil glands, sweat glands, pores, and hair follicles. Dead skin cells need to be sloughed off so that they do not clog those pores (which can contribute to hair loss, if you needed another good reason to brush your hair). Additionally, brushing actually cleanses the hair in much the same way as brushing suede lifts dirt particles from it. We have veered from these simple basics, becoming conditioned to reach for a hair care or styling product as an immediate fix. Meanwhile, a more natural, effective, and economical solution has been around all along. The act of brushing became viewed as obsolete as products became more advanced. But when women did not have the luxury of all these wonderful conditioning products, they simply brushed their hair daily.

THE RULE
Never brush curly hair.

THE RULE BREAKER: In my experience, when women say that they
hate their curly hair, it is usually because it is not healthy but dry and frizzy. It feels rough and looks dull. So many women have described their hair texture by saying to me, "It's just not a 'good curl.'" Nightly brushing would help to alleviate this and change the way they feel about their natural texture. But women with curly hair almost never brush it. Many have never even owned a brush! And yet they are the ones who would benefit most from it. I have worked on so many women who have beautiful ringlets underneath and a frizzy texture on the top. This damaged exterior is exposed to the elements and perhaps to the heat of a curling iron or a diffuser, not to mention chemical treatments. It then gets loaded with silicone-filled frizz-fighting products that build up and dull the hair. Brushing will help to even out those textures and add shine by removing some of that residue.

Most of those who have curly hair think that brushing it will make them look like Diana Ross in the 1970s movie *Mahogany* or perhaps Barbra Streisand in *A Star Is Born*. And it definitely will. This is why you should brush before going to bed and rinse your hair in the shower the next morning (warning your husband or partner is also recommended).

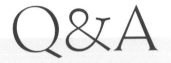

Q&A

Q: *Does rinsing with cold water make the hair shinier?*

A: Yes, it is a good idea to finish your shower with a cool rinse. A hot steamy shower raises the cuticle, while a colder temperature makes it contract. A flatter cuticle has a smoother surface that reflects light and looks shinier.

Q: *Is a two-in-one shampoo and conditioner as effective as using them separately?*

A: Perhaps because of the money- and time-saving aspect of using one item instead of two, these types of products are popular. But shampooing and conditioning have very separate functions. The typical shampoo/conditioners are less effective for conditioning and are not beneficial for dry or color-treated hair. To me, these products have always felt like oilier shampoos that leave a residue in the hair to make it feel as if it has been conditioned. The concept is similar to that of mixing your facial cleanser with your moisturizer. You would not sufficiently cleanse or moisturize.

THE MOST COMMON HAIR PROBLEMS AND SOLUTIONS

It can be scary when you experience an adverse change in your hair. There could be one or several elements at play. To cover all the bases, it helps to have a keen awareness of what is going on in your body and your life. Refer to the checklist on page 105 when you encounter a hair problem to help narrow in on the possible cause(s).

While split ends, dry hair, and frizz are usually telltale signs of external abuse, your hair is also a reflection of your inner health and should be viewed as a valuable clue to what is going on inside your body. For example, hair loss may be linked to a thyroid disorder or anemia. Additionally, a hair problem you are experiencing now could have been caused by something (stress, new medication, illness, or surgery) that happened several months ago. Because hair grows on average about half an inch per month, it may take some time for a side effect to appear. When reading about the following hair problems, refer to the chapters on haircutting, coloring, and styling for the culprits that cause external damage. In chapter 9, "Beauty from the Inside Out," I will talk about treating these conditions through nutrition and lifestyle changes.

Dry Hair

Dry hair is usually the result of using the wrong products (or lack thereof), external damage, or diet. If your hair is color treated and chronically dry, talk to your colorist about using an ammonia-free colorant on it. Also, choose more hydrating hair care products and hydrate from the inside out with the right nutrition and supplements.

Breakage

If you have healthy, strong, shiny hair at the root area but are experiencing breakage from the midshaft to the ends, that is usually a sign of external damage. Breakage closer to the scalp, however, is most likely induced internally. It could be stress-related, hormonal, or nutritional. I have seen clients with such damage after a divorce, an illness, or a death in the family. I even experienced it myself during a very difficult time in my life. If that is the case for you, the problem should subside once your body recovers.

Split Ends

Split ends occur when the hair has been compromised by external damage or simply because it desperately needs a trim. Remember that hair is quite old near the ends and the strands split in a way similar to fabric fraying from constant wear and tear (like the hem on a pair of jeans that becomes

BEAUTY SECRET

Create a liquid barrier on your hair before swimming

Before you swim in a chlorinated pool or take a dip in the ocean, saturate your hair with clean water. The hair will absorb less of the chlorinated or salt water if it's already wet. (Like a sponge, it can absorb only so much liquid.) While salt water is not as damaging as chlorine, it is still dehydrating to the hair. When I go swimming, I also apply natural oils to my hair, which creates a protective barrier against the water and keeps it from drying out.

ragged after months of dragging on the ground). Over time, especially with frequent use of heat from drying and ironing, this fraying is likely to happen to your hair. Regular brushing helps to prevent this by conditioning the hair, while using a thermal protection product before heat styling shields the ends. Although you can temporarily smooth the ends with hair oil or a silicone product, or smooth them under with a round brush to look more presentable, ultimately this is only camouflage and does not solve the problem. The only real remedy for split ends is to cut them off.

Frizz

The hair problem I am asked about most is frizz. Women usually chalk it up to the weather, heredity, or a curse, but it is more often induced or exacerbated by poor hair care habits, improper heat styling, bad haircuts, and negligent hair coloring (as explained in chapters 1 and 2). Other than that, treating the hair roughly, in general, can create frizz even without heat. For instance, aggressive towel drying lifts the cuticle, even before you begin to style the hair. It may even lead to breakage and/or split ends over time. Be gentle with your hair: blot it dry by softly squeezing it with your towel.

Climate is another trigger: humidity expands the cuticle of the hair. On curly or coarse textures this can be an inescapable formula for frizz. Applying an antihumectant product such as a smoothing serum temporarily coats the strands to counteract the effects of humidity. Ultimately, however, this kind of product can build up, weighing down the hair and dulling its shine. What you really need is consistent moisturizing to keep the cuticle smooth. An effective way to achieve this is through regular brushing. Another is by applying a conditioning hair mask once a week.

If you take proper care of your hair and still battle with frizz, or if you just want a quick solution, you can try getting a keratin treatment at a reputable salon. These treatments took the industry by storm around 2009, suddenly becoming all the rage. Since keratin is a protein that the hair is made of, this process coats the hair, thus smoothing the cuticle and making it lie flat. Keratin treatment formulations vary in strength, from those that act as a relaxer to the milder versions that remove frizz without significantly affecting the natural hair texture and wave pattern. The end

CHECKLIST

Causes of hair damage or loss:

- Heredity
- Illness
- Hormonal changes
- Medication
- Emotional or physical stress
- Nutrition and diet
- Environment
- Home styling and care
- Salon chemical services, cutting, styling

Natural Remedy

Oils for scalp conditions

There is an array of essential oils with strong healing powers for the skin and scalp. Keep in mind that these remedies will not immediately cure the problem, so give them a few weeks of consistent use to see improvement.

- Rosemary oil has cleansing properties that make it especially effective for treating dandruff.
- Neem oil is cleansing and purifying for the scalp and conditioning for the hair. It is good for treating a dry, flaky scalp.
- Lavender is ideal for treating an oily scalp because it has antibacterial properties and calms the skin, helping it balance natural oil production.
- Tea tree oil has natural antiseptic properties and is an effective remedy for a number of scalp conditions, such as itchiness, flaking, and dandruff (keep in mind, however, that tea tree oil can strip synthetic hair color).
- Borage oil applied topically has been found to cure cradle cap, a form of seborrheic dermatitis that affects infants. For adults, it helps to heal eczema and other scalp conditions.

result typically lasts three to four months. Prices for these treatments are all over the map, depending on where and how they are done. As always, the success of a chemical service has to do with the expertise and care of the professional. The blow-dryer and the flat iron have to be used correctly, and the hair should be taken in thin sections for the best results. A flat iron with a temperature gauge is necessary. If the heat of the iron exceeds the recommended temperature, the hair can be damaged. For a stylist, this is a painstaking process that must be done meticulously and cannot be rushed through.

The technology behind Keratin treatments is still in a state of infancy, and there has been a good deal of controversy about the safety of their active ingredient, which is formaldehyde or a derivative of it. Therefore, you will often see technicians, as well as clients, wear masks during the service to prevent inhalation of the product. The stronger the treatment, the more formaldehyde it contains. Hopefully, through technological advancements, formaldehyde will be replaced with a more innocuous active ingredient in the near future.

Oily Hair

Oily hair is caused by an overproduction of sebum. Remember that the skin and scalp are one, so if your skin is oily, it is likely that your scalp is, too. For teenagers who have excessively oily hair, the problem is most likely hormonal and will pass. In the meantime, anyone with oily hair should simply follow common sense and shampoo more often, but not more than once per day. You can also use a clarifying shampoo more frequently, perhaps twice a week, to deeply cleanse the excess oil and residue that are weighing the hair down. In addition, since brushing cleans the hair, it will actually help loosen dirt and oil, so the hair does not look so flat.

Flaky, Dry Scalp

A flaky scalp is not necessarily dandruff. It can be a symptom of extremely dry skin, just as flaking occurs with dry skin on the body. It can be caused by something seemingly innocuous like the dry heat in your home during winter months, in which case a humidifier can be used to add moisture into the environment. If you notice that your scalp feels itchy and begins to flake a day or two after having your hair colored, you may have sensitivity to that specific color line. This is definitely a topic to discuss with your colorist, who may suggest trying a gentler coloring agent or a demi-permanent formulation. You can also try a different color line altogether. If you color your hair at home, do a patch test on your skin before applying the color. It is also possible that you may be sensitive to a shampoo or another hair product. Additionally, many women suffer from dry skin all over the body due to low levels of estrogen during menopause.

NATURAL REMEDY

A milk rinse to soothe the scalp

Whole milk can be a very healing, natural remedy. The lactic acid and the richness of the milk are soothing, especially to irritated, sensitive skin. Pour milk over the hair after shampooing and rinse about five minutes later. We sometimes use a milk rinse at the salon (a pint of whole milk for one application) after chemical services for women who have especially sensitive scalps.

BEAUTY SECRET

How to keep oily hair from going flat

Even with a diligent cleansing routine, many women with oily scalps complain that their hair looks limp by the end of the day. Try using a dry shampoo as a styling product to prevent your hairstyle from collapsing. It helps absorb the oil that inevitably emerges by midday. After blow-drying and styling your hair, mist the dry shampoo (most come in a spray-on powder form) at the root area and gently brush it through the hair. Women with fine, oily hair love this beauty tip. Another method is to use a salt-infused styling product, often referred to as a "beach spray," which helps dehydrate the scalp a bit and give volume to the hair. I have found that this works better than a mousse or gel on fine or oily hair, because it does not weigh it down.

A simple, natural remedy for dryness or irritation of the scalp is borage oil. You can open a capsule and massage the oil onto your scalp. One of my clients was suffering from eczema around her hairline and found that applying borage oil directly to the area significantly helped to heal the flaking, itching, and dryness. Even better is to take borage-oil supplements in addition to the topical application, to hydrate the skin from the inside and out. Remember, regular brushing helps exfoliate the scalp and feels fantastic, especially if it is itchy. We never think of exfoliating our scalps, but dry-scalp conditions can occur because of a lack of stimulation. A woman recently emailed me to say that she had suffered from psoriasis on her scalp and once she had started brushing her hair every night, the psoriasis cleared up on its own!

Dandruff

A flaking, itchy scalp may not be due to dry skin, but be caused by one of two scalp conditions: a fungus (*Malassezia furfur*) or an inflammatory disorder of the skin called seborrheic dermatitis, which accelerates skin-cell turnover. This is characterized by larger, often greasy flakes and may be accompanied by redness and irritation of the scalp. (The flakes from dry skin are typically tinier and dry.) A doctor can prescribe a medicated shampoo to control the fungal condition, and seborrheic dermatitis can be treated with a topical medication. Be aware that these medications can be effective in curing the scalp condition, but they do a real number on your hair color and the health of your hair. Dehydration, brassiness, and frizz are a few of the side effects. I generally recommend using such medications as a last resort and trying the available natural remedies first, or using prescription shampoo just once a week, which still yields positive results and is less damaging to the hair. Keep in mind that although over-the-counter dandruff shampoos may be less harsh, they still tend to strip the scalp of natural oils, drying the hair without treating the source of the real skin disorder. Some of the active ingredients in these shampoos are meant to exfoliate and clean the scalp (salicylic acid and zinc are two), but this can be also achieved more holistically with natural oils and regular hair brushing.

Hair Loss

Hair loss is a very emotional issue because our sense of femininity and beauty is so tied to our hair. Culturally, we have grown up with iconic images of beauty associated with gorgeous, shiny, healthy hair. It plays an enormous role in how we feel about ourselves. When you start to lose your hair, it can trigger anxiety and send you into a complete tailspin. It is alarming and frightening, but understanding the condition you are experiencing and what may be behind it will help you to deal with it more effectively. You should know that there are numerous ways of treating hair thinning and hair loss, depending on the underlying causes.

For starters, we lose 50 to 100 strands of hair a day. If this sounds like a disturbing amount, remember that we can have more than 100,000 strands on our heads. On a healthy head of hair, some fall out and new ones grow in as the new hair pushes the old strand out of the follicle. This hair growth cycle occurs in three stages: the anagen (active growth stage), the catagen (transitional phase), and the telogen (resting phase). A shock to the system, such as surgery, hormonal changes, or extreme emotional and/or physical stress, can cause the growth cycles to reset. This can result in more follicles going through the resting phase (shedding), and, therefore, hair loss.

Menopause and childbirth can elicit temporary hair loss or shedding. I have also known young women in their twenties who experienced hair

Professional Technique
Cutting and styling to mask hair loss

Something as simple as changing your haircut or parting your hair differently can create an illusion of fuller hair and help to mask hair loss. For example, try cutting your hair a couple of inches shorter to make it less weighed down and allow for more lift. A side part or a side-swept bang also helps to mask a thinning hairline.

loss as a side effect of taking oral contraceptives. Other factors that can cause hair loss include hormonal disorders such as an underactive thyroid (hypothyroidism); medications such as blood thinners, antidepressants, and those for high blood pressure, arthritis, heart problems, or seizures; extreme stress that compromises your immune system and sets off a domino effect in your body. The growth cycle may be interrupted after a physical or emotional trauma, but that clock will reset again once the body has recuperated and normal hair growth will resume. (Clearly the body does not treat our hair with the same priority as we do.)

If you feel that you are shedding more than the normal amount of hair, you should make an appointment with your dermatologist for a checkup. He or she can assess the density of your hair per square inch to tell you just how much hair you are losing and refer you for a few simple blood tests to discover why this may be happening. Your doctor may also suspect a hormone imbalance and recommend further testing from an endocrinologist (a hormone specialist).

You should also be mindful that when your hair is already in a compromised state, you must be extra careful with how you treat it. Hair color, bleach, and chemical straighteners stress weak hair and can make the problem worse. The way you style your hair can also be a factor. Using ceramic or metal brushes when heat styling can break, pull, or burn the hair. It is better to use a soft natural-bristle brush. There is even a rare condition that causes women to compulsively pull and twist their own hair, resulting in traction alopecia. I have a few clients who suffer from this. They do it subconsciously and ultimately create bald spots.

Managing Hair Loss

Whether the treatment for and management of your particular condition should involve topical medications, nutritional supplements, a change in diet or lifestyle, prudent hair care and styling, or a combination thereof depends on the cause(s) of the problem. I mentioned that brushing helps stimulate circulation at the scalp and exfoliates the skin to unclog the hair follicles. Women whose hair is shedding are understandably terrified to brush it. Some have told me that so much hair comes off on the brush that they want to cry. But brushing does not have to be aggressive to be effective. You can lightly set a soft natural-bristle brush (not one with mixed bristles) on top of your head and gently move it in small circular motions. You can even give yourself a nightly scalp massage with your fingers to help increase circulation.

Stress management and nutrition are other crucial components of healthy hair growth. Eating disorders or continual dieting can result in hair loss due to a deficiency in essential vitamins and minerals. Even if you do not have an eating disorder, you may not be eating healthfully enough while trying to lose weight. While supplements should not replace whole foods, they can help repair hair when integrated into a balanced diet to create a powerful healing force.

Styling, Extensions, and Wigs

I have talked about haircutting and coloring techniques, as well as products that make the hair look thicker. In chapter 4, "Hairstyling," I will discuss styling for fine hair. Depending on the severity of your hair loss, you can apply these methods, experiment with lightweight extensions that do not stress your hair, or even invest in high-quality hairpieces or wigs. I often order and custom cut and color beautiful human-hair wigs for my clients who are experiencing more severe hair loss. Remember that when it comes to wigs, your stylist is usually the best person to find the right one for you and especially to create the haircut and style. A well-made and expertly cut and colored human-hair wig can look completely natural and even better than your own head of hair.

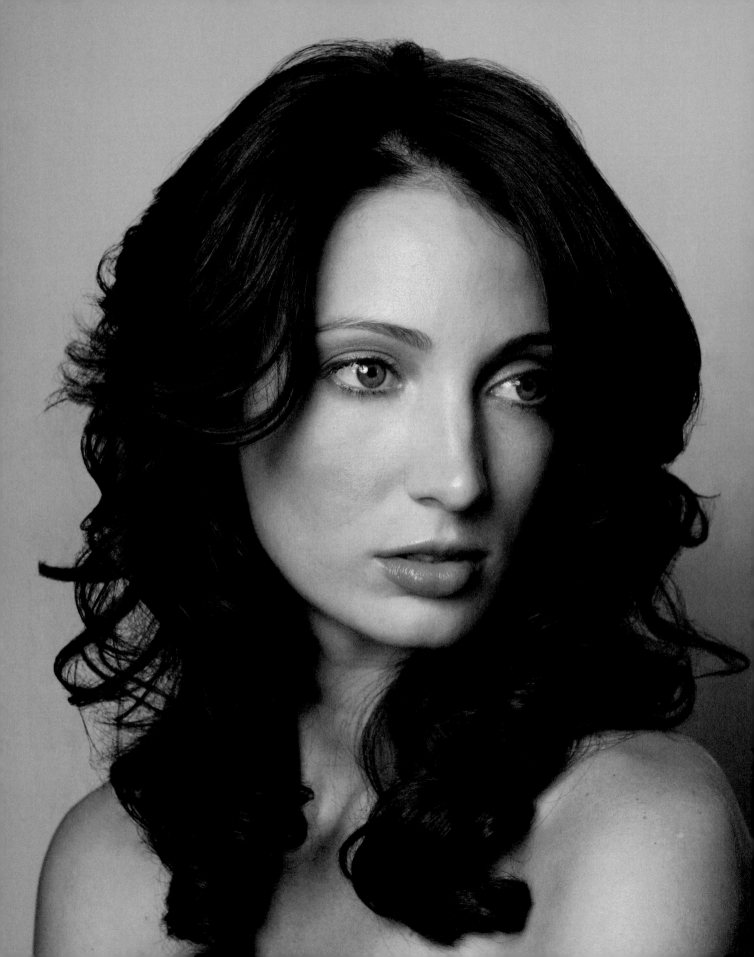

4

HAIRSTYLING

The details are not the details. They make the design.

—Charles Eames, American designer, filmmaker, and architect

No one rolls out of bed with phenomenal-looking hair, unless you are in a sex scene on a film set. Movie stars and fashion models are usually featured with hair that is far from how it looks in their everyday lives. However, women tend to judge their own looks against these unrealistic images and to feel inferior if they do not measure up. I have worked with actors, celebrities, models, and thousands of other gorgeous women, so trust me when I say that beauty comes with some effort. Styling ties together everything you have just read about hair. It is a skill that you can learn under the right tutelage. I know firsthand that it takes solid techniques and a little patience to have a good hair day. This section will put you in charge of your hair and empower you with professional know-how to make it look great every day.

While cutting and coloring are in the hands of your stylist, the everyday maintenance and styling are up to you. This final presentation is what maximizes your investment in a great cut and color. Imagine spending the time and effort to cook a beautiful meal and then serving it on a paper plate; your guests would underestimate the work and care that went into creating it in the first place. It is the finishing touches that make the meal so appealing and appetizing. The same goes for styling your hair.

A good hairstylist may seem like a magician because he or she makes your hair look fantastic with seemingly little effort. But we are not just born with this ability—professionals hone these skills with years of daily practice. Mastering a few basic styling techniques will save you time and your sanity as you get ready in the morning or for a special occasion. It can make the most of a good haircut or help mask the flaws in a bad one. It all starts with the right tools and techniques.

TOOL SCHOOL

If you want professional results, you need to use professional implements such as high-quality brushes, combs, and hot tools. Even well-made bobby pins make a big difference when you are putting your hair up. The investment in superior equipment and products gives the return of better-looking hair, as well as saved time and frustration.

The Brush Guide

Brushes come in a variety of shapes and sizes to produce different looks. Knowing how and when to use them is the secret to successful hairstyling. I work with many kinds of brushes and may use up to three different types during one blowout. Every woman needs to assemble her own brush wardrobe.

Before buying your brushes, consider the look(s) you want to achieve. Are you aiming for bouncy and sexy or smooth and straight? If you like both, depending on the day and occasion, it is worthwhile to invest in two or more kinds of brushes. Styling is based on a feeling that you want to create, which, together with the texture, density, and length of your hair, will determine what you need.

Flat Natural-Bristle Brush

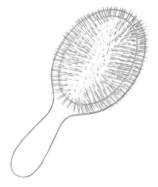

Flat, natural-bristle brush

This is the essential brush that pulls your natural oils through the hair shaft, exfoliating the scalp and improving circulation. It is also excellent for styling bangs and creating straighter, smoother looks. After you use a round brush during the blowout, a flat brush polishes the hair for a gorgeous finishing touch. Going over sections with a blow-dryer and the flat natural-bristle brush makes them shinier and a bit straighter, guaranteeing a perfect, long-lasting blowout.

Round Brush

You are probably accustomed to seeing professionals use this brush at your salon. This is because the densely packed bristles firmly grip each section of the hair, producing tension to easily pull the wave or curl out of it. Combined with the slight turning action of the wrist and the heat of the dryer, it also helps to give amazing shine to the hair. In addition, depending on the way you manipulate it, a round brush can create more volume and lift at the crown. Round brushes come small, medium, large, and extra-large.

1. Small is typically used on short hair and is good for straightening the hair at the nape or the finer hair around the face. The small size is especially good for blowing out kinky, curly hair, even if it is longer, because you can get better tension. (The more tension, the easier it is to mold the hair.)

2. The medium size works for midlength hair and on the shorter layers of longer hair (such as bangs and the sides of the face).

3. A large or jumbo round brush is best for long hair and can also be used to polish and touch up a blowout on the second day.

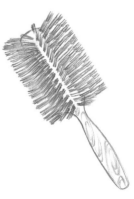

Round brush

Paddle Brush

The body of this brush is flat and usually square. The majority are made with plastic ball-tipped bristles and are safe and effective for detangling thick wet hair. (If there are tips missing, however, the bristles can snag the hair and cause breakage.) This brush is also great for blowing out straight hair (where you don't need the tension from a round brush), to polish the ends of the hair after a blowout with the help of some shine serum, and to blend the subsections that have been dried with a round brush. While a flat natural-bristle brush can achieve the same effect with even greater shine, the paddle brush is quicker and easier to use.

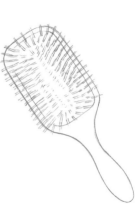

Paddle brush

Vent Brush

This brush has widely spaced plastic bristles attached to a hollow, vented body. The holes allow the heat from a dryer to pass through. This unique construction is good for producing the maximum amount of body in very fine hair, whereas using a regular round brush on such hair can smooth

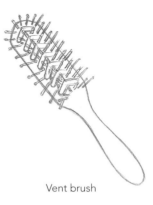

Vent brush

Kendra's hair styled with a flat brush.

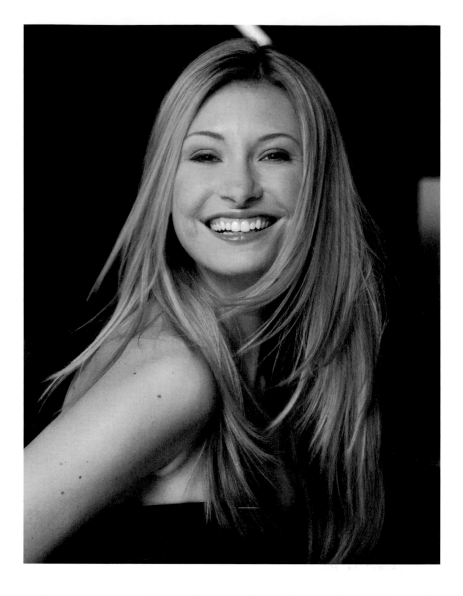

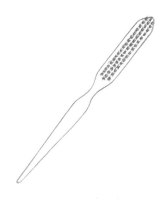

Teasing brush

and compress it to where it becomes limp. The vent brush also works well on short hair to create a soft, natural look, while a small round brush can mimic the look of a roller set and make it too "done."

Teasing Brush

This thin brush is made for teasing the hair to create more texture and lift. It is a gentler alternative to a teasing comb, as the tighter tease created with a comb is difficult to brush out (trying to do so can also break the hair). Personally, I prefer to use a small (travel) flat brush to tease the hair because its width produces a slightly softer look.

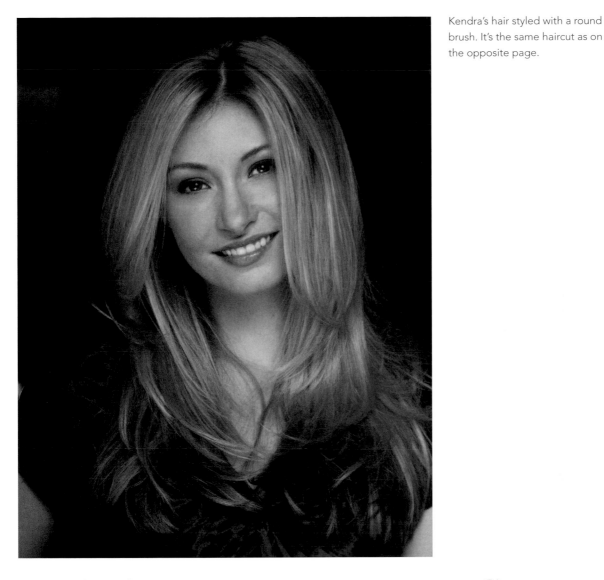

Kendra's hair styled with a round brush. It's the same haircut as on the opposite page.

Thermal Brush

The body of this typically round brush is a conductor of heat, as it is made of either ceramic or metal. It acts like a large curling iron when used with a blow-dryer during styling. I do not advise the daily use of a thermal brush. It is fine on special occasions when you want more curl or lift in your hair, but you should pre-dry the hair as much as possible. If used for the entirety of the blowout, a metal brush can really stress the hair. Many women with fine hair find that this brush is the only thing that helps them achieve more lift, body, and curl. If your hair is short and regularly trimmed, it may be able to withstand

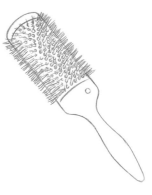

Thermal brush

such heat more frequently. Long hair, however, will start to look and feel dry from regular use of a thermal brush.

Travel Brush—Natural Bristle

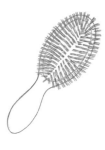

Travel brush

This mini flat brush is a smaller version of the full-size natural-bristle brush. It is great not only for travel but for styling. The petite size makes it easier to blow out bangs or to softly tease the hair at the crown of the head, and is perfect for putting your hair up or into a ponytail. This is also a wonderful brush for kids and men.

How to Buy a Brush

It pays to purchase high-quality brushes. The design details of the brush are vital, down to the length of its bristles. Any brush is much more effective at smoothing and straightening the hair if the bristles are at least three-quarters of an inch long. If you use a round brush now and feel that your hair could be smoother, or if you notice that the bristles are not able to get through and grab the hair, they are probably not long enough. The bristles should be able to clear the hair and come out the other side of each section. If you cannot see them popping out, either your sections are too thick or the bristles are too short.

If selecting a paddle brush or vent brush with plastic ball-tipped bristles, make sure that the bristles and the rounded tips are one seamless unit. On some cheaper versions, those tips can fall off, leaving the exposed ends to snag and break the hair. (European-made vent and paddle brushes are generally the best quality.)

Ask your stylist what he or she prefers to use. Many salons carry the same products and tools as used by their hairstylists, and working with them sets you up for a greater chance of success on your own.

The Care and Cleaning of Your Brushes

Once you have invested in high-quality brushes, treat them with care. They will last for years and perform better if you do. Store them upright, with the handles down and the bristles exposed. I like to place mine in a large cup or a wide vase on the vanity. Because dirt, oil, and product residue can break down the bristles, try to clean the hair out of your brush after each use and wash the brush every couple of weeks. You can do this in your bathroom sink with a drop of shampoo added to warm water. Gently rub two brushes together to remove the buildup from each. Rinse them well and dry facedown on a towel. If you use a plastic paddle brush in the shower, wash it weekly because mold and mildew can settle onto the bristles and body. Since the bristles are spaced farther apart, you can simply use your fingers to scrub and clean between them.

When to Replace Your Brush

Round brushes should be replaced when the bristles wear down. In addition to styling products and your natural oils, the heat of a dryer breaks down both plastic and natural bristles. If you use a round brush almost daily, think about investing in a new one every two to three years. On natural bristles, this deterioration creates an uneven depression in the brush, which reduces its effectiveness. Whether you notice this change in shape, are no longer getting a smooth finish, or struggle while blow drying, it is likely to be a result of using old, broken-down tools.

OTHER STYLING TOOLS

Combs

Out of the myriad of combs on the market, there are two that most women need: a wide-toothed plastic comb to detangle and distribute conditioner through hair in the shower and a basic, traditional comb for sectioning before styling. European-made tortoiseshell combs tend to be the most gentle and highest in quality. Stay away from metal combs, which can pull and break the hair.

Clips, Pins, and Elastics

Longer metal clips called "duckbill clips" (so named because they look and operate like the bill of a bird) hold sections of hair out of the way during styling and help to mold damp hair.

Women with heavy, long hair often have a difficult time holding sections in duckbill clips. I have discovered amazing Japanese-made clips

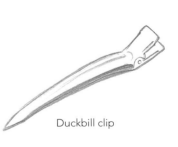

Duckbill clip

Japanese clip

Indecent exposure

A butterfly clip is perfectly fine to use during the styling process to help pull a large section of hair out of the way as you blow out another. It also serves to keep your hair pulled back while you are cooking or washing your face. However, this is not an accessory and should never be worn in the professional world (going to the gym or a yoga class with one is fine, but that's about it).

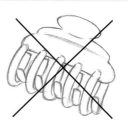

The dreaded butterfly clip

designed especially for long and/or thick hair to use for sectioning during blow-drying.

There is a big difference between a bobby pin and a hairpin. A hairpin is U-shaped, while the prongs of a bobby pin are closed to tightly grasp a section of hair for a more secure hold.

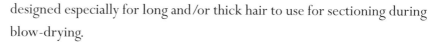

Hairpins may seem a relic from a bygone era, but professionals use them all the time to gently and discreetly pin hair in place without making a big depression.

We use both types of pins to create an updo: first, bobby pins to firmly anchor the hair, then hairpins to make subtle adjustments and refine the shape of the upsweep.

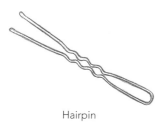

Bobby pin

Hairpin

Covered elastics (thin fabric encasing a rubber band) are the safest to use for ponytails because the smooth cord does not snag the hair. However, any type of ponytail holder will cause breakage if removed carelessly. Many women yank them off in one motion, snapping off hairs in the process. Instead, gently unwind it the way you created the ponytail, layer by layer.

Velcro Rollers

Ideally, Velcro rollers are best used on dry hair after blow-drying to add more lift and body, especially in the crown area. For a stronger set and longer-lasting results, you can mist a bit of hair spray onto the section of hair before wrapping it around the roller and then heat it with a dryer for a few moments. (With this method, use rollers that have a metal core, since they conduct heat more effectively.) With or without heat, rollers should be left in the hair for at least ten minutes. (I suggest you do your makeup and finish getting ready in that time.)

Removing Velcro rollers can be tricky. If you are not careful, the self-gripping mesh on the roller can easily snag the hair and create a tangled mess. To avoid this, it is important not to wind the hair around the roller too tightly and to carefully unroll it (rather than pull it out) to release the hair. If you find that Velcro rollers are always getting caught and pulling your hair, do not use them. Some hair, especially if it is bleached, tends to get caught more easily.

HOT TOOLS

Heat makes the hair malleable enough to mold and shape with tools or even just your hands. Almost like candle wax, your hair will hold the form once it cools. Even more so than with other products and tools, the quality of these hot tools can mean the difference between quick and effective styling and wasted time and frustration, poor results, and even damage.

Blow-dryers

Ionic dryers dry the hair more effectively and rapidly than conventional ones and are therefore healthier for the hair. They give off negative ions, which break up water molecules, making them evaporate faster and drying the hair in half the time. If you spray your bathroom mirror with water and dry it with an ionic dryer, you can actually see the droplets breaking down. The beads of water splay out like a starburst on the mirror before disappearing. With a regular dryer, that water will run down the mirror and dry at a much slower pace.

Look for a professional dryer that is ergonomically designed. These are made for hairdressers to hold comfortably as they work with them all day long. You can purchase a professional ionic dryer at many salons or find one online.

Dryer Attachments

Be sure to use a plastic nozzle attachment on the end of your dryer. All good blow-dryers come with one. This concentrates the heat and directs the airflow in one area, which helps smooth the cuticle to reduce frizz and increase shine. These attachments have a tendency to come off during use. A good way to secure one in place is with electrical tape. For curly hair, a diffuser attachment can be used instead of a nozzle to reduce the amount of airflow from the dryer and moderate frizz. This attachment does not ordinarily come with the dryer, so make sure to purchase one that fits its brand and style.

Irons

Irons take molding of the hair to the next level with direct heat. They can be used after a blowout to get the hair even straighter or to create curls and waves and eliminate frizz. Even if your hair is naturally straight, an iron can enhance its shine. The flat iron or curling iron you purchase should be ceramic. It conducts heat more evenly than metal, which tends to create hot spots along the iron. Ceramic also emits negative ions, neutralizing the positive charge in the hair that otherwise causes static and frizz. Extinguishing that energy makes the hair smoother and shinier. Most of today's flat irons have narrower plates (one inch or less) to get around the hard-to-reach hairline and bang area without burning your skin. Curling irons come in a variety of sizes and each creates a different-shape curl:

- ⅜-inch barrel to add definition to kinky, curly hair
- ½-inch for tight ringlets
- ¾-inch for medium-size curls
- 1- to 1¼-inch for more relaxed, looser curls
- 1½- to 2-inch for big luscious waves

Crimping Irons

In fashion magazines there has recently been a resurgence of wild, sexy, big-hair looks with brushed-out crimped hair. The crimping iron has zigzag plates that give the hair a very different and avant-garde texture. The hair does not have to be 100 percent crimped; just a few sections here and there will create a fun, edgy look that is perfect for a photo

PROFESSIONAL TECHNIQUES

USING YOUR HANDS AS A STYLING TOOL: You can use your hands and a blow-dryer to shape the hair. Pulling a section taut or lifting it at the root is a wonderful method of pre-drying the hair before styling it with a round brush. If you have short hair and some pieces around your face are not long enough to get around a brush, you can smooth and pull them with your fingers into the style and shape that you want.

CURLING IRON: If your hair is naturally curly, the iron can be used to make the top layer as curly as the bottom. My hair looks best when I use a curling iron on just a few pieces around my face and a couple on the top of my head to better define the curl pattern. If you have more time, try alternating small and medium-size irons to produce a head full of gorgeous, natural-looking curls.

HOT ROLLERS: Starting on dry hair, take a subsection no bigger than the width of the roller, wind it up to the scalp, and secure it with a roller clip. If your roller set tends to turn out too curly, try leaving out the ends of the hair. Start by positioning the roller one to two inches from the ends of each section, then roll toward the head and secure with a clip. To further modernize a set, apply a dab of pomade or wax and run it through the hair. It will look more relaxed and separated, and give you that sexy, slept-in look.

shoot or going out dancing (but probably not for a meeting at the office). A nice variation of this look is made by pulling the crimped hair into a ponytail.

Hooded Dryers

As old-fashioned as it sounds, a hooded dryer is generally the best choice to dry curly hair. If you are not a fan of air drying and a diffuser does not work for you, this may be heaven-sent, since it dries curls with beautiful form and no frizz. Apply some leave-in conditioner or a curl product, twist a few sections of hair around the face and the top of the head, and sit under the dryer while working, reading, or watching television. Your hair will be completely dry in about fifteen to twenty minutes, as opposed to the hours it can take to air dry. This type of dryer can be ordered online and is compact enough to be stored in a closet.

Hot Rollers

These plastic rollers are encased in a soft material so as not to pull or snag the hair. (Be careful, though: the U-shaped metal pins that hold these rollers can lose the rubber grips at the ends of their prongs and end up snagging the hair.) Rollers can be easier for some women to use than a curling iron. It really depends on your preference. Roller sets can give more lift and body in the base of the hair but can often make the ends very curly. An iron creates a more uniform curl but it is typically not as long-lasting because the roller set sits on the hair longer with a lower level of heat. Some women, however, love the more retro, coiffed look of a roller set, reminiscent of old Hollywood glamour.

STYLING PRODUCTS

When it comes to styling products and tools, most people simply don't know what to buy or how to properly use it. There is a dizzying array of products to choose from, and while they may all seem similar, each type serves a different purpose. Some are made to help straighten your hair or make it curlier; others calm frizz or pump up volume. Every hour of every day I am asked by women and men which products would work best for them. I always ask what they already have at home and hear the same response: "I have so many products!" People keep buying so much because they simply do not know what they need, and end up with a stockpile of things that don't work for them. They become frustrated from not being able to achieve the look they want, but even a hairstylist would have difficulty working without the right products.

Applying Product—The Right Way

When women tell me that a product is too heavy on their hair, I usually learn that it is because of how they apply it. It is easy to use too much product, which makes the hair oily and heavy. As with shampoo and conditioner, a common mistake is to apply a styling product first to the front and top of the head, which can result in an oil slick in the front and not enough in the back. Instead, start from the back, where the hair is thicker, and work the product through the sides and then the top of the head. Even if you apply too much, your hair will not be weighed down near your face or at the crown. It is also better to add small amounts of product, section by section, rather than all at once.

The amount of styling product necessary to make your hair behave can be a barometer of its health and the quality of the cut. The healthier the hair and the better the cut, the less product you should have to use. Relatively healthy short hair usually requires a dime-size amount of product for the entirety of the hair; a nickel-size amount is adequate for medium lengths and a quarter-size for long hair. With a heavier, oil-based pomade (such as a wax), you should need even less. When applying mousse, I like to use a small dollop on each section of the head. With serum, one to two pumps will be plenty for the entire head. Again, start with just a drop—you can always add more. The key is to apply the product in small amounts and in the right order.

Since each product has a specific purpose, do not dilute one's functionality with another. When washing your hair, you would not combine the shampoo and conditioner together or use a rich conditioner first and then shampoo it out. With styling products, follow a similar logic: first lift the hair where you want volume, then add something to smooth the ends or shape your curls. Finally, when the hair is dry, add the appropriate finishing product. The sequence can be broken down into four steps:

1. Foundation spray to prepare the hair.
2. Volumizer for body and lift.
3. Smoothing product to remove frizz and polish the ends.
4. Finishing product to add texture and/or hold the shape.

Step One: Preparing Your Hair

Everyone needs a foundation spray to prime the hair for other styling products. This is an essential first step because it adds a fine layer of water-based moisture to even out the porosity of the hair (remember that hair is more porous toward the ends). I apply a foundation spray on all my clients' hair before I style it. Your styling spray, cream, or whatever other product you put on next will lie more evenly and be more effective. For instance, hair that is dry at the ends will not overly absorb product and become weighed down. Foundation spray is similar to a makeup foundation that evens out your skin tone, or a base coat for your nails. It also lets you comb through the hair and detangle it more easily. And on weekends, you can just use the foundation spray by itself. It is so lightweight that even those with oily hair or who generally find styling products too heavy will love it. They may even choose to use it as their primary styling product.

Step Two: Creating Lift and Body

The second step is building height and fullness into the hair by choosing one of the products listed below. Using a small amount, start where you want the most lift, and move the product through the hair. For fine hair, apply more evenly throughout. If you have a lot of volume naturally, you may want to skip this step.

GEL: Gel typically gives the strongest hold. On straight hair it produces body, and on curly hair it provides some structure to hold the curl shape. On straight hair, apply it just in the root area for lift in the crown, which creates a prettier overall head shape. On curls, it can be distributed throughout the hair before applying a cream-based product to the ends, which prevents the gel from becoming too stiff if air drying.

MOUSSE: Mousse has a light, foamy feeling when initially applied, which is why women with fine hair tend to like it. Ironically, though, if left to air

PROFESSIONAL TECHNIQUE

Properly distributing product

If not properly distributed, a product can just sit on top of the hair. I like to comb styling products through after each step. This works especially well if you are blow-drying your hair straight. When you use the right products in the right way—one step at a time, like the pros—you will get better results.

dry, it can make the hair feel hard and dry. I am not a big fan of mousse without the use of a blow-dryer, which keeps the hair soft, as the product is broken down by heat. Generally, products that create a firm feel to the hair are more effective when used with a blow-dryer, which also steams off the excess residue.

STYLING SPRAYS: A volumizing spray gives lift, shape, and hold to the hair. By leaving a thin film on the hair, it works in two ways: the extra layer of product makes the strands feel and look thicker, while the formulation gently swells the cuticle. Some sprays have wheat bran and other ingredients that help to make the hair appear fuller. They are best used with heat, which instantly increases their efficacy. However, even if you let your hair air dry, they are still effective, as they "beef up" the hair strands.

STYLING CREAM: This product is creamy or opaque like a moisturizer but it can be just as strong as a gel. It adds emollients that smooth the hair and give it body. Its refined, modern formulation helps create lift at the root when combined with heat, while protecting your hair from it. A styling cream is used to create maximum hold with a lighter and softer feel to the hair than you get with a gel or mousse.

Step Three: Smoothing

No matter how much volume is desired, everyone's hair looks shinier and healthier when the ends are polished. For this reason, smoothing products are usually applied midlength and through the ends. A few drops or a pea-size amount before blow drying will do.

STRAIGHTENING SERUM: Products with descriptions such as "smoothing," "straightening," or "relaxing" help remove frizz as well as straighten and smooth the hair, since they contain antihumectant agents, which repel moisture. For example, you can use a gel in the roots for some lift, then layer a bit of serum to smooth the frizz. Even on curly hair, a few drops help smooth the ends and tame frizz without disturbing the curl.

CURL CREAM: A curl cream is formulated to encourage springier, bouncier curls. It enhances the wave pattern and helps to minimize frizz by hydrating the hair and smoothing the cuticle. Some formulations include fruit enzymes, which have been found to promote a prettier curl shape.

BEAUTY RECIPE

Instant root lift

You can make your own dry shampoo using talc and cornstarch. Mix equal amounts of the two, put them through a sifter, and store the powder mixture in a small plastic or glass jar. To apply, take a few pinches in your palm and rub it between your hands, then tilt your head forward and apply the powder to the root area, massaging it in with your fingertips. Brush the hair to remove any excess.

CHECKLIST

At-a-glance styling product guide

- **Step 1:** *Foundation Products:* Detanglers, porosity equalizers, vitamin-and-mineral-infused waters, foundation sprays.
- **Step 2:** *Lifting Products:* Styling milk and creams, gel, volumizing spray, mousse, salt-water spray.
- **Step 3:** *Smoothing Products:* Straightening and smoothing serums, curl creams, heat-activated thermal creams or sprays.
- **Step 4:** *Finishing Products:* Shine serum, shine spray, hair spray, pomade, wax.

LEAVE-IN CONDITIONER: While a curl cream helps to promote more curl, a leave-in conditioner is lightweight and provides only moisture, which is what many women with curly hair are lacking because they rarely brush. Leave-in conditioner is often used as a styling product when air drying curly or wavy hair. It hydrates the hair, smoothes the cuticle, and enhances the natural texture. For straight hair, some women like to use a pea-size amount on the ends before blow-drying, which helps protect against split ends.

HEAT-PROTECTIVE PRODUCTS: In addition to smoothing, these products are designed specifically to protect the hair from hot irons and blow-dryers. They come in the form of serums, sprays, and creams and contain anti-thermal ingredients that form a protective film on the hair.

Step Four: Finishing Product for Hold or Shine

This is your last step and the finishing touch: a product applied once the hair is dried and styled to add whatever ingredient you might need. It could be a drop of shine serum on the ends if they still look a little fuzzy, a dab of pomade to calm the flyaway baby hairs around the face, or a hair spray to hold your style in place.

SHINE SERUM: A serum helps to eliminate frizz on dry hair because it typically contains silicone to coat, smooth, and flatten the cuticle.

SHINE SPRAY: This is basically serum in a spray bottle. A shine spray appears to be lighter-weight because of how it is dispensed. However, you need only a small amount, and if too much comes out at once, spritz one pump on the palm of your hand instead of directly onto your hair. Rub your hands together, then graze them over the outer layer of the hair to calm frizz and flyaways and add shine.

POMADE AND WAX: These products generally fall into two categories: water based and oil based. Water-based pomades are lighter and more matte, and can be rinsed out with just water. Oil-based waxes are heavier, shinier, and have to be washed out with shampoo. They help create a "piecey" texture in shorter haircuts but can also be used to play up the layers of a longer cut. The key is to use a very small amount (about the size of a pea) and emulsify it by warming it between your palms before working it into the hair. Apply it more toward the ends, using your fingertips. A little bit of wax is the perfect way to tamp down baby hairs for a smooth ponytail or to eliminate a halo of frizz. A matte or dry formulation is incredible when used in the root area for volume or to prepare your hair to be teased. But be aware that waxes can quickly make the hair look dirty, so you may need to wash it more frequently when using them.

HAIR SPRAY: Hair spray has gotten a bad rap over the years as a dull, stiff product used for old-fashioned hairdos. However, there are actually two types of hair spray: working spray and finishing spray. A working spray, usually specified by "light hold" or "flexible hold" on the label, can easily be brushed out of the hair. It is lightweight enough to mist onto roller sections or to spray on the hair before using a curling iron to create a stronger set. Working spray is what session stylists use on photo shoots to quickly and easily change hairstyles on the models.

A finishing spray gives a stronger hold to a hairstyle and is used as the final step when you want to hold the hair in place. It is also great on short hair to maintain the textural effect from wax or pomade.

STYLING LESSONS

The secret to effective styling is that there is no secret! You just have to learn the proper techniques, practice, and take your time. This is a skill set that everyone can hone. There is a methodology to styling, whether blow-drying the hair or pulling it into a chic ponytail. Here, I will simplify professional techniques and empower you to accomplish them on your own.

COMMON MISTAKE

Blow-drying your hair in a hot bathroom

After a shower, your bathroom is about as humid as a jungle. There is no way to escape so much steam in a small room. Give your blowout a head start and a much better chance of success by working in a moisture-free environment. If you are not able to set up a proper vanity, try creating a temporary hairstyling station at your desk or kitchen table. In warmer months, it is also a good idea to turn up the air conditioner. The room must be cool to achieve a blowout without frizz.

The Ten Biggest Blow-drying Mistakes

1. NOT SECTIONING THE HAIR FIRST

Before starting to blow-dry, have your brushes, clips, and products within reach. Begin by sectioning your hair. Although most women skip this important step, it makes blow-drying much easier. (Refer to the illustration at the bottom of page 133.)

2. STANDING UP AS YOU BLOW-DRY

One of the best pieces of blow-drying advice I can give is to have a seat. You will not believe the difference this makes. In a comfortable seated position, you have much more upper-body strength and will be less likely to tire out and rush through the blow-dry.

3. HOLDING THE BRUSH IN THE WRONG HAND

A big mistake women make is holding the brush in their weaker hand and lifting the dryer with their dominant one. Although it feels instinctual to hold the heavier dryer in the stronger hand, you need the dexterity and coordination of that hand to manipulate the brush, making it easier to twist, turn, and pull. Even many professional hairdressers learn this incorrectly.

4. OVERTWISTING THE BRUSH

Many women start twisting as soon as the brush gets near the scalp. This is how a brush gets stuck in the hair. At the base of a section, make just a one-quarter turn with a slight shift of the wrist to grab the hair and initiate tension. Next, smooth the section by pulling the brush away from the head to the midpoint of the hair length (for shorter to midlength hair, approximately two to three inches from the head). This is where you can start making more quarter turns. When you get to the ends you can do more twisting without the brush getting snarled in the hair (refer to illustration C on page 134 to see correct positioning for quarter turns with the brush).

5. PULLING THE HAIR DOWNWARD AT THE CROWN

Most women direct their brushes downward, pulling the hair toward the floor to get it straight. This will not give you the lift at the top that comes from a professional blowout. Instead, pull your hair up, toward the ceiling. Identify the recessions of your hair (near the temples) and picture the area between them and over the top of your head as a horseshoe. Everything in that horseshoe gets directed straight up with the round brush. (This is another great reason to be sitting down.) Bangs are the exception to this upward direction. The hair below that horseshoe is pulled straight down. You can even use a flat brush for this lower part as you would a round brush. The finished look is more modern, with lift at the top and sleekness around the sides and back of the head (refer to illustration C on page 134 for correct positioning of the brush underneath the horseshoe).

6. HOLDING THE DRYER TOO CLOSE

Women tend to smash the end of their dryers into their hair, which happens frequently when in a hurry or thinking that the extra-close proximity will dry the hair faster. Some also use the dryer to hold each section of the hair in place while styling it. This causes damage to the hair (as well as to the brush) that will be even more extreme if a plastic nozzle is not attached. The nozzle should be kept at least one inch away from the hair as it follows the brush along the hair shaft.

7. HOLDING THE DRYER IN THE WRONG POSITION

Not holding the nozzle parallel to each section can result in flyways, since blowing your hair around irritates and raises the cuticle. Instead, use a polishing technique to dry the hair directionally: angle the dryer to direct the heat from the nozzle alongside the hair section to smooth and flatten the cuticle (refer to illustration B on page 134 for correct positioning of the blow-dryer parallel to the section).

8. KEEPING THE DRYER MOTIONLESS

Professionals never hold the dryer completely still over a section of hair, but move it very slightly back and forth with the wrist to prevent concentrating too much heat on one spot. This is a real trick of the trade that few women know about. To a stylist this is second nature and we do it almost subconsciously. Conversely, most women do the opposite and end up frying their hair with the dryer.

9. GOING WAY TOO FAST

Perhaps it is the noise of the dryer that amps people up, but women often blow-dry too fast, as if they are in some kind of panic. This is not a race against time. On the contrary, slow down the process; be more methodical and careful. You will have a much better outcome if you section your hair, remain systematic in your technique, and keep your dryer one to two inches away from the hair. I recommend keeping a spray bottle with water nearby to rewet your hair if part of it has prematurely dried or if you make a mistake. Water acts like a magic eraser, allowing you to start over and restyle a section.

10. NOT DRYING THE HAIR *COMPLETELY*

If your hair begins to frizz right after styling, it is probably because you did not dry it 100 percent. Sometimes the hair looks completely dry, but if it feels cold to the touch, there is still water in it. Your hair should be room temperature after blow drying. If there is even a trace of moisture left, it will frizz or curl in a few hours. Hairdressers go over each section numerous times not just to flatten the cuticle and create a more polished finish but to remove any remnants of water.

THE ART OF BLOW-DRYING
(The Right Way!)

When first learning to blow-dry your hair properly, expect some awkward fumbling, many mistakes, dropped brushes, and probably some cursing. But this is a technique worth practicing and perfecting—and you *can* do it.

Pre-dry (Before You Blow-Dry)

Pre-drying can cut the blow-drying time in half. The extent to which you should pre-dry your hair depends on how curly it is and how much body you want. You should implement the brush when very curly hair is more wet to give yourself extra time for stretching and polishing it smooth. Wavy hair should be about 50 percent dry before you begin working with a round brush. Straight hair can be pre-dried 70 percent or more.

Pre-drying is easy because you use only your hands and the heat of a blow-dryer, but there is a technique to it. You are not just haphazardly

HAIRMARE

blowing your hair around, as if in a wind tunnel (as you have already learned, that roughs up the cuticle and creates frizz). Using your fingers, pull the hair in the top horseshoe area of your head taut and directed straight up to the ceiling. By doing so, you start the lifting action before even implementing a round brush. Direct the hair down where you want it to be flatter. Now, if you want a lot of body (and I mean *really* big hair), you can pre-dry it all over the place and throw this sectioning method out the window. You can even throw your head forward and rough up the roots with your hand, which is good for those with very fine hair. You have to try these techniques for yourself to gauge what works best. If you have curly hair or just a texture that tends to frizz, it is best not to pre-dry or to pre-dry only a section at a time as you move up your head.

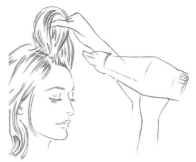

Pre-drying

Sectioning the Hair

Sectioning will help keep your work organized and prevent you from going over the same sections repeatedly and dehydrating the hair. Use clips to separate the hair into four sections: the top horseshoe, the bottom section from the occipital bone to the nape, and each side section from recession to the ear. If you have bangs, separate them into a fifth section. Within these four main sections, take one-and-a-half-inch subsections that should fit in the center of the brush, leaving a little room on either side. A section that is too wide will spill over the side of the brush and cause tangling. (You don't want to end up in a situation like my aunt Jan!)

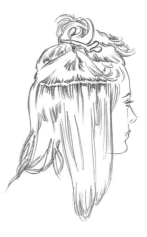

Sectioning

THE PERFECT AT-HOME BLOWOUT

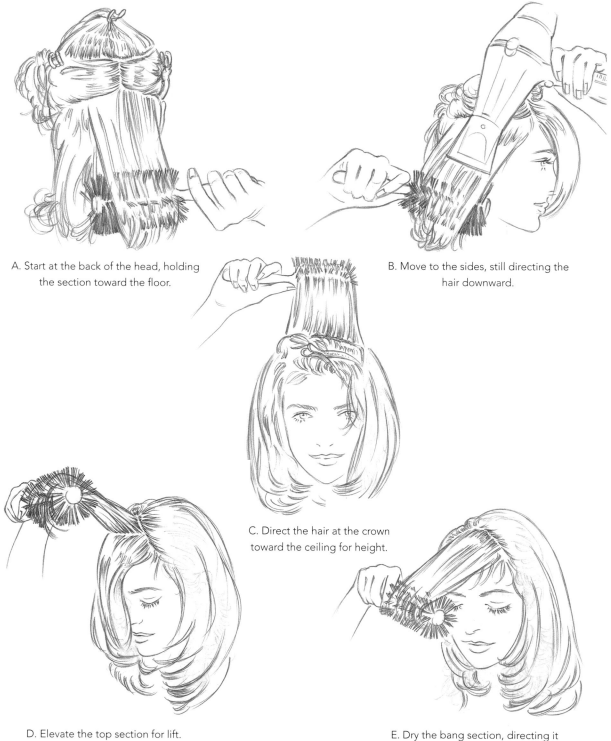

A. Start at the back of the head, holding the section toward the floor.

B. Move to the sides, still directing the hair downward.

C. Direct the hair at the crown toward the ceiling for height.

D. Elevate the top section for lift.

E. Dry the bang section, directing it straight ahead, toward the mirror.

Get straighter ends

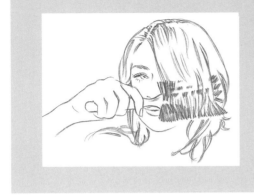

To ensure smoothness, the brush must have good traction in the hair to pull any wave out of it. When you get to the ends, pull the hair just enough so it stays in the bristles, take the dryer away, and let the hair cool on the brush for a few seconds before you release it. This technique can change the vibe of your blowout completely—from "mumsy" to chic.

MAKING YOUR BLOWOUT LAST
Getting to Day Two and Beyond!

There are two steadfast rules for extending the life of a blowout: (1) use small amounts of product on your hair and (2) stay away from water in all forms, including steam and humidity. I am not saying that you should forgo bathing or skip the products altogether. If you eliminate the crucial step of protecting your hair from direct heat, it will be adversely affected over time. Mist a foundation spray and apply a minimal amount of styling product (a few drops of smoothing serum can be best for smoothness and heat protection).

Moisture is the mortal enemy of a blowout. The faintest hint of dampness (from humidity, steam, water, or perspiration) can instantly create frizz and make the baby hairs around your face and the nape of your neck curl. Do your best to be conscientious, if not paranoid, about avoiding water if you want your blowout to last. First of all, be sure your hair is absolutely bone dry after blow-drying it. When trying to preserve a blowout, it is wise to skip showers in favor of warm (not hot) baths. Steam is a sneakier form of water and will make its way under your shower cap. If you are just not a bath person, wear a terry-cloth headband to cover your hairline under the shower cap. Immediately blot any moisture from the hair after bathing. (Washing your face without getting water on the hairline can be tricky. Prepare your hair beforehand by pulling it back off your face into a ponytail and using a headband over the hairline.)

If a little bit of moisture touches your hair when you are bathing or washing your face, or from perspiration, touch up the blowout in those spots only. Dampen the section and blow-dry it with a brush or just use your fingers, pulling the hair away from the head to smooth the hairline.

PROFESSIONAL TECHNIQUES

Hair spray: Apply in light layers

If you use a heavy hand with hair spray, it will end up weighing everything down. Even if an aerosol makes it seem light, it is still a liquid that works better when applied in a fine mist. Wait half a minute for it to dry before applying another spritz and you will have a much better hold than if you do it all at once.

Curly hair secret: Volumizing spray as a finishing product

It may surprise you that a volumizing spray is one of the best finishing products for curls. Mist this on as a last step when your hair is dry, instead of a hair spray, then gently caress the curls with your hands. Since these products are water-based but still give hold, they create a softer look while enhancing the hair's natural waves for more lifted, gorgeous curls, while helping to remove that "halo" of frizz.

Second-day revival: Water as a styling product

Dampening the hair with a little water reactivates any product already in the hair and allows you to "touch up" your blowout in minutes without having to start over. Just mist some water from an atomizer bottle around your face and a few sections on the top of your head, then dry your hair as you normally would using a flat or round brush. You will be surprised at how great your hair looks without shampooing.

Reinvigorate your wave or curl

Foundation spray is a magic potion to mist on your hair at midday if it looks a bit frizzy. It also works well if you do not have time to wash your hair in the morning, by providing the perfect amount of moisture to bring your curls back to life. Just spray six to eight pumps onto the exterior of your hair and caress the ends, gently squeezing and pushing the product in with your hands. This also works well to make static and flyaways vanish.

PROFESSIONAL TECHNIQUES

Using the cool button to set a perfect blowout

After finishing the blowout, switch the setting on your dryer to cool and go over the entirety of the hair. You do not even have to use a brush; just blow-dry freestyle. This contracts the cuticle, similar to a cool rinse of water on your hair in the shower. Heat from blow-drying makes the hair malleable, and in that state strands can bend. A shot of cool air sets the smooth shape you have created to help ensure the longevity of your blowout.

How to get more body

Think of a round brush as a big roller. (In fact, blow-dryers and round brushes have mostly replaced the rollers and hood dryers of the past.) The round brush mimics the roller when you wind the hair around it. If you want more lift after a section has been blow-dried, roll the brush from the end of the section to the scalp and hold the heat on it as if the brush were a hot roller. After a few seconds, take the dryer away and allow the section to cool while it is still wrapped around the brush, or apply cold air by pressing the cool button on your dryer, then unravel the hair (A and B). If you want straighter ends, you can leave them out and roll the brush down from the midshaft to the scalp. This will give you some volume and fullness without the curl (C).

A   B   C

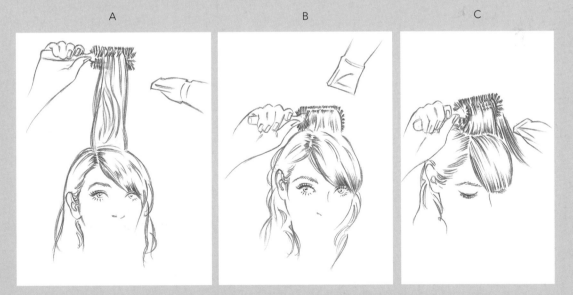

A and B: Using a round brush like a roller for volume.
C: "Bumping" the root area of the hair with a round brush for added lift.

PROFESSIONAL TECHNIQUE

The curly blowout

The goal of a blowout is not always stick-straight hair. Sometimes a woman with naturally curly or wavy hair would like her curls to look like loose waves, or her waves to look smoother, without completely straightening her natural texture. This technique is for achieving a bouncier, more voluptuous blowout (think of Sophia Loren's sexy hair). It provides a more polished look for curly hair, while taking advantage of its natural lift and wave. This is also a great way to touch up a blowout, giving it fullness and bounce on day two or three. What makes this curly blowout so special is that it works with the natural waves, so you can style only the sections that need more smoothness and skip the ones that don't.

1. Allow the hair to air dry as much as possible (ideally until it is 80 to 90 percent dry) to maximize the natural body and root lift.

2. Wrap sections, one by one, around a medium-sized round brush from the ends to the scalp with the brush in a vertical position; heat them with the dryer for five to seven seconds; allow to cool (A).

3. Untwist in a spiral pattern (B). You are not straightening the wave completely, just smoothing sections and removing some of the frizz to create big bouncy curls (C).

A	B	C

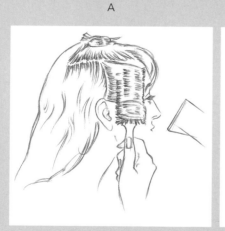 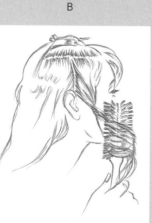 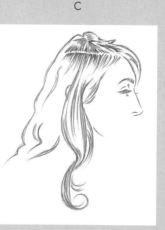

Take vertical sections for a wavy blowout. Roll the hair toward the scalp while drying, then allow to cool.

Using a circular motion, unwind the hair.

The end result.

PROFESSIONAL TECHNIQUES

Do not apply styling product to fine hair until it is more than halfway dry

If you have fine hair, whether curly or straight, layering product into it when wet weighs it down. You will get much more lift if you first allow the hair to dry 70 to 80 percent, which is when it begins to lift off the scalp. Since curly hair has a natural bend, it will have more volume if some of the wave at the root area is utilized. Then you can use a foundation spray, followed by a volumizer or a salt-water spray to expand the cuticle.

Adding polish to your hair when you're running late

It is comforting to know that a blowout does not have to be all-or-nothing. You can concentrate only on certain areas of your hair, like smoothing the front pieces around your face, even if you use your hands to pull on those sections. You will be surprised at how this simple technique improves the shape of your hair. It is a very modern way of blowing out the hair: smoothing just the outer perimeters and working some of the natural texture into the overall style.

Styling Bangs

Typically, it is best to use a flat brush to style bangs because a round brush can make it too bubbly and round. Bangs generally look better if they are flatter at the base, near the scalp. Refer to the illustrations on the following page.

1. Separate the triangular bang section from the rest of the hair.
2. Separate a one-inch horizontal subsection and secure it with a clip. If the front of the hair dries before you get to it, spritz it with water or style the bangs first.
3. Angle the dryer nozzle with the heat directed down at the root area and dry that part first. Using a flat natural-bristle brush, blow-dry the lower section flat and smoothed down toward the face.
4. Take the next section above the one you just dried and slightly elevate it with the brush, directing it toward the mirror in front of you. This creates a bit of lift so the bangs are not plastered to the forehead.
5. If you have a third top section, lift straight to the ceiling.

6. When finished, use your brush to grab the entire bang section and go over it one more time with forward elevation to integrate all of the sections. If you have longer side-swept bangs, use the same technique but direct the sections at an angle, aiming more for your cheekbone than your nose. Since the fringe is longer, you may want to use a round brush to get more lift and body.

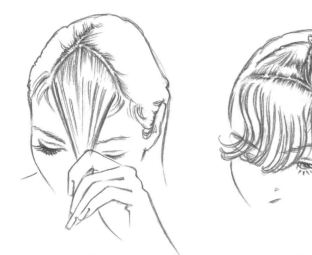
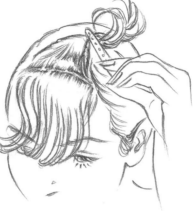
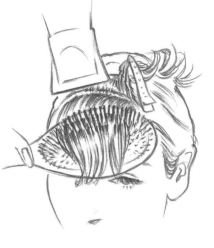

Step 1

Step 2

Step 3

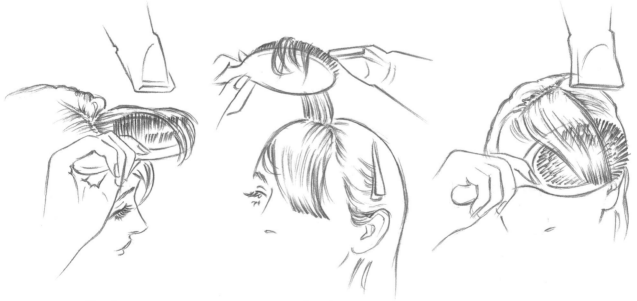

Step 4

Step 5

Step 6

FLAT IRON TECHNIQUES

Like all hot tools, flat irons damage hair not so much because of the tool itself but from how it is used. Most women rush through the process without first sectioning their hair. They randomly grab and iron large sections, inevitably going over the same hair more than once. To avoid this, clip the top sections of your hair out of the way and start with the bottom layer. Iron one-inch sections, making sure you go over each section only once. When you are finished with the lower half of your hair, work your way through the top layers—again, one section at a time. If it feels as though you have to re-iron your sections to make them straight, they are probably too thick or you are going over them too quickly the first time around.

DIFFUSER TECHNIQUES

A diffuser can be a great time-saver for women who like to wear their hair naturally curly but cannot wait for hours to let it air dry. Many complain that a diffuser makes their hair frizzy, but that is usually a result of improper use. As with regular blow-drying, correct use is often a lesson in what *not* to do.

1. *Do not* keep the dryer on the highest heat setting. Adjust it to medium heat or alternate between medium and high.
2. *Do not* aggressively attack your hair with the diffuser or with your hands. This is meant to be a gentle way of drying.
3. *Do not* lean your head over and pile the hair right onto the hot diffuser. This will burn the ends and make them frizz. Instead, keep the attachment an inch away from your hair as you tilt your head back and let the curls pour into your hand.
4. *Do not* scrunch your hair while drying it (despite what you may have heard). This breaks the natural curl pattern. Think of caressing your curls, cupping the ends in your hand and gently pushing them toward the scalp in an accordion-like motion. Heat a section for a minute, then take the dryer away and let it cool in your hand. Remember, heat makes hair malleable and cooling it sets the shape.

HANDS-ON TRAINING
Get a Blow-dry Lesson from Your Hairstylist

You can learn a lot just by paying close attention to what your hairdresser is doing during your blow-dry. But if you are having a hard time getting the hang of styling your hair, you will benefit from an actual lesson. Ask your salon if it offers group blowout classes (some do), and if not, book an appointment with your hairstylist for a private lesson. It may cost a bit more than a blowout but is totally worth it. The stylist will walk you through the process step by step, then let you try it yourself. He or she will adjust your form and make sure that you are holding the brush and angling the blow-dryer properly, correcting any mistakes you might make. However, make sure that your stylist uses the correct form himself. Many don't. If you notice that he or she is doing things like smashing the blow-dryer into your hair, not only should you not take a lesson from that person, you should find a new stylist altogether.

AIR-DRYING TECHNIQUES

Being able to let your hair dry naturally (and have it look good) is a true test of its health and how well it is cut. Since you are not relying on the manipulation from heat and a brush, a strong and well-balanced hair shape will do most of the work for you. As the health of your hair improves, you will notice that air drying becomes a more feasible option. Someone with dehydrated, frizzy, and damaged hair is not likely to be happy without the aid of heat styling. However, if frizz is part of your natural texture, rather than a result of damage, there are still effective ways to create a polished look with air drying. Again, "natural" does not mean doing nothing—products and technique are very important.

Allowing naturally straight hair to air dry is not as easy as one may think. You still want volume in the root area and smoothness throughout the ends. A stronger styling product at the base and a few drops of shine serum on the ends will help compensate for the lack of heat styling. In addition, letting the hair dry on top of the head (held up with a clip) can prevent gravity from pulling it down and making it go flat. This is where the dreaded plastic butterfly clip can come in handy. If your hair is too short to be piled on top, apply the product combination recommended for longer hair, but comb the hair into place, the way you want it to set. In general, it is helpful to naturally dry your hair with some form. If you want it to dry smoother around your face, comb the hair straight down with the fine-tooth side of a comb. If you want it to dry off your face, comb everything back and away.

Molding naturally curly or wavy hair into place while air drying takes some skill. Since this happens to be my natural texture, I have perfected these techniques over the years. Keep in mind that when it comes to curly hair, every head is different, and what works for another may not necessarily work for you.

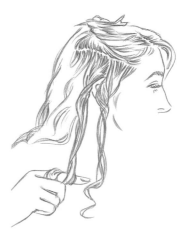

Twisting the hair to enhance its natural curl.

HAIR-TWIST METHOD FOR CURLY HAIR: Gently finger-comb the wet hair (using a wide-tooth comb can stretch some of the natural wave out of the hair). Apply foundation spray, then either a leave-in conditioner or a curl cream, and rake the products throughout your hair, using just your hands. Divide your hair into the usual four sections. Next, twist one-inch subsections, some toward your face and some back and away from it. If you prefer the hair around your face to be smoother (wavier rather than curly), take larger sections or smooth and clip against the head.

Duckbill clips or tiny butterfly clips are used as molding tools to hold or lift the hair and help produce volume at the top of the head and wherever else you need it. When your hair is about 80 percent dry, slip in one or two duckbill clips near the part, about an inch from the base. Leave them there until your hair is completely dry.

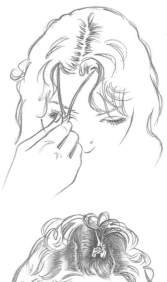

(Air drying can take hours, so, after molding the desired shape into your hair, you can take a diffuser to it or place a hooded or bonnet dryer over it to speed up the process.) Once the clipped hair has been released, you will have instant lift!

When your hair is completely dry and the clips have been removed, place your fingers at the scalp and shake the hair from the roots. You can even tilt your head forward to help release the curls. If some of the wave is too curly, you can relax it by using the warmth of your hands to gently stretch the hair (it will also fall a bit on its own). Just be careful not to completely break the curls apart and create frizz by raking your hands

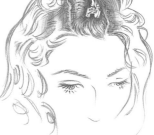

Using duckbill clips in the part to create volume and lift.

like combs through your dry hair. A broken curl is a frizzy curl, so don't ruin the shape and form you just created. You can carefully apply a couple of drops of shine serum to remove any halo of frizz that may have formed.

AIR DRYING LONGER HAIR: This method works best for longer lengths to create light, loose waves in the hair. Apply foundation spray and leave-in conditioner (if your hair has a natural wave) or some curl cream (if your hair is straight and you want to create more texture). Separate out two-inch sections around the hairline and blow-dry them smooth using a round brush. Smoothing the hair around the face will give you a more polished overall look. After these front sections are blown out, dry the rest of the hair 70 to 80 percent using the pre-drying method. Smooth the hair all over with a natural-bristle brush and secure it into a French twist. When you release the hair after it has air dried, it will be smoother and have a soft wave.

BUNS ARE NOT JUST FOR THE OVEN: Drying the hair wrapped in buns overnight can produce tousled waves while you sleep. Divide your hair into four sections when it is just slightly damp (leaving out the bangs if you have them). Twist each section into a doughnut-like bun and secure on your head with a pin. I must admit that it is a bit challenging to find a way to position the four buns so that you can sleep comfortably, but you will soon figure out the right placement. When you wake up in the morning and release the hair, it will "naturally" fall in beautiful, smooth waves.

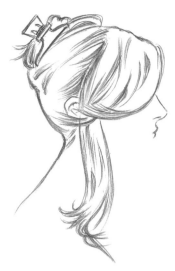

Air-drying longer hair: blow-drying the hairline and air-drying the back.

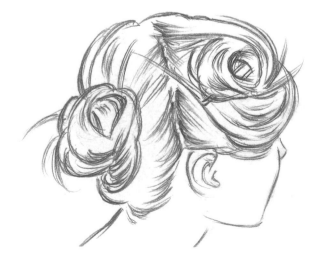

The bun technique. Loosely pin hair up and allow to dry. When dry, release the hair for soft, loose waves.

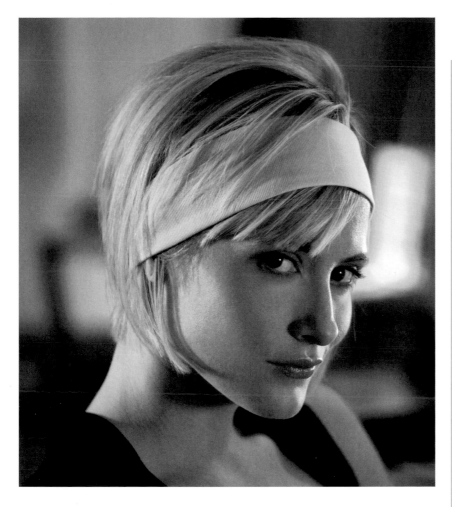

BEAUTY SECRET

Freshen your bangs when you wash your face

If your bangs seem to get oilier or feel dirtier than the rest of your hair, you can wash them separately when washing your face. You then have to restyle only that one section. Separate the bangs and pull the rest of the hair into a ponytail; wet the bang section and massage in a drop of shampoo; rinse it out well. This is particularly helpful for those who have oily skin or thick hair that is exhausting to blow-dry daily in its entirety.

Styling tips for wearing a hairband

A hairband can enhance the definition of a hairstyle, especially an up-sweep. It makes a ponytail or a bun instantly look fresh and modern. This stylish finishing touch is like dressing up a beautiful outfit with a scarf around your neck. When wearing a band with an updo, place it around your neck first, then style your hair before pulling up the band.

Wearing a hairband is also a chic styling option for women whose hair is too short to be pulled back. The trick is to keep the band closer to the face, near the hairline. This is a more contemporary way of wearing it and more flattering to the shape of the head, creating height at the crown. For a soft lift, tease a few sections using a brush, which gives everyone that sexy, girly look.

PROFESSIONAL TECHNIQUE

The sexy ponytail

All hairstyling requires technique, even a simple ponytail. It all goes back to details. A ponytail should not always be a last resort when you don't want to deal with your hair. When done with skill, it is a classic, polished style. The placement of a ponytail is a matter of personal preference. Some like it higher on the head, while others prefer it lower, close to the nape of the neck. Experiment with what is comfortable for you and which look you like best.

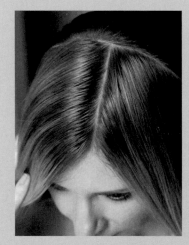

1. Part the hair from ear to ear, separating the front section from the back.

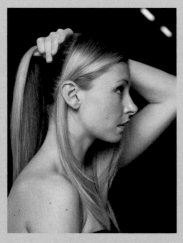

2. Gather the back section of the hair into a ponytail and secure it with an elastic band.

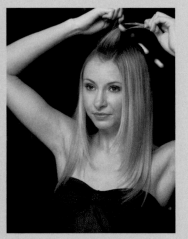

3. Take a Mohawk section and secure it with a duckbill clip.

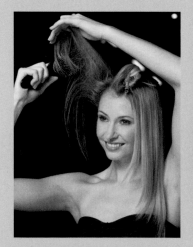

4. Gently tease each side of the hair.

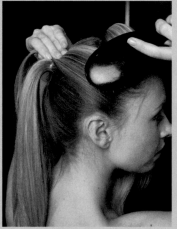

5. Brush one side section back and smooth it over top of the ponytail.

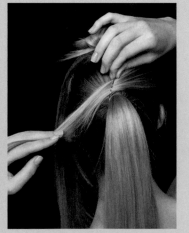

6. Secure it with a bobby pin just above the base of the ponytail.

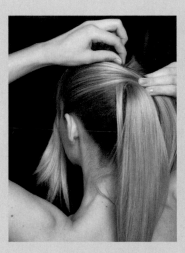

7. Repeat steps 4, 5, and 6 on the other side. The sections from the two sides should crisscross each other.

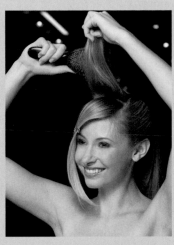

8. Tease the top section.

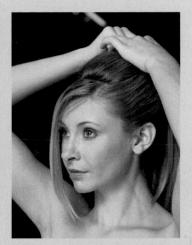

9. Smooth it, and pin it on top of the previously pinned sections (the bobby pin must be pointed straight down to stay hidden).

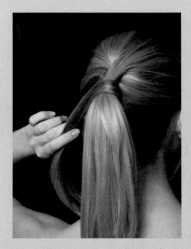

10. Take a half-inch section from the bottom of the ponytail and wind it around the base to hide the three sections you just pinned.

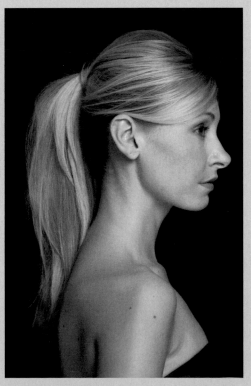

11. For the finishing touches: If you have side-swept bangs or shorter pieces in the front, you can leave them out for a softer look around the face. To make sure the baby hairs around your face lie flat, warm a tiny dab of pomade in your hands and use your fingertips to tamp down flyaways around the hairline.

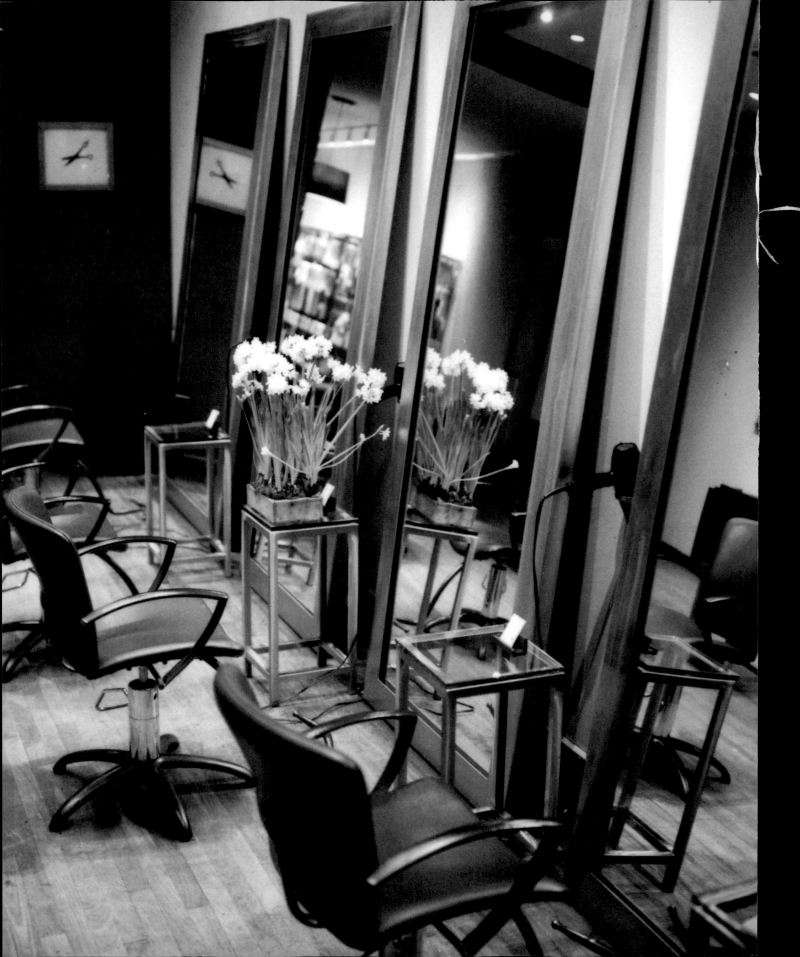

5
SALON CONFIDENTIAL

By lifting the veil that has long covered this industry, I will help you to get the most out of your salon experience and give you a better chance of having your expectations met. Despite the gossip, hearsay, and crazy reality shows, this information has not been presented to the public in a truthful and meaningful way. Therefore, I will share some of my insight and lessons I have learned to help you bridge the communication gap with the professionals.

This is a unique, exciting, and complicated business. I have had my own salon since I was in my early twenties, but it was not until I expanded my one-woman show into a larger enterprise that I truly understood the challenges that people face trying to find the right stylist while sifting through the gossip and the smoke and mirrors that are so prevalent in this industry.

Salons are filled with colorful, creative, and crazy characters who range from talented, interesting, and passionate to downright disturbing. While most choose this craft because they are inspired by beauty and the art of transformation and love to connect with people and make them happy, others do so mainly because they have artistic tendencies and don't fit into a professional environment. I have had every kind of personality work for me over the years, including those who inspired me with their

Personal Story

Having done this for so long, I still love nothing more than being in my salon, surrounded by my team and our clients. When I come to work each morning, I am greeted with smiles and questions—so many questions! I patiently answer them, whether they are about a color formula or a personal problem. I feel genuine warmth and generosity toward my staff and want them to be happy and successful. When I look around the salon, I also see smiling customers in all the chairs—it all goes hand in hand. I walk over to my stations where two clients are patiently waiting while my assistants comb out their hair and make sure that they are comfortable. Day in and day out, I come to this positive and bustling place. Sometimes it is as hard for me to believe as it is for others that it began nearly twenty years ago out of a fourth-floor walk-up apartment. Before, I was only an artist with an innate ability to connect with people. Today, I'm a craftsman, entrepreneur, mentor, and leader . . . learning more every day.

skill or a sincere desire to learn and helped motivate me to grow my company, and others who made me reflect wistfully on the simpler days in my cozy little three-chair salon.

So who becomes a hairdresser and how? What separates the best from the rest? Finding the right one for you comes down to three basic elements in addition to talent: good taste, the right education, and a professional attitude.

BASIC TRAINING . . . AND BEYOND

I am frequently asked to recommend a stylist in someone's hometown. However, usually I can do so only if there happens to be a stylist whose work I have seen personally (or who was recommended to me by someone I trust). The only way to evaluate a hairstylist is by his or her work. A cosmetology license is necessary but meaningless when it comes to one's skill, as is duration of one's experience. Anyone can get into beauty school and the bar for obtaining a cosmetology license is extremely low. There are no advanced degrees in this business (not counting training-seminar certificates), making it almost impossible to judge a stylist on his or her credentials.

I struggle to think of another industry that requires a practitioner's license where the differences in the quality of work can be so dramatic.

It is no secret that there are those who will completely butcher your hair, those who can positively change your life with their work, and everyone in between. The biggest mistake many young hairdressers make is going right from beauty school to taking clients as a practicing stylist or colorist with no real supervision or further training. It's a dangerous proposition for both the professional and the customer.

The real education comes *after* beauty school. Generally, schools focus on teaching subjects that are mandated by the state, such as theory, bacteriology, and anatomy. Since the stylist works so closely with the scalp, this basic safety knowledge is important, but it certainly does not make for a skilled hairstylist. Most of the practical education is built around basic roller sets, perms, and generic layered haircuts that were popular decades ago. Some schools teach more progressive techniques, but these schools are quite rare. Regardless of the school, however, there is only so much that a student can learn over the course of approximately eight months, which is what it takes to graduate, especially if much of that time is spent studying textbooks and practicing techniques on mannequin heads (that do not have opinions about their hair).

This is why going through an apprenticeship program at a reputable salon is critical for a stylist's future. Of course, there are exceptions, and some people have become good without ever apprenticing, but from my experience they are few and far between. It takes a great deal of dedication and initiative for a young stylist to learn this craft correctly on his or her own. Unfortunately, many learn to do things the wrong way, either by observing others who also lack training or simply by following the motions that feel comfortable and natural but often are incorrect. Once learned, and especially if practiced over the years, bad habits are very difficult to break.

There are advanced-training seminars available, and although this education can be invaluable, the amount of learning that takes place in the course of a few hours to a week is limited. More important, because attendance is discretionary, many stylists go through their entire careers without ever attending such training or having a strong mentor. Even some of those who do partake do not apply themselves to continue practicing what they just learned, eventually forgetting it. This is why you

BEAUTY SECRET

What's in a name?

Professionals in our industry are referred to interchangeably as "hairdressers" and "hairstylists." Is there a difference between the two? Back in the old days, a hairdresser's primary role was quite literally to dress up hair. They would create beautiful and complicated styles using rollers to direct and shape the hair (which is why rollers are still so popular in beauty schools). Women were not liberated from rollers and hooded dryers until the mid-twentieth century when Vidal Sassoon began to create different shapes and styles with the haircut itself. That is when the term hairstylist became mainstream.

cannot judge a stylist's skill solely by how long he or she has been doing hair. Although stylists usually regard their years of experience as a testament to their skill, those who never properly learned the technical aspect of this craft have simply become more accustomed to doing things wrong. I have seen plenty of young people with just one or two years of *proper* training who can run circles around such highly experienced stylists when it comes to haircutting, coloring, styling, professionalism, and attitude.

In the end, it's about a hairstylist's personal commitment to the craft and the integrity with which he or she treats it. Education must be a lifelong pursuit, and any stylist who stops learning inadvertently stops caring. No design is ever completely finished or is as good as it could possibly be—whether it's fashion, your home, or a haircut or color. There are always improvements that can be made, or adjustments that keep the design current. I have clients who have been coming to me for twenty years and are thrilled with their hair, but each time I try to do something a little better than the last. I know that perfection will never be achieved by any stylist. I am the harshest critic of my work and I plan to continue getting better until the day I stop doing hair.

I am happy to see that as our industry evolves, more dedicated and talented people choose this profession, and not for a lack of other opportunities. Many of the stylists who work for me went to beauty school *after* college. Others started with me at a very young age, as soon as they could legally hold a job. I hope that they all become the next generation of industry greats and never stop learning.

FINDING THE RIGHT STYLIST

I wish that I could give you the formula for finding the right stylist or colorist, but no such thing exists. However, there are ways to narrow your search, or maybe you will even get lucky on your first try. Unfortunately, the methods on which so many rely can be quite misleading. Many look for press mentions in beauty magazines about the latest and greatest associated with some celebrity's hair. Others scour through online reviews. But remember, until you have personally seen or experienced someone's work, it is nearly impossible to judge.

For this reason, the best way to find a good stylist is to approach someone whose hair you admire and is similar in texture to yours. She will most likely be flattered and only too happy to recommend her person. This is how many of my clients found out about me when I was first building my business, whether working out of my apartment or at a small, obscure salon with no walk-in traffic. I was consistently busy because my clients were like walking billboards. I did not start using a publicist until I opened my first full-service salon and had to build a clientele for an entire staff.

PERSONAL STORY

A salon owner's perspective

Finding the right stylists is even more important for salon owners because our businesses depend on it. When it comes to creating a great environment for the clients, nothing is as vital as having the right people on your team. In the beginning, I based the hiring process on what an individual brought in the way of skill or clients, but over time I learned to balance that with what someone might take away. One may be a very good hairdresser but not have the right personality or attitude, which will adversely affect everyone's experience. Such a person cannot possibly contribute enough financially to compensate for the damage. Maintaining a happy and healthy environment is my daily commitment. It is as critical an element as the quality of the work.

BEAUTY SECRET

Try out a potential haircutter with a blowout

If you would like to try a stylist without committing to a full haircut or color, schedule a blow-dry first. This is a terrific way to see how she works with your hair and how she listens. If you specify that you like your hair blown out with some body and bounce but leave with poker-straight, sleek hair, you might want to rethink this choice of stylist.

Keep in mind, however, that a recommendation is only a starting point, not a guarantee of success. Stylists can be very personable and charming, and women tend to get so caught up in loving their personalities that they sometimes overlook the quality of the work. Additionally, as in any relationship, the chemistry between the two of you is important. One person can have great chemistry with a hairstylist who may totally "get" her hair, while another's experience with the same stylist can turn out the opposite. In the end, there is no sure thing, so the goal is to improve your odds.

PICKING A SALON OR STYLIST
Most Frequently Asked Questions

Over the years, women from all walks of life have asked me about this business. They are curious about hairstylists and salons that they have read about in magazines and seen on television. Rumors and gossip spread like wildfire in this business, especially around prominent hairstylists. I have heard shockingly untrue stories about myself and have held some misperceptions about various industry peers based on rumors. When I finally meet them in person, however, I am often surprised to find that they are completely wonderful (maybe they are thinking the same thing about me!). It comes down to the fundamental lesson of not judging people until you meet them yourself. I hope my answers to some of these common questions help to make your decision process easier.

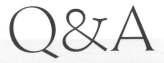

Q: *Are some hairstylists better at cutting than coloring, or vice versa? Do I need to find a different person for each?*

A: As opposed to specializing in a certain type of hair, cutting and coloring are very different skills and art forms, which is why most professionals are stronger at one than the other. Working as a colorist is very right brain and feminine, filled with subtleties and nuances. Although the chemistry behind formulating color is precise, what the colorist attempts to create is based largely on a feeling. Cutting hair is more left brain: structural, technical, and masculine, like architecture. In most salons, it is commonplace for hairstylists to cut and color hair, but one has to work very hard to do both equally well. Often the best work comes from a focus on one or the other.

When I was first starting out in this profession, I had to learn to do everything, since few hairdressers in the Midwest specialized at that time. That range of expertise gave me the invaluable ability to personally train my staff in all facets of beauty. These days it is common, especially in the larger cities, to find hair colorists who do not cut hair and stylists who don't do color. You will often see this kind of departmentalization at higher-end salons. This allows apprentices to focus and become proficient enough in one skill set to begin taking clients. Ultimately it depends on the talent of the professional and his or her ability to work in two different modalities.

Q: *I struggle with my naturally curly hair. Do I need a stylist who specializes in cutting this texture?*

A: Many women with curly hair believe that skillfully cutting it requires some elusive expertise that the average hairdresser may not possess. Understandably, this perception usually comes from frustration with bad haircuts and years of struggle with one's hair. Although cutting curly hair well does not require "special" expertise, it does require expertise at cutting hair whatever the type and texture. Each has its own challenges, and a good hairstylist can and should work with all of them equally well. Although the technical methodology may stay the same, cutting curly hair is different from cutting straight hair, just as cutting short hair is different from cutting long hair. Probably the most common mistake that stylists make with curly hair is pulling on each section too much and stretching it during the cut, only to find that the shape looks very different from what was intended when the curls bounce back. The "secret" to creating beautiful and accurate curls is to cut the hair with very little tension. Any experienced and skilled stylist should know this.

Even though some hairstylists feel particularly passionate about working with a certain type of hair, in most cases it should not be their entire repertoire. In addition, the majority of women enjoy wearing their hair in different ways—sometimes naturally curly and at other times blown out straight. Cutting the hair to be worn only straight or curly does not allow for such versatility. The term *curly hair specialist* is a label with which the media likes to brand certain stylists. Although such labels are limiting, they can also be great marketing gimmicks. People, in general, tend to pigeonhole artists as being good at only one thing: "Blondes are his thing" or "She's great with brunettes." I have personally witnessed this in women with long hair who felt that I would better "understand" their hair because my hair is long. However, I have always had just as many short-hair clients. The bottom line is that a hairdresser should specialize in doing great hair, not just one type of hair or haircut.

Q: *So many famous hairstylists are men. Do male stylists have a better perspective on how to make a woman's hair look beautiful?*

A: Historically, women have looked to men for validation, having more respect for their opinions than for those of other women. This was particularly telling in hairdressing. It took a man, gay or straight, to make a woman feel beautiful. Although times are changing, this attitude is still quite prevalent in our industry.

Another reason why men have traditionally been the ones in the limelight has much to do with the physical strength and stamina required to execute the job. This is a very artistic profession, but many do not realize that it is such a physical one as well. You are standing all day with your arms lifted: cutting, brushing, ironing, holding up a hot blow-dryer. It takes a tremendous amount of physical and mental fortitude to work in a salon and perform with a smile. You are onstage all day long and it is showtime every single hour when the next client arrives. A female hairdresser has to do the same taxing physical job as her male counterpart for anywhere from seven to ten hours a day, but usually in less comfortable shoes. I always recommend that the women I train in my salon (my salon is actually female dominant) go to the gym to increase their endurance and strength. I often say that I feel like an athlete in high heels!

Q: *Is it worth paying extra for an appointment with the salon owner?*

A: As with any stylist, the answer depends on the skill and attitude of the owner. Anyone can open a salon, but most salon owners take great pride in their business and the work that comes out of it. If the salon has a good reputation, it is usually for a reason. The owner sets the tone for every client's experience. Anyone working in my salon is a reflection of my brand and directly affects my reputation.

The owner is usually the primary teacher who has mentored many of the other stylists. This technical and artistic legacy helps to ensure quality and consistency. Any of the stylists hired or personally trained by me have my seal of approval. I know they are some of the best in the business and I am sure that other salon owners feel the same way about their staffs. As long as you choose a salon with the right type of owner, it is less important to see the owner herself. If she is out of your budget, make an appointment with another stylist at that salon who apprenticed under her.

Q: *Why is the hairdressing profession still looked down on by many?*

A: Unfortunately, bad behavior and drama are as much a part of the salon industry as cigarettes and gum. Although I cringe with embarrassment when watching salon-based reality shows, I know that there is much truth in these portrayals. It is sad to me that in this day and age of the sophisticated consumer, our industry has yet to move past the stereotypes that have plagued us for decades. Thankfully, many salon owners and stylists are becoming better businesspeople and are taking customer service and professionalism more seriously. There is no room for the arrogant attitudes that are still so prevalent in some salons, or the inappropriate clothing and unprofessional behavior. Remember that you are a paying client and no one is doing you a favor by working on your hair. So, if you go to a salon where the front desk staff is not friendly and accommodating, where stylists act as if your experience is about them and not you, or where you can see G-strings (or worse) peeking out above low-rise jeans and are forced to listen to loud conversations about the stylists' relationships, ailments, or other personal matters, my advice is—find a different salon. As long as you accept such behavior, it will go on.

Q: *Are celebrity hairstylists that much better than other stylists?*

A: The idea that a hairstylist has to work with celebrities to be considered great is unfortunate because there are so many talented professionals who are overlooked as a result. Hairstylists feel forced into this trap of having to claim celebrity clients to get press and build their business. I use the term *clients* loosely because the claims are often grossly abused. A common example is when a stylist works with a celebrity once on a photo shoot, a television show, or a movie. The stylist was probably hired by the production company or the publicist and could have just blown out the celebrity's hair or powdered her forehead. But suddenly the celebrity becomes this person's "client," whether or not they ever worked together again. Another example is someone famous walking into a salon for just a manicure, and immediately becoming a "client" of the salon. There have even been cases of celebrities serving salons with cease and desist orders to stop using their names for publicity.

It is a way of getting recognized in our celebrity-obsessed culture, but the fact that you need to have a celebrity name attached to yours to be considered a top stylist is unfair and sad. Without a celebrity to leverage, a talented hairstylist will have an extremely hard time getting his or her name in the pages of fashion magazines or finding an agent, no matter how beautiful the portfolio. (It is also why most celebrities do not even pay for salon services.) Generally, the media is interested in featuring only hairstylists who have celebrity clients because that is what readers find credible and is what sells magazines. As a result, even many of the best stylists become identified by their celebrity clients rather than establish an identity of their own. I have been featured in countless magazines and articles over the years, but until I became more prominent in the industry, the beauty editors' qualifying question was nearly always about my list of celebrities. If I had not had any to give them, it is highly doubtful that I would have been included in most of those articles. Likewise, numerous publications have wanted to include other hairstylists from my salon in articles or "best of" issues, but they rarely make the cut without one or two famous clients to offer.

To me, the true artists are in the salons, working hard every hour, doing transformative work on people from all walks of life—not just celebrities. There is nothing wrong with going to a hairstylist whose work you have admired in magazines, but it is more important to look at stylists' professional philosophy than their client list. You can be assured that there are many great hairstylists across the country who do not work with movie stars but who do beautiful work that you would be thrilled with, and who will appreciate you as a client that much more.

Q: *Are well-known salons mostly based on good PR?*

A: No, because you cannot buy success. It has to be earned. A great ad man once said that good advertising is the fastest way to kill a bad product. It means that by effectively promoting yourself or your company, you heighten expectations and create a perception of value that stimulates customer trials. If your product does not measure up, the customers will not return and negative word of mouth will spread, thereby destroying the product.

In our business, if you are in a big city and it seems that you have something special to offer, a good publicist can usually get beauty editors and maybe even celebrities into your chair. But these are the most fickle customers who can go to the best salons for free and see almost any stylist they want. Beauty editors, in particular, have usually been to most of the good ones. Unless they are truly impressed, they probably will not write about you, will never return, and will even tell other beauty editors (it's a small community, although they work for competing publications) not to waste their time or risk their hair. You have only one shot to impress them, especially in the beginning.

If you do manage to start getting magazine mentions, you also build higher expectations from the customers who read them. Maybe you have even raised your prices. If you do not impress these new clients as you did that editor, your fame will be short-lived. Assuming you have passed these first hurdles, your reputation may continue to grow along with customer expectations. You had better keep up and continue to improve and impress.

Q: *Are online reviews a good way to find a salon or stylist?*

A: Although the idea of online reviews seems logical (word of mouth en masse), the participation in and reliance on such websites have proliferated to the point of absurdity. What makes them so popular is the very thing that makes them misleading—anyone can post an anonymous review. That includes the salon's owners, employees and their friends, disgruntled former employees, and every other person with an opinion. It is the easiest and cheapest way to either promote or trash a business. Of course, many reviews are perfectly valid, but many are not. However, even with reviews that are not posted by impostors, you simply do not know the source or whether the claims are accurate. Perhaps the most onerous element of salon reviews is that they are usually based on an isolated experience with one stylist who may not be representative of the business and may even no longer be there.

THE FIVE GOLDEN RULES OF CLIENT ETIQUETTE

How to Be a Better Client and Get the Best Service at a Salon

The way to get the most accommodating treatment and assistance in a salon is not so much a trade secret as basic good manners. If you follow these five golden rules of thoughtful salon conduct, you will have a more positive salon experience and get a better haircut and color in the process.

1. BE ON TIME FOR YOUR APPOINTMENTS. IN FACT, SHOW UP EARLY.

You have learned the importance of dry cutting and finishing work. Try not to compromise that by being late. Busy stylists rarely have time to spare between appointments. By being even five or ten minutes late, you risk losing precious time at the end from the blow-dry or even the important dry cut. Unless the stylist is great at multitasking and has a few assistants to help take over (most do not), that time is going to come out of your appointment if there is another client directly behind you. (I actually tell clients who are notoriously late that their appointments are fifteen minutes earlier.)

COMMON MISTAKE

Choosing a stylist on the basis of looks and personality

Showmanship is such a big part of our industry that it can be difficult to see through the act. Sadly, some stylists are more concerned with being good performance artists than with doing good work. While theatrics can be fun to watch, they distract your and your stylist's attention from your hair, as does a lively conversation during the service. Remember that appearance, charm, and an air of grandeur cannot make up for a lack of skill. Unfortunately, many women easily become smitten and fall into this trap. Meanwhile, a far superior stylist who happens to be more serious, quiet, and focused on the work at hand is often overlooked. Although your experience should always be a pleasant one, do not forget why you are there. Focus on the stylist's expertise, education, and dedication to always giving you the best haircut or color possible. Don't be cajoled into choosing someone who will simply keep you entertained.

2. TRY NOT TO CANCEL AT THE LAST MINUTE.

If you have to cancel your appointment, call the salon twenty-four hours beforehand or at least first thing in the morning. Many salons will charge you the full amount of the service if you do not show up for an appointment and a portion of it if you cancel the same day. (Of course, emergencies do happen and the salon should be accommodating in such cases.) This strict policy might sound harsh, but it was put in place because some people chronically abuse the situation, which affects everyone. Late cancellations and especially "no shows" cause the stylist to become understandably frustrated and angry, since he or she could have booked another client for that time slot.

3. PREBOOK YOUR NEXT APPOINTMENT.

Prebooking the next appointment before you leave the salon helps you stay on plan with trims and especially color touch-ups, not to mention allowing you to reserve a time of your preference. It helps to ensure that your hair always looks its best and prevents a panicked plea of "Can you just squeeze me in?" once your roots are totally apparent and you realize that your colorist is booked for the next several days. The salon should call or email to remind you of your appointment so that you can reschedule if you need to.

4. DO NOT RUSH YOUR STYLIST.

It is a good idea to budget extra time for a scheduled service in case it takes longer than expected. Sometimes this happens, especially with color. If you rush your stylist because you have to pick up the kids, get to a meeting, catch a flight, or make a dinner reservation, you risk compromising the quality of her work (not to mention driving her crazy). If the stylist does not have enough time to do her job properly, you may unfairly judge her work on the basis of that experience, and/or have to spend more time by returning for a redo. This is especially important when you see a stylist for the first time or return to an old faithful after going to other salons.

5. BE GRACIOUS TO EVERYONE.

A salon experience should be pleasant for everyone involved, including the people who work there. There are clients who go out of their way

BEAUTY SECRET

Do not ask to be "squeezed in" to a stylist's booked schedule

There is no such thing as "fitting someone in." It really means cutting your service short, and possibly that of the people before and after you. When you plead for an emergency appointment, the salon will want to accommodate you, but this starts a domino effect that continues throughout the day. It creates unnecessary stress for the hairstylist, who is now running behind, which makes it more difficult for her to be at her creative best, so you are not getting the full service in terms of time and energy.

to be friendly and sweet to their hairstylists but take out their frustrations on the assistants or receptionists. Treat others as you want to be treated—the ultimate golden rule! You will have a much better time and get better service.

In addition, when it comes to scheduling, no salon can operate like a machine. We work with people and unexpected situations occur, sometimes affecting the exact time when your service begins. Perhaps the client before you was new to the salon and the haircut or color turned out to be more time-consuming than expected. Or maybe she did not read rule number one and was late.

At a well-run salon, the front desk will call the client if her stylist is running late, but it is not always possible to foresee this. However, if you go to a salon where this happens too frequently, I can certainly understand the frustration. You should discuss this with the manager, and you can always call prior to the appointment to see if your stylist is running on schedule.

EXPRESS YOURSELF

How to Communicate Better, Set Boundaries, Complain Effectively, and Have a Successful Relationship with Your Hairstylist

The salon environment and the relationship a woman has with her hairstylist are fascinating—they both straddle the line between personal and professional. Psychologically, it has been shown that we maintain a three-foot boundary of personal space around us to feel safe. Our families and others with whom we have intimate relationships are the only ones we comfortably allow into that space. The moment someone uninvited crosses the line, you feel that the person is too close for comfort. Your hairstylist becomes one of the chosen few who have your permission to enter that space, to touch you and groom you. This is why people feel a false sense of intimacy with their hairstylists and why personal subjects and secrets are discussed too freely in salons. Women share confidences with us that they would tell only their best friends (I often learn that a client is pregnant before her family does!). I think another reason why it happens is that this unique relationship has a safe sense of disconnection. Think about it: much of the time you are looking at and talking to the stylist in a mirror, even though he or she is right next to you. Do you have any other conversations in this odd manner? It is almost as if you are not talking to a real person, and when the appointment is over you can walk away from it as if the conversation had never taken place.

Although it can be so easy to tell us anything as we work on your hair, it is also wise to remember that you are the client paying for a service at a business and your needs have to be met. For this reason, you should set some boundaries. Becoming too close with your hairstylist can spoil the safe intimacy between you. The stylist may feel guilty if she cannot squeeze you (or your friend) into the schedule, or you may be afraid to hurt the stylist's feelings by expressing dissatisfaction with her work. It is hard to say that you don't like something about your

BEAUTY SECRET

The strategy for silencing a chatty hairdresser

Trust me—clients are not the only ones interested in having a social session at a salon. There are plenty of chatty hairstylists who are too busy gabbing to give you a precise haircut. Don't let that go on. A good way to get them to focus is to open a book or a magazine, or get out your BlackBerry or iPhone (as long as you are typing, not talking!). You should sit up straight with your legs uncrossed to be in a balanced position. Tell the hairdresser that you have to get some work done or that you are just going to relax and read. He or she will get the hint. You can always add, "Just let me know when you want me to put my head up."

cut or color when it feels that the person working on it is your good friend. Everyone will be happier if both the client and the professional can separate their feelings from the actual service. If the relationship is kept on a business level, albeit a friendly and personal one, the lines of communication can remain open.

Another reason not to become best buddies with your hairstylist is that you may actually get second-rate service because the stylist is more focused on chatting with you than on your hair. He or she may also feel too comfortable and confident in knowing that you will be happy or will forgive mistakes, and not focus enough or not try to improve on the work with each visit. The emphasis must be kept on the job at hand. Cutting the hair with precision or coloring it with accuracy requires concentration. Too much chair talk can be distracting. Imagine trying to work on your computer while having a full-blown conversation with someone who is telling you all about her day or her marriage. Obviously, you would make typos. To get the best, most attentive work from your hairdresser, I recommend that you not talk while he or she is working, or at least for the first half hour of the cut. Forming a relationship is important, but it is best not done while cutting. Talk during the consultation, or even during a single-process color or a blowout, when the stylist's actions are more mechanical and demand less concentration.

Speaking of not speaking, please be considerate and turn off the ringer on your phone, and try not to talk on it during your service. Besides being annoying, talking on the phone causes your head to shift and move and can throw off the accuracy of the haircut (as can chewing gum).

HOW TO COMPLAIN EFFECTIVELY AND DIPLOMATICALLY

I am continually surprised by how scared most women are (perhaps due to their fear of confrontation) to share directly with their stylist or the salon owner that they are unhappy with their hair. Many people avoid this conversation at any cost and would rather walk away from the hairstylist and the salon forever than address an issue head-on. This causes everyone to lose out in the end. Good communication is even more important when you hit a bump in the road.

Unfortunately, many creative people are insecure and misperceive a complaint about their work as a personal attack. They react by making the client feel uncomfortable or intimidated. This is a huge mistake that too many professionals make. Not voicing your unhappiness actually does a disservice to your hairdresser, who is then not given the opportunity to fix the problem or to learn and grow from it. To be successful, stylists must focus on their weaknesses, not just on the things they do well. But too often hairstylists reach an acceptable level of proficiency within a narrow range of haircuts or color and stagnate. Meanwhile, their clients are too concerned about hurting their feelings to say anything.

As with all relationships in our lives, the most effective way to deal with a problem is to speak directly, clearly, and calmly to the other person. If you are unhappy with your cut or color, express how you feel directly to your stylist (face-to-face, not in the mirror). When you tell him or her exactly what you do not like about it, a solution can usually be found right away. Often, just a subtle alteration can fix the whole problem. If you realize later, when you get home, that you do not like something, call the salon and schedule an appointment to return for an adjustment. Say something like, "I would like my color to be more this way or my haircut more that way." If this is done politely and discreetly, you should not have to worry about hurting that stylist's reputation or feelings. Of course, if you absolutely hate your hair and are afraid to return to the same person, you should ask to speak with the manager or owner and request a different stylist who may be more adept at working with your hair. Remember that hair is very personal and subjective. This happens from time to time at all salons, so never think that you are being "difficult" when politely expressing your dissatisfaction.

The least effective recourse is to later become outraged, call the salon, and complain to the receptionist. She simply may not know how to handle the problem effectively, and it can be embarrassing for your stylist. I completely understand the desire to take your anger out on someone. Hair is a highly emotional issue: you are disappointed and have had your expectations dashed. Speaking directly to the stylist will usually help to resolve the crisis easily and harmlessly.

Role-Play: Communicating Your Distress the Right and Wrong Ways

You are the client paying for the service, so your feelings about the color and cut are more important than ours. But remember that every artist has a fragile ego and your complaints have a better chance of being heard if they are conveyed diplomatically. It is all in the delivery. The following two role-playing examples might help if you find yourself in a sticky salon situation. You have learned many cutting and coloring terms in this book, and now you can use that professional language to communicate more effectively with your stylist. My best advice: remain calm and always start any complaint with a compliment.

DON'T DO THIS:

Client: "My hair looks like I cut it myself with a pair of kitchen scissors!"

INSTEAD, DO THIS:

Client: "I like the cut, but it feels too choppy. I'm not sure it fits my personality. I'd like something a little bit cleaner and more classic."

DON'T DO THIS:

Client: "I hate this color. This blond is so fake, I look like a stripper!"

INSTEAD, DO THIS:

Show the colorist a photo of the color you wanted and then say:
Client: "This is the blond that I was going for, something buttery and warmer. This is pretty, but I feel that it's too light for me. I want a more sophisticated color. I wonder if this could be taken down a notch with some lowlights or a glaze?"

Divorcing Your Stylist—Guilt-free

Divorce not only occurs in one's personal life but can happen between you and your stylist and often for exactly the same reasons: lack of communication and growing apart as your needs change. In fact, some of the most common questions I am asked have to do with changing stylists. Often, a breakup is caused not by one particular situation but by an over-

COMMON MISTAKE

Expecting your hairdresser to bat a thousand

If you have been going to one stylist for a while to maintain the same haircut, you may believe that it is simple for him or her to re-create that look each time. However, it actually takes the same amount of concentration and focus as the first time (or at least it should). Just as a painter cannot create two identical paintings, each haircut is always slightly different from the last, even if you don't notice it. Therefore, if your hairstylist has always given you great cuts in the past and messed up once, it is likely that he or she will go back to doing a great job once you explain the problem. You may simply have caught the stylist on a bad day.

Bullies are not just on the playgrounds

An unfortunate part of our industry is the beauty bullies who make their clients feel intimidated, insecure, and terrified to see another stylist. I often witness this fear in women who confide in me that they are not really happy with their haircut and/or color but could not imagine going elsewhere because they have been seeing their stylist for so long. They're afraid of how he or she would treat them and make them feel as a result. This big mistake, which too many stylists make, most likely stems from insecurity in their work and ability to retain clients. If you see a stylist who makes you feel this way, make no mistake: you are in an abusive relationship. Fortunately, it is one that you can walk away from at any time. The other type of beauty bully is one who does not come across like a bully at all but keeps you hostage through the "tyranny of weakness." This stylist is just so darn nice and sweet that you can't bear the guilt of hurting his or her feelings by going to someone else. Regardless of which scenario you may find yourself in, make decisions based on your needs and not those of your stylist.

all sense that you and your stylist no longer share the same aesthetic, or that you simply want what is outside his or her expertise. This hairdresser may not be bad, but is no longer the right match for you. Whether trying a different stylist in the same salon or leaving an old faithful for greener pastures, it pays to remember that you are not in a committed relationship with your hairdresser. But because this is an intimate business relationship, it can feel as though there is an awkward personal separation.

Try to keep it in perspective. As a paying customer, you should be satisfied with the service. If you love your salon but have fallen out of love with your stylist and want to try someone new there, it is your right as a client. One approach is to be brave and have that conversation directly with the

PERSONAL STORY

Many women consider their time at the salon to be not only beautifying, but therapeutic and healing. A few years ago, a regular client arrived at my salon in an ambulance! Although a bit groggy, she generally seemed okay, so I inquired about her unusual means of transportation. She explained that earlier in the day she had had a low-blood-sugar attack and fainted in the subway station. After spending several hours in the hospital, she was released and the ambulance was supposed to take her home. Not wanting to miss her four o'clock hair appointment, she requested to be dropped off at the salon instead. "I just told the paramedics that I'll be better taken care of at my salon than at home—that I can have some tea and biscuits, get a nice scalp massage, and just relax," she told me. Despite hospital rules requiring that patients be dropped off only at home, the paramedics gave in to her persistence. She had a lovely couple of hours at the salon, after which I asked one of our assistants to walk her home. This heartwarming scenario made me proud that our clients felt this way about our salon environment.

stylist you currently see. You can say something like, "You have been wonderful and I so appreciate your taking extra time with me, but I feel we are misunderstanding each other. Is there someone else at the salon who you think would get the challenges I'm having with my hair?" (Your hairstylist might actually be thinking the exact same thing and be relieved to suggest another person. We know each other's work so well, and can usually recommend someone else who may be perfect for you. It's a horrible feeling to realize that you are just not able to make a client happy, and no one wants to remain in such a relationship.) You can also speak about this with the owner or the salon manager. This acknowledgment and honesty are so much better for everyone involved than if you walk out frustrated, never to return. Finally, keep in mind that switching stylists probably makes you feel much more uncomfortable than it does your former stylist, who most likely has many clients and may not really care that you are in someone else's chair. Things move very quickly in a salon and are therefore quickly forgotten.

The other scenario that women wrestle with is leaving a longtime stylist for a different salon. I know women who dodge and hide from former stylists years after they have stopped going to them. Seriously, they avoid eye contact by pretending not to see them, hide behind cars, or quickly turn into a store if they spot them on the street. They are afraid to run into them because they never explained why they left the relationship. You can separate on good terms by sending a simple note to say good-bye and thank you. Thanking a hairstylist for years of creativity and service will not only leave the door open if you decide to come back, it will eliminate all that guilt and awkwardness when you run into this person. I treat my clients as true customers who can come into and out of my salon at any time they want, no questions asked. I have had clients leave because they just wanted a change and then return a few years later. A true professional will not harbor resentment toward former clients. On the contrary, a client who decides to move on should be made to feel that she would be welcomed back at any time.

GRATITUDE

Writing this chapter has been a particularly gratifying and personal experience for me. However difficult or painful some of my experiences in this business may have been, I have learned to feel gratitude for them. Without them I would not be who I am today, or be in a position to reach others through this book. Gratitude is what turns lemons into lemonade and makes the good times even sweeter. If my stylists complain about being exhausted because they had such a busy day, or about having to stay late to accommodate a client, I tell them to feel gratitude rather than resentment that they are in such demand. It can be the difference between feeling happy or miserable about the same situation—tired or elated.

In this business and particularly in my role, I feel special gratitude for having a unique opportunity to touch and influence people's lives. I am so grateful for all the cards and emails that I have received over the years from clients telling me of the impact that my work has had not only on their appearance but on their self-esteem and even on their relationships, or from listeners of my radio show who have been able to improve their overall well-being by following my advice. But I'm especially inspired and moved when I affect young people, or people who are close to me, sometimes without even realizing it.

A few years back, a particular client would bring her two daughters along when she came to me for haircuts. The girls were about fifteen and sixteen at the time. I thought it was cute how intently both of them watched me cut their mother's hair, although they never got haircuts themselves. Not long ago, two sisters came to my salon to interview for assistant positions. They were around nineteen or twenty, had just graduated from beauty school, and were so excited to get started. Since I needed only one additional assistant at the time, I hired one of them but did not make the connection until a month or two later when she shared with me how I had inspired her and her sister to choose this profession when they watched me cut their mother's hair.

Just recently, one of my colorists shared another personal story. Having recently moved here from another country, she started working for me as an assistant when I first expanded to my larger salon in 2003. This was a second career for her and she passionately wanted to become a great colorist. In the beginning, it was difficult for her to learn a new language, not to mention all the intricacies of hair color. One day, her five-year-old daughter asked me, "Is my mom a good colorist?" I smiled and replied, "Of course, she will be one of the best!"

Seven years later, through perseverance and dedication, she has in fact become one of the best and busiest colorists in New York City. In her earlier years, whenever she came home distressed from a difficult day or a challenging color situation, her daughter would remind her, "Eva said that you're one of the best colorists there is!" (It was the way she remembered my comment.) I realized how I had unwittingly made a little girl believe in her mother, and how the girl in turn helped her mother to believe in herself, making an instinctive remark to a five-year-old a self-fulfilling prophecy.

BEAUTY SECRET

Salons are the "golf courses" for women

In a man's world, golf courses are not just for sport; they are where relationships are built and business is done. For women, that place is the salon. I cannot begin to count how many fruitful introductions I have purposely or inadvertently made in my salon. I will often sit clients next to each other and introduce them if I know that there is business synergy between them (I may also do it if I just think that they will hit it off and become friends). Many business deals have actualized as a result—from someone getting a nanny referral or being hired for a job to real estate and fine-arts transactions. The salon is a woman's world and we should make the most of it!

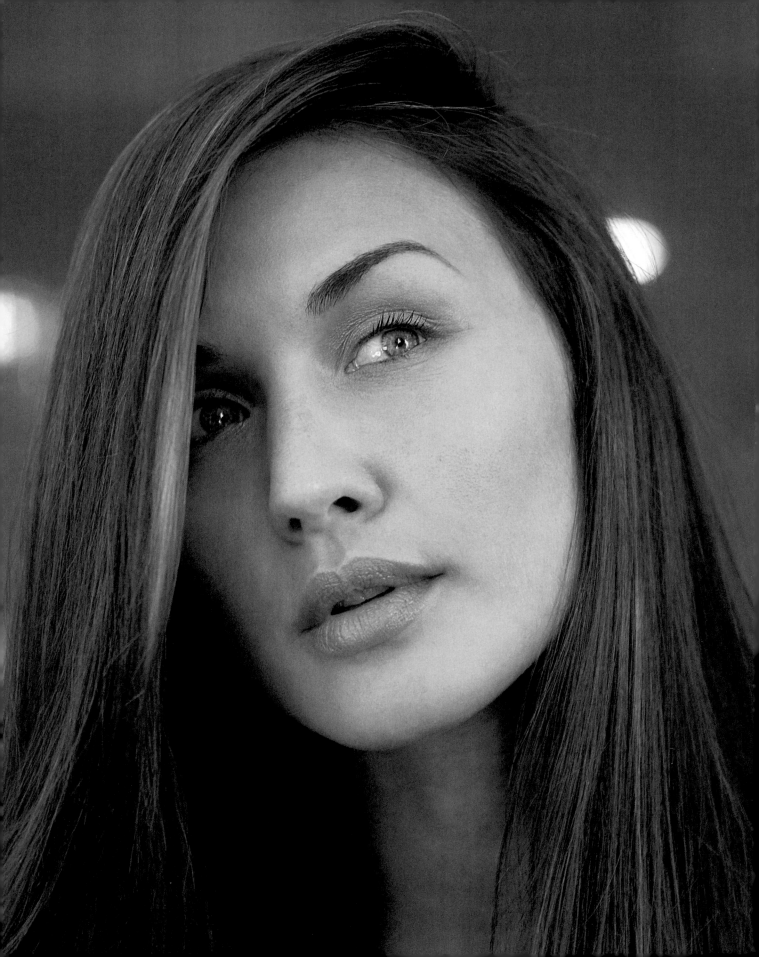

6

SKIN CARE

As a makeup artist, I have to be an expert on skin care, which also happens to be a great interest of mine. Over the past twenty years, I have studied this subject and have experimented both on myself and on my clients. A woman's skin is her canvas and makeup is the art. You have more control than you may think over how your skin looks. With the right products and home-care routine, facials, and dermatology, along with proper nutrition and lifestyle, a radiant complexion is within the reach of nearly every woman. But no one thing can make your skin beautiful and I am sure that you intuitively realize that its appearance is largely a reflection of your health. For example, you may have noticed how much better your skin looks after you've been exercising and how dull and pallid it is when you have not had enough sleep or have been sick.

When a body is out of balance, the symptoms can show up in the form of acne, fine lines, loss of color, inflammation, and excessive redness. Skin is the largest organ in the body, as well as the largest instrument of absorption and elimination. Therefore, it mirrors what is happening on the inside. You have to take a whole-body approach to caring for your face and a holistic attitude toward skin care in general. Receiving all your advice from a single expert, be it an aesthetician or a dermatologist, limits your scope of knowledge and the benefits you could receive from other resources. Many people also focus on just one avenue of skin care and neglect others: they buy firming creams but neglect diet; try countless acne medications but never see a dermatologist; or use a prescription medication for a skin condition without researching the underlying cause that may be triggering it, such as a hormonal imbalance or an allergy. The key is to take a closer look at your daily routine and realize that everything you do has an impact on your skin.

The adjective *anti-aging* is slapped onto countless products and is overused in magazine articles and books about skin care, diet, exercise, fashion, and beauty. It is a catchy term and one that is obviously marketable. It has become ingrained in our society that getting older is a bad thing—that youth is beautiful and aging is to be resisted at all costs. Perhaps our culture's anti-aging obsession stems from the fundamental fact that aging is scary. Looking in the mirror is a daily reminder of our mortality and of time passing. Admittedly, this can be jarring, so we try to fight it or deny it completely. But I believe that the objective should be to look your best at every stage of your life, as opposed to trying to look the way you did twenty years ago. My skin does not look as it did in my twenties, but that does not mean it looks bad. We have to stop thinking that the natural changes in our faces are negative or that we are powerless over them. Aging gracefully does not mean giving up on how you look. It is much more liberating to accept the aging process and the subtle shifts that occur in our faces, bodies, and skin, while realizing that we can take care of ourselves and improve our appearance along the way.

The media loves to categorize women by chronological age to define their skin care routines, as well as how they should dress and wear their hair and makeup. "This is what you should do in your thirties, your forties, your fifties," and so on. This is true only to an extent. One's complexion does change over time, and the planes of the face shift gradually with the pull of gravity and the loss of collagen and fat. But this does *not* mean you should be resigned to looking "old" at a certain age. I have read countless magazine articles and books that state that a woman should look a certain way when she approaches forty, but I don't resemble that stereotype. Despite having gone through intense stress during certain periods in my life, I do not see obvious signs of aging, because I have taken care of my skin and my health (I also started using my mother's eye cream when I was only thirteen). I have seen women in their forties who look as though they are in their early thirties because they have been conscientious about their skin care and overall health. I have also seen women in their thirties with sun spots and crow's-feet starting to form because they have not.

My mother has had a beautiful complexion for as long as I remember, but it is due to her disciplined skin care regimen. She suffered from acne as a teenager, so she took incredible care of her skin as an adult. On the other hand, *her* mother had naturally flawless skin but never took care of it. Her skin aged prematurely as she got older. My mother enjoyed the daily and nightly ritual of skin care. She would bring a basket of products into the living room and sit in front of the TV at night while she removed her makeup, applied toner, and put on different creams and lotions. She passed this lovely ritual, this practice of taking care of herself, down to me and my sister. Beauty is a legacy my mother gave to me, and the lessons she taught me about caring for my skin are gifts that I continue to give to myself on a daily basis.

I believe that our image of "old age" is actually what results from a lifetime of neglect, as opposed to an inevitable fate for which we are all destined. Although everyone's face will change and lose some firmness, we do not have to lose the clarity, color, and smoothness of the skin. The good news is that even if you have neglected to take care of your skin up to this point, you still have the power to change it for the better, starting now.

There is an overwhelming amount of information available about skin care. This chapter sums up what I have learned over the years from my research and practical experience, as well as from many experts in both the beauty industry and the medical field. This is what works for me, for my family, and for my clients. Because I have the unique privilege of seeing my clients on a very regular basis, usually every four to eight weeks, I am able to observe the difference in a woman's complexion after she embarks on a new skin care regimen or to see if a particular product is effective. I hope the information in this chapter empowers and motivates you to begin, or continue on, your own path toward better skin care and a more proactive approach to your complexion and health.

BEAUTY SECRET

YOUR SKIN CARE STRATEGY
Night and Day Routines

Prevention is the most effective way to care for your skin. Therefore, the sooner you learn good habits, the better your skin will look throughout your life. No matter what kind of skin you have now—whether it is dry or oily, red and/or sensitive, losing its elasticity or breaking out—a diligent, smart skin care regimen will improve it. The following nighttime and daytime routines are ones that I try to follow. We all have those nights when we get home late, exhausted, and are barely able to remove our makeup. In a perfect world, I would complete each step nightly, get eight hours of sleep, exercise daily, and eat a well-balanced diet. Be realistic and try to do your best. Being as conscientious and consistent as possible can lead to amazing results.

NIGHTTIME ROUTINE

Step One: Cleanse

Cleansing makeup, oil, dirt, and perspiration from your face at the end of the day should be a two-step process:

1. Remove makeup with a cream-based cleanser. I like to use a non-comedogenic cream cleanser, which will not clog the pores, so even someone with oily or acneic skin can comfortably use it. Massage the cleanser onto dry skin with your fingertips, then continue with gentle circular motions, using a damp cotton pad (made of 100 percent organic cotton) instead of a washcloth. Cotton is an amazing and gentle exfoliant that can replace an abrasive scrub. This is especially good for those with rosacea or sensitive skin who may find most exfoliants irritating. It is also more hygienic, since you throw away the cotton when you are done (unlike a washcloth, which can harbor bacteria unless immediately laundered).

2. After rinsing off the creamy cleanser, wash your face again with a foaming cleanser. Your skin will be radiant and clean after following this two-step process.

Step Two: Tone

Now that you have thoroughly cleansed your skin and exfoliated it with a cotton pad, apply an alcohol-free toner to soothe and hydrate. Many dermatologists consider toner a superfluous product, but I believe it is an integral step. Toner helps to calm the skin after cleansing, which can reduce inflammation and redness caused by general skin sensitivity. Look for a toner that contains essential oils such as lavender, rosemary, geranium, or rose, which also calm, heal, and hydrate. Essential oils can actually penetrate the skin, making toners more effective. Toner can be sprayed on, applied with a cotton pad, or blended over the face and neck with your fingers.

Step Three: Nourish

Think of serums as topical vitamins for the skin. They are the concentrated ingredients found in most creams and lotions and are beneficial for all types of skin. Some hydrate dry skin with humectants like hyaluronic acid, while others brighten the complexion and help to prevent or correct environmental damage with antioxidants such as vitamins C and E. Serums made for acneic skin contain antibacterial, antiseptic, and anti-inflammatory ingredients that calm redness and help to prevent clogged pores. Use one to two pumps or six to eight drops of serum for your face and neck.

BEAUTY SECRET

Applying toner over makeup

I love to mist a spray-on toner over my face throughout the day. This is great for rehydrating the skin and refreshing the makeup midday, since the fine mist will not disturb it. The subtle moisture allows you to lightly blend and touch up concealer or foundation that has settled in the creases around your eyes and laugh lines.

Common Mistake

Relying on a foaming facial wash to remove cosmetics

Most women completely bypass the important first step of removing makeup with a cream-based cleanser. (Unless you are using 100 percent water-based makeup, there is some amount of oil in all cosmetics, even in powder.) Oil and water don't mix, so lathering your face for a few seconds with a soapy product literally is not going to cut it. Have you noticed that when you swipe a cotton pad with toner over your skin right after washing it, the pad looks dirty? That is the residue of makeup and oil that your facial wash did not remove. (Toners became very popular for this very reason—they help remove the makeup that foaming cleansers cannot.) Because oil breaks down oil, the most effective way to emulsify makeup is with an oil or cream. Think of this first step as breaking down the product that clogs pores and leads to blemishes. For many women still struggling with breakouts in their thirties and forties, this could be the culprit. When they start using this method of makeup removal, their skin begins to clear up.

CHECKLIST

P.M. routine

- Remove makeup with a cream-based cleanser.
- Wash the face with a foaming cleanser.
- Calm skin with toner.
- Nourish with a serum.
- Moisturize with a lotion or cream, including eye cream.

If you line up your products next to one another, you can do this routine in less than three minutes.

Step Four: Moisturize

A moisturizing cream or lotion utilizes emollients—agents that seal moisture in the skin and create a protective barrier—and lightweight humectants, which attract water to the skin. A commonsense approach is best: if the skin feels dry, use a richer cream that contains ingredients such as squalene, coconut, shea butter, or jojoba oil. For normal skin that may become oily in the T-zone (forehead, nose, and chin), choose a moisturizer with lighter humectant properties such as hyaluronic acid and glycerin. If your skin is oily, try using an oil-free moisturizer. If that still feels too heavy, try using just a serum, which may sufficiently hydrate. You also don't have to put moisturizer all over your face. For example, if the skin on your forehead or chin tends to break out, you can avoid those areas.

Eye Cream

The skin around the eyes is thinner, more delicate, and has fewer oil glands than the rest of the face. As a result, this area can become more easily dehydrated and prematurely wrinkled. Although many women do not use eye cream, to me this is an essential part of moisturizing. At night, I like to use an eye cream that is more emollient and contains a mild over-the-counter retinoid. Apply it just in the circular dip around the eye, above the cheekbone, and under the eyebrows. It will migrate, so there is no need to have it too close to the lash line. Some women find that eye cream irritates their eyes, which is probably because they are applying it too close (and which can also cause puffiness in the morning). If your eyelids are naturally oily, it may not be necessary to apply eye cream to them.

GENTLE RESURFACING

While manual exfoliation (such as facial scrubs or cleansing with cotton pads) helps to get rid of dead skin cells that dull your complexion, there are numerous products that take this a step further to improve the texture of your skin. By removing the surface layer, they also enable nourishing and moisturizing ingredients to penetrate better. There are many exfoliating agents: alpha-hydroxy acids such as glycolic acid (best for reducing the appearance of fine lines) and beta-hydroxy acids such as salicylic acid (best for acneic skin). Natural fruit enzymes like those found in pumpkin and papaya also make effective peels. Retinoid creams not only exfoliate the skin but encourage collagen production and cell turnover, which slow down with age.

Retinoid Creams

A prescription retinoid (a derivative of vitamin A) can be very effective in making your skin smoother and clearer. It helps heal and prevent acne and minimize fine lines. But remember that this is a prescription medication. Women often use a retinoid cream incorrectly, applying too much, as if it were a moisturizer. Just a pea-size amount is sufficient for the entire face.

It is most effective when applied to clean skin, and it is normal for the skin to feel a bit dry after application. You can add a moisturizer or a few drops of serum on top, but first allow twenty to thirty minutes for the retinoid to absorb into the skin.

One more word of caution: begin with a low-dose formulation when starting to use a retinoid cream. Some have to build up a tolerance for it, and it may even be wise to wait two to three days between applications. Many enthusiastically start applying a retinoid every night, only to find that it is too aggressive for their skin. They assume that the product is just too harsh for them and discontinue using it. You have to build up a tolerance for it and start slowly. Although a retinoid does not have to be applied daily, for some people such frequent use works well. I personally use it every other night. Those with sensitive skin can get wonderful benefits without irritation by applying it just twice a week.

Q&A

Q: *What is the difference between natural botanical extracts and essential oils?*

A: Serums frequently contain either botanical extracts or essential oils. These two terms are often used interchangeably, but there are distinctions between them. *Essential oils* get their name from embodying the distinctive properties and fragrance of aromatic plants or flowers. They are produced through a steam-distillation process, and typically only a few drops of essential oil are harvested from pounds of raw plants. Rosemary, lavender, peppermint, and eucalyptus are common examples. *Botanical extracts* also come from plants. They are not distilled like essential oils but are left in their natural state. These botanicals have powerful medicinal properties for calming and healing the skin and are often added to skin care formulations for their antioxidants. Examples are green tea and echinacea.

Q: *Will essential oils cause breakouts?*

A: This assumption may understandably stem from the word *oil*. An essential oil is not a heavy, greasy substance; it is a highly concentrated liquid essence distilled from a plant. Essential oils do not clog the pores. In fact, lavender and tea-tree oil are two of the best antibacterial agents for acneic skin. Essential oil molecules are small enough to penetrate the pores without obstructing them. The extracts are very potent and can be too strong if applied directly to the skin, which is why they are combined with other ingredients within a serum or a moisturizer. This base formulation also acts as "carrier" to allow the oil, with its healing properties, to be used without causing irritation. Many essential oils for daily moisturizing of the body or therapeutic massage are blended in a primary base of carrier oil such as jojoba, sunflower, or avocado. Products that clog the pores usually contain mineral oil, not essential oil.

Q&A

Q: *Do I need a separate moisturizer for my neck?*

A: Even if your face is normal to oily, your neck most likely is not. Therefore, you will need to use something more emollient. Keep in mind that the skin on the neck is thinner and has fewer oil glands (much like the delicate skin under the eyes), which is probably why these two areas are the first to display fine lines and wrinkles. Even when a woman's face looks great, her neck can be a sign of her real age (along with her hands). Overlooking these areas when it comes to moisturizing and protecting the skin surely contributes to the effects of aging. Treat your neck and décolletage as part of your face when cleansing, toning, applying serum, moisturizing, and protecting with sunblock. I never fail to apply the same moisturizing serum that I use on my face, along with a neck cream (that is richer than the one I use on my face), to my neck and upper chest. You can use a retinoid cream here as well, but be aware that the skin is more sensitive.

DAYTIME ROUTINE

Step One: Rinse

Unless your skin is oily, there is no need to wash your face in the morning. Skipping the cleansing step helps to maintain the moisture balance in the skin—especially important if it tends to be dry. (If you have oily skin or simply feel better washing it with a gentle foaming cleanser in the morning, then by all means do so.) Splashing tepid or cool water over the face (approximately twenty splashes) is fabulous for the skin and a refreshing way to wake it up. This splashing technique is essentially hydrotherapy, which invigorates the face and improves the color and clarity of the skin. It is a simple therapeutic treatment that dates back centuries and has been an integral part of the European spa tradition, which is based on the curative benefits of water.

Step Two: Tone

This awakens and lightly hydrates the skin. It is also refreshing and gives a light cleansing if you gently wipe your entire face and neck with toner on a cotton pad.

BEAUTY SECRETS

How to store skin care products

Many skin care products contain preservatives that give them a longer shelf life. Even so, after a year or two, or if a product starts to smell different, it is time to toss it out. Once it begins to go bad, a product becomes ineffective. Since heat and sunlight accelerate this process, keep your skin care products in a dark, cool place to increase their longevity. It is also important to clean any product remnants from around the top of the container and keep it tightly shut to prevent bacteria and air from getting in. You can even refrigerate your creams and lotions to keep them fresh longer. At the end of summer, for example, I put my sunblocks and self-tanners in a sealed plastic container in the back of the refrigerator.

Essential oils actually last much longer than most creams or lotions. I have kept them for up to three years, but I also take good care of them. Most essential oil products come in dark glass containers to protect them from sunlight. They should be sealed tight and stored in a cool, dry place. Therefore, the medicine cabinet in a steamy bathroom is not the best place to keep them.

Keep your products in sight

If you tend to forget to put on moisturizer or sunscreen before leaving the house in the morning, keep your daily essentials outside the medicine cabinet and readily accessible. If they are attractively displayed on a small tray at your sink and in plain sight, you will be more likely to use them.

Step Three: Nourish

Apply three to four drops of serum to your face and neck.

CHECKLIST

A.M. beauty routine

- Rinse with tepid to cool water (cleanse if you have oily skin)
- Tone
- Nourish
- Moisturize
- Protect with a sunblock

Step Four: Moisturize

Apply moisturizer over your face and neck. We all have our favorites. I prefer something lightweight that's compatible with makeup. If you have combination skin, try a water-based formulation. If your skin is drier, use something more emollient and wait a few minutes for it to absorb before applying your makeup. For skin that is on the oilier side, skip this step and use your serum to hydrate.

Step Five: Protect

After moisturizing the skin, protect it with a sunblock. I do not recommend using a sunblock in place of your moisturizer, although you can apply a smaller amount of both. Most women do not get enough moisture on their skin and a sunblock is not a sufficient substitute.

I have oily skin that tends to be dry on the surface. This is a frustrating and contradictory problem that is common for women over the age of thirty. You want to prevent wrinkles by moisturizing, but are afraid that it will cause breakouts. Most women end up drying out their skin to get rid of blemishes, causing it to become red and irritated. After much experimentation, this is what has helped my skin to improve dramatically. After my two-step cleansing, I apply an alcohol-free toner with essential oils that help hydrate and soothe my skin. To prevent fine lines, I add a serum that is lightweight and noncomedogenic. Lavender, rosemary, and calendula are ingredients to look for in serums, which also help calm the skin and prevent breakouts. After serum, I apply a pea-size amount of water-based moisturizer. The key is not to apply too much of any one product; just a small amount of each.

FACIALS

A spa facial is an incredibly therapeutic and restorative treatment for your face and overall sense of well-being. It thoroughly cleanses the skin through steaming and manual extraction of blackheads, increases circulation through facial massage, and exfoliates with a professional-strength peel. The AHA (alpha-hydroxy acid) and beta-hydroxy-acid solutions at spas are of a higher concentration than what you can get over the counter. These are essentially light peels that must be applied by a licensed and trained aesthetician (stronger chemical peels require a visit to the dermatologist). The application of steam during a facial makes the peel stronger and more effective, which is also why you should discontinue the use of topical prescription medications for the face up to a week before a facial. If taking oral prescription medications for acne, forget the peel altogether.

Extraction (manual removal of blackheads) is a controversial topic. Many dermatologists feel that it is unnecessary or unsafe, because an unskilled aesthetician can end up damaging your skin. Again, success depends on the expertise of the person performing the service. When safely and skillfully done, I believe that extractions are about the only way to eliminate stubborn blackheads. A blemish will eventually go away, but a clogged pore can last for years.

PROFESSIONAL TECHNIQUE

How to give yourself a facial at home

A do-it-yourself facial may not incorporate professional-strength peels or the theraputic benefits of massage, but it can still be a relaxing way to treat yourself and take better care of your skin. To do this effectively, make sure that you have at least thirty minutes of uninterrupted time to yourself.

1. CLEANSE AND EXFOLIATE YOUR SKIN. Emulsify your makeup with a cream cleanser, then wash your face with a foaming cleanser. You can use a cotton pad to exfoliate while you cleanse, or use a facial scrub as an additional step. Rinse well with tepid water and pat dry.

2. STEAM YOUR FACE. Soak a couple of hand towels in hot water, carefully wring them out, and apply to your face. Make sure that the towels are not too hot (they should feel comfortable on your skin) and avoid the eye area. A few drops of your favorite essential oil added to the basin of hot water makes for a wonderful aromatherapy effect while the towels are steaming your skin. Wrap one towel in the shape of a horseshoe, centering it at your chin and up both sides of your face. Let it sit for a few minutes, then change the towel and repeat. Lying down is the easiest way of keeping it in place.

3. MASSAGE. See the page opposite on how to perform a facial massage. This can be done for one to five minutes, depending on how much time you have. You can use your favorite moisturizer, applying a bit more than usual to give your fingertips some slippage. When you are finished, wipe off the remaining cream with the wet towel.

4. APPLY A CLAY MASK. Now that your pores have been steamed and your facial muscles relaxed, put on a clay mask to purify and deeply cleanse your skin. A wonderful tip is to add a pea-size amount of your facial moisturizer to the mask (just blend the two products in the palm of your hand). This will keep the clay active and moist and prevent if from hardening to the point where it starts to crack. The mask will be just as effective, but more comfortable to keep on and easier to rinse off. You can also mist a clay mask with toner to keep it moist. Relax with the mask on for ten minutes. For a nice spa-like touch, place chilled cucumber slices or chilled chamomile tea bags over your eyes and lie down.

5. APPLY A HYDRATING MASK. Rinse off the clay mask and apply a hydrating mask for ten minutes. It should contain ingredients that have humectant properties such as aloe vera, glycerin, or sodium hyaluronate to bring moisture to the skin, and emollients such as shea butter or other natural oils to lock in that moisture.

6. MOISTURIZE YOUR SKIN. After rinsing off the hydrating mask, finish by applying serum, moisturizer, neck and eye creams, and lip balm.

PROFESSIONAL TECHNIQUE

Facial massage

Facial massage is not only relaxing but detoxifying and therapeutic. It improves the tone of the skin and reduces puffiness. These massages for toning and lymphatic drainage can be done on yourself one after the other. The *toning massage* helps to give the face a mini workout by increasing the circulation and stimulating the facial muscles. The *lymphatic massage* has been practiced by aestheticians for years to reduce fluid retention, help minimize eye puffiness, and relieve stress.

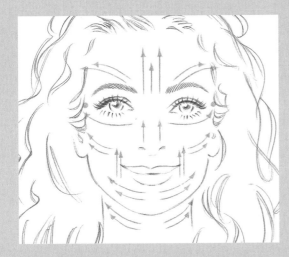

TONING MASSAGE

1. Massage with the pads of the fingers, using upward sweeping strokes, for 20 to 30 seconds in each area. Start at the neck, going from the center toward the jawline.
2. Move to the chin, using upward strokes toward the ears, then straight up at the sides of the mouth to help stimulate the laugh lines.
3. Continue from the cheekbones toward the hairline.
4. Starting with both middle fingers on either side of the nose, move straight up to the tops of the cheekbones, in a semicircle under the eyes, and toward the temples in one fluid motion. Repeat 10 to 20 times.
7. Take a few moments to press on the temples to help relieve stress and headaches.
8. From between the eyebrows, slide your fingers toward the hairline, alternating left and right hands.
9. Finish by moving from the eyebrows to where the hair naturally recedes above the temples.

   By doing this for a couple of minutes each day, you should see a difference in the tone and color of your skin.

LYMPHATIC MASSAGE

1. Rest your elbows on a solid surface and press with both middle fingers on pressure points at the center top of the cheekbones, just below the under-eye area. Massage in small circles for 10 to 20 seconds.
2. Move to pressure points just below the cheekbones, an inch to the left and right of the nostrils. You can massage longer here to relieve sinus pressure.
3. Repeat at pressure points half an inch from the corners of the mouth.
4. Slide your fingers to the corners of the jaw and repeat.
5. Move your finger tips across to the top of the jaw, just above the bone. This also helps to relieve stiffness related to TMJ.
6. Finish at the temples, near the hairline.

Repeat these six steps three times for the full effect.

Why facials are important

If getting a facial every month is not possible, try getting one at the end of each season. It can be something you do four times a year to deeply clean, exfoliate, and moisturize your skin. Especially at the end of the summer, a facial can be the most effective way to remove the buildup of sunblock that can obstruct the pores and cause breakouts. Your face also takes a beating during a cold, windy winter, and a facial can help to replace the lost moisture or calm any redness and inflammation.

Another important element of a spa facial is massage for lymphatic drainage and stimulating circulation to the skin. A skilled facialist is also a body worker and a good facial should be a true spa experience with restorative benefits from head to toe. While your mask is on, the aesthetician should be massaging your neck and shoulders to further relax you and stimulate blood flow to your face, or working pressure points on your feet. She should not leave the room during that time to attend to other business.

DAMAGE CONTROL
Skin Conditions and Solutions

While we all want immediate solutions to get rid of an acne flare-up or alleviate dark under-eye circles or puffiness, it is also important to have a more holistic approach to find real solutions with long-lasting results. You have to be somewhat of a detective in order to determine why a skin condition is occurring. Often, a pharmaceutical prescription alone will not eradicate a problem. Dermatology tends to treat the topical symptom rather than the underlying cause. A topical medication may only mask the symptoms instead of addressing the real problem. For example, if you have an allergy with symptoms that are showing up on your skin, applying cortisone cream to the affected area acts only as a bandage. Unless you discuss your dietary habits, sleep patterns, and stress level with your doctor, the real issue may go undiagnosed.

We need to treat the body as a whole rather than compartmentalize the skin and hair as separate entities. If a problem is showing up on your face, take a closer look at all the products in your life. A rosacea-like condition could arise from something simple, like sensitivity to the laundry detergent or fabric softener used to wash your pillowcases. Similarly, chapped hands can be caused by household cleaning products.

The following skin problems are the ones I am asked about most frequently, and you may be struggling with some of them yourself. However, you have more control than you may think. Here are some simple solutions that can help alleviate these conditions, as well as some of the possible underlying causes.

Dark Circles

Since the skin in this area is thinner, dilated blood vessels become more apparent. We tend to notice dark circles more when we don't get enough sleep, which causes the skin to appear paler and the pigment underneath more visible. Dark circles can also be a result of inflammation in the sinus cavity. Most people with chronic sinus problems accept this as a way of life, but it is a serious issue and should be addressed by an ear, nose, and throat specialist. For example, you may have a deviated septum or polyps. Both can be corrected with outpatient surgery.

WHAT YOU CAN DO: After being tested for allergies or a possible vitamin deficiency, see a sinus specialist. Decrease or eliminate your intake of caffeine (particularly from coffee—tea is much better), which is believed to worsen dark circles and can negatively affect your sleep patterns. Yoga inversions (standing on your head or lying on the floor with your legs raised up against a wall) is an excellent way to get the blood flowing in the opposite direction and help flush out some of that discoloration from the under-eye area. I have also found that one of the best topical remedies for dark circles is the application of an eye cream containing rosemary, which stimulates circulation under the skin.

Exfoliate your lips

Most people use a lip balm, but few exfoliate their lips. I recommend doing this weekly to make them soft and smooth. Buy a separate, soft toothbrush to use as a lip scrubber. Put a drop of natural oil such as jojoba, avocado, or vitamin E onto damp bristles, and gently scrub your lips. Afterward, rinse off the dead skin. Apply a layer of lip balm when finished. Always use a balm made with natural ingredients, since it will be ingested whenever you lick your lips, eat, or drink. Additionally, balms that are not natural can actually make your lips feel more dry.

Puffiness

Puffiness can be the result of fluid retention in the tissue under the eyes, which may be exacerbated by eating processed foods with high sodium content, as well as by dehydration. The inflammation under the skin could also be due to an allergic reaction, perhaps to a fragrance in a skin care, cosmetic, or household product. You may even be allergic to the down in your pillow. As with dark circles, a sinus condition also contributes to puffiness under the eyes, which tends to be worse when you wake up in the morning due to accumulation of fluid from the forces of gravity and being still for hours. Once you are up and your head is elevated, the swelling usually begins to diminish.

WHAT YOU CAN DO: While drinking six to eight glasses of water per day should prevent dehydration, splashing cold water over your face twenty to thirty times helps to reduce swelling and inflammation. An eye cream that contains rosemary is also effective for treating eye puffiness as well as dark circles. To increase its benefits, refrigerate the cream so that it is chilled when you apply it. You can also apply a thick layer to the semicircular areas under the eyes (but not too close to the lash line) for about ten minutes. Placing cold slices of cucumber or chamomile-tea bags (that have been steeped and then chilled) over the eyes will also take down the swelling. The cold constricts the blood vessels, while both chamomile and cucumber have anti-inflammatory properties. A pack of frozen peas also works well as a cold compress. Another effective solution is the lymphatic facial massage (see the illustration on page 183) to help move the fluid away from the eyes. This is especially beneficial for people who suffer from sinus pressure that may be contributing to the puffiness. A wonderful and natural way to keep your nasal passages clear and help reduce allergies, no matter the cause of the problem, is with a neti pot. This is an ancient ayurvedic remedy that allows you literally to wash your sinuses with salted warm water. Neti pots can be found in many health food stores.

Rosacea

Rosacea is a form of acne and is a commonly misdiagnosed condition. Many people think that they suffer from it when they simply have red, irritated skin. A doctor will sometimes label the problem rosacea and treat it with a topical cortisone solution without addressing why the symptoms are occurring in the first place. Rosacea-like flushing and inflammation can be triggered by things such as sun exposure, dehydration, and certain foods. This condition is a prime example of how your own detective work, lifestyle changes, and thoughtful skin care, *combined* with a diagnosis from your dermatologist, provide the best answer.

WHAT YOU CAN DO: Stay away from the triggers that irritate your skin, whether sun exposure, hot baths or showers, or spicy foods, and limit your caffeine and alcohol consumption. Make sure that the redness and irritation do not stem from something simple like dry, irritated skin. I have seen women's skin become instantly calmed when hydrated with the right serum and moisturizer. Look for anti-inflammatory ingredients in these products, such as chamomile, calendula, and cucumber. Rose water is wonderful for healing and calming the skin, and even whole milk has therapeutic benefits when applied topically as a cold compress for five to ten minutes. Its lactic acid calms inflammation and the fat moisturizes. Spices like turmeric and ginger have amazing anti-inflammatory properties and are great to use in cooking, to drink as an herbal tea, or to take as a supplement.

Natural Remedy

Aloe vera—the magic moisturizing plant

Fresh, pure aloe is a miracle product for the skin. It has amazing anti-inflammatory and humectant properties and is transformative for dry or sensitive rosacea-type skin. It reduces inflammation and helps heal injuries such as burns, as well as rashes. The best way to get pure aloe is from the plant itself. Keep one in your kitchen or bathroom. You can clip off part of a leaf and apply the gel inside it right onto your skin. I regularly use pure aloe as a moisturizing mask, especially if I have a photo shoot that day or if I am traveling. Keep the mask on while checking email in the morning or in the evening while reading or watching television (I leave it on for up to an hour). If you have chronically dry skin, applying this moisturizing mask daily will transform your complexion.

Acne

Acne can become a problem even for adults who were never plagued with breakouts as teenagers. When a pore is clogged, oil and bacteria build up inside and a blemish is produced. This can be caused by not removing your makeup well and not cleaning your makeup brushes or powder puffs regularly, as well as by frequently touching your face. Blemishes can also be an inflammatory response to a product that has irritated your skin. Additionally, you could be breaking out because of hormonal fluctuations during your menstrual cycle or menopause, or because of emotional stress that releases cortisol in the body, which in turn increases oil production.

WHAT YOU CAN DO: If you suffer from a condition that is more serious and chronic than a few occasional blemishes, you should seek the help of a professional. Many people feel embarrassed by this problem and try to take matters into their own hands, or fear that seeing a doctor will entail a big financial investment. Most dermatologists accept health insurance and you can ask your primary physician for a referral. A dermatologist may be able to clear up the entire problem with a topical or oral antibiotic. A retinoid medication can also help heal acne by exfoliating the skin and preventing congestion in the pores. That being said, I know women who see a dermatologist regularly and still cannot get a handle on their acne. If dermatology is not working, you need to find the source of the problem. Your skin is trying to tell you something. Your body may be overloaded with toxins that are literally coming out through your pores. It can take time to figure out where this imbalance is coming from and why, so be patient.

Over-the-counter solutions can also be effective for treating blemishes, especially if the condition is on the mild side. Benzoyl peroxide helps to reduce bacteria and dry out the pimple. Products containing salicylic acid keep pores unobstructed by gently peeling the skin. A clay mask can also double as an acne medication, since it is an excellent drying and antibacterial agent. Use a cotton swab to dot the mask right on the spot and leave it on overnight.

Q&A

Q: *Is there a way to make the pores on my nose and chin look smaller?*

A: A prescription retinoid cream is effective, since it not only exfoliates the skin but refines the pores. A salicylic-acid product is also good. You can apply it just to the nose and chin areas rather than treat your entire face. This would also be a good time to schedule a professional facial. An aesthetician will apply a peel and do extractions to cleanse the clogged pores, making them appear smaller almost immediately.

If products and/or prescription medicines are not solving the issue, take a close look at your diet (more on this in chapter 9). Additionally, don't forget to consider external factors. Breakouts can occur from not cleaning your phone or changing your pillowcase frequently enough. Perspiration and oil from your skin, along with the residue from your hair products, remain on your pillow. Therefore, if you are prone to breakouts, buy extra pillowcases and change the one you sleep on daily (or as frequently as you can).

Dull Skin

A lifeless, dull complexion can be due to a lack of exfoliation: the dead-skin-cell layer is covering the fresh skin underneath. Internally, it can be an indicator of dehydration, lack of sleep, lack of exercise, or possibly a vitamin deficiency.

WHAT YOU CAN DO: As we get older, our skin does not renew itself as efficiently as it used to, and daily exfoliation with a gentle scrub can do wonders to brighten the complexion. One of the best solutions for dull skin is exercise. Breaking a sweat cleanses the pores and makes your skin appear instantly brighter. Dehydration could also be the underlying cause. Drink more water throughout the day and supplement your diet with omega-3 oil, borage oil, and/or flaxseed oil. An equally important factor is your emotional well-being. When someone is overwhelmed or exhausted, you can actually see it on her face.

BEAUTY SECRET

The stubborn blemish

If a blemish is too deep or is infected, trying to extract it may only further irritate it and make matters worse. My advice is to see a dermatologist for a cortisone shot. It is the best remedy for a big problem that feels more cystic and painful. It will reduce the redness immediately and dissolve the monster on your face within days, which is worth a trip to the doctor.

BEAUTY SECRET

Try mineral sunblocks

I actually prefer to use a mineral sunblock that contains titanium dioxide and/or zinc oxide, rather than one with chemical sunscreen ingredients. Some people are also allergic to these chemicals and find that wearing sunscreen irritates their skin. Others are afraid to use it daily because it makes their skin break out. In such cases, a mineral-based sunblock can be the answer. I have found that it does not clog the pores (this is different from mineral oil). In chapter 7, "Mastering Makeup," I will talk more about using mineral makeup.

Hyperpigmentation

Brown spots that show up on the face, chest, arms, and legs are due to years of sun exposure. Therefore, prevention is the key. Even if hyperpigmentation has already started to appear, wearing sunblock and protecting yourself with a hat and other clothing will help to prevent further discoloration. Women get sun spots in their thirties and forties (so let's stop calling them age spots!). The bottom line: no one wants dark spots on her face or body at any age.

WHAT YOU CAN DO: Prescription lightening creams have been found to be effective, but some contain controversial ingredients with long-term side effects that may not be worth the short-term results. Ask your doctor what is safe and how to use it. A retinoid is frequently prescribed to slightly fade sun spots by accelerating cell turnover and encouraging peeling of the skin. However, since retinol creams also make the skin more sensitive to the sun, protecting it becomes even more imperative to prevent further hyperpigmentation. Over-the-counter (OTC) products that contain natural lightening agents such as kojic acid (a by-product of the fermentation of rice during the manufacturing of sake, Japanese rice wine) and licorice extract can be effective for the less pronounced spots. Laser treatment is currently by far the most immediate and effective solution, and may be worth the investment so you can just stop thinking about the problem.

Fine Lines, Crow's-Feet, and Loss of Elasticity

When fine lines begin to appear, your skin is starting to lose some of its elasticity. Like a crease that an iron makes in fabric, once there, it is difficult to erase.

WHAT YOU CAN DO: The key to treating lines and wrinkes is to approach the problem from a few different angles. You have to plump, hydrate, and protect the skin. To plump it, you need to stimulate collagen production, which can be aided by products containing retinoids and peptides (the building blocks of protein), along with a healthy diet. Humectants such as hyaluronic acid are ingredients to look for when buying a moisturizer or serum. Moisturizing the skin instantly rejuvenates it and softens the appearance of fine lines. Nourish it with a serum containing vitamin C, which is proven to repair the skin from free-radical damage (which causes wrinkles) and increase collagen production. And remember to apply sunblock daily.

I am also convinced that sleeping on your side or stomach makes creases more pronounced. Look in the mirror and compress your face with your hands to see what this does to the laugh lines and crow's-feet. Over the years, I have trained myself to sleep on my back. Seriously, I make a mental note before going to sleep to turn on my back if I happen to shift to my side while sleeping. This gentle reminder sneaks into the subconscious and your body responds. It really does work.

BEAUTY SECRET

How to keep your skin hydrated on a plane trip

The recycled air inside airplanes is very low in humidity and is therefore dehydrating to the skin. I like to pat moisturizer on my laugh lines and around my eyes during the flight. Sample-size moisturizers are perfect to travel with. I also keep a small spray bottle of alcohol-free toner with essential oils to mist on my face every half hour or so. For this reason, I usually wear very minimal makeup on the plane—just a bit of eye makeup and lip balm. When preparing to land, I will apply a little foundation, powder, and blush. I also try to use a moisturizing mask the night before and the morning of a flight, as it provides a boost of moisture to the skin before you travel.

SKIN CARE ALTERNATIVES
Cosmetic Procedures and Plastic Surgery

The term *plastic* originates from the Greek word *plastikos,* which means to form or to mold. Decisions regarding cosmetic procedures or plastic surgery are very personal. You have to determine what (if anything) may be right for you, and when. We live in an age where lines on the forehead can be magically erased, laugh lines can be filled, and chemical peels and lasers can resurface the skin. Facial rejuvenation no longer means a full face-lift. Fillers and injectables have replaced many surgical procedures, although to date plastic surgery still remains the most effective solution for sagging skin on the neck or bags under the eyes. Many people think that such procedures are an all-or-nothing deal, but there is a world of options in between. It no longer means looking like a different person or even as if you have had something "done." As always, the expertise of the professional is the key to success, and in the hands of the right surgeon a medical procedure can make someone look more refreshed, rested, and youthful.

As a woman ages, she sometimes looks in the mirror and sees a person who looks very different from how she feels on the inside. I hear many women say that they do not want to start down the road of cosmetic procedures. I completely understand that point of view and think that it is a healthy attitude to have, as long as your physical image does not adversely affect how you feel about yourself. Otherwise, a simple dermatologic procedure, and even plastic surgery, can enhance not only your looks but your psychological well-being.

There is no shame in doing something that dramatically improves how you look and makes you feel better about yourself. If injectables are done conservatively and correctly, they can bring a woman back to looking like the person she remembers. So, if you agonize over the bags under your eyes and they are all that you see when looking in the mirror, you should know that there are solutions. You don't have to see yourself in such a negative light. Do some research and discuss your options with a plastic surgeon.

It is also important to recognize that some people are overzealous when it comes to cosmetic procedures and plastic surgery. They may get too much done, have procedures too frequently, or start too young. I truly believe that it is better to look a little older than risk looking crazy, which is what happens when you go overboard. We have all seen people who no longer look like themselves, or even like normal human beings, because they are too pulled, frozen, or filled up. They do not necessarily look young; they just look like they have had too much work done (which, ironically, makes a person look old). I cannot begin to count the number of times I thought people were being rude to me when they actually had so much Botox injected that they were unable to change their facial expression to acknowledge me! It should not be about trying to look thirty at fifty, but about looking like a great fifty. As with everything in life, moderation and good judgement are key.

BEAUTY BELOW THE NECK, AND BELOW THE BELT

Skin care should not stop at the neck. Your routine should incorporate basics such as moisturizing and exfoliating the body and hair removal. There are simple ways to make the skin on your body look healthier and more beautiful with added color and luminosity from products like a self-tanner, body oil, and shimmer.

Exfoliating

Many women feel that no matter how much they moisturize the skin on their bodies, it is always dry and rough. If this is the case, you should exfoliate daily in the shower with a natural-bristle brush or a sea sponge. Such a scrubbing tool will remove the dead cells that dull the skin and clog the pores and might otherwise lead to blemishes and ingrown hairs. Exfoliating the body has the same benefits as exfoliating the face.

Moisturizing

We tend not to moisturize our skin enough, on the face or on the body. In a rush to get ready in the morning, many do not apply enough (or any) body lotion after a shower. Don't be stingy with a moisturizer. You should slather on a generous amount from head to toe. In fact, sometimes one application is not enough, especially on particularly dry areas such as the knees and elbows. Reapply moisturizer if your skin still feels dry after the first layer has been absorbed.

HAIR REMOVAL

Shaving

The secret to getting the smoothest shave is to do it like a man. Guys shave their faces daily and have perfected the practice. We might as well take a lesson from them. First, use a high-quality tool. Do not bother with those pink plastic disposable ladies' shavers. I use a man's razor with sharp, multiple blades to get the closest shave. Second, you will get a much better result by using shaving cream, as opposed to lathering with soap. Shaving cream softens the hair and lifts it from the skin so that the razor can do its job more effectively. It also protects and lubricates the skin, helping the razor to glide across it to avoid nicks and razor burn. You will get a more comfortable and safer shave by taking shorter strokes (two to three inches) rather than rushing through the process. For highly sensitive areas that are especially prone to ingrown hairs, such as the bikini line, it is much less irritating to shave in the direction of the hair growth and to repeat the process if necessary.

Shaving the legs can present a particularly awkward and dangerous challenge in a stall shower. Clearly, these showers were not built with women in mind, and we have all had to suffer through the unattractive experience of hoisting one leg up on the side of the wall to shave it (I once threw my back out that way!). For a typical stand-up shower, have a small but secure shelf installed onto the tiles, so that you can rest your foot on it when shaving. Being comfortable is more conducive to getting a good shave and not hurting yourself in the process.

Waxing

Whether on your face or body, waxing is a job better left to a professional. The results will be much more reliable and the experience less painful (in more ways than one). It is important to go to a reputable spa or waxing salon and to find an experienced aesthetician who specializes in waxing

BEAUTY SECRET

Hair conditioner for shaving

If you suddenly run out of shaving cream, a basic hair conditioner is a great alternative. Since conditioner is designed to soften the hair, it will do the same for the hair on your legs, in addition to providing the necessary slippage. You may even find that you prefer it to conventional shaving cream altogether.

Managing ingrown hairs

Topical solutions can be effective in dealing with razor bumps and minor irritation. For more serious situations, the best remedy is to remove the hair. If you cannot see the hair and/or it is too deep to be plucked out, see an aesthetician (or a dermatologist if the aesthetician is unable to remove it). You risk scarring yourself if you take matters into your own hands.

(as opposed to another type of beauty technician who also knows how to wax). You want someone whom you can trust and feel comfortable with. It is also a good idea to go to one person consistently, as she will tend to wax in the same pattern, which prevents folliculitis (inflammation of the hair follicles). An ingrown hair occurs when a pore becomes blocked with dead skin, not allowing the hair to grow out of the pore. In that case, it curls back inward and continues to grow under the skin. A hair can also just miss the pore altogether, which happens frequently after waxing. Body brushing and exfoliating the skin daily with a gentle scrub or a body wash containing salicylic acid will help prevent this.

Request that your aesthetician use a hard wax for sensitive areas like the upper lip and the bikini line. This wax is thicker and more emollient than the kind that gets removed with a strip of fabric. Once it has cooled and hardened on the skin, it can be peeled off along with the hair. It is gentler on the skin, is much less painful, and helps to minimize the breakouts and irritation that can result from waxing.

It is wise to discontinue using glycolic or salicylic acids and retinoid products on your face or body one week before getting waxed. These products remove a layer of skin, making it more sensitive and vulnerable to a mini-disaster such as ripping the skin off with the wax and causing a painful burn or scar.

Laser Hair Removal

Laser hair removal is worth the investment, since over time it eliminates stubble, razor burn, and ingrown hairs. Today, it is the ultimate option for removing unwanted hair on the body. I used to wax under my arms until I graduated to laser. Once the process is complete you are permanently hair-free. No more monthly waxing or daily shaving under the arms. Even the toxic deodorants and antiperspirants become unnecessary. With the hair gone, you do not sweat (or smell) as much—it is truly emancipating! This is also a great solution for those who get ingrown hair from waxing. Laser is done at a dermatologist's office or at a spa that specializes in hair removal. It typically takes a series of six to ten sessions to make the hair go away almost completely. One session is done about every six to eight weeks. After completing the series, you may have to return for the occasional touch-up—a small commitment compared with the time, money, and inconvenience of daily shaving.

Although generally safe, laser hair removal can be less reliable on the face, depending on the pigmentation of the hair. Laser light is attracted to dark pigment, so if you have light peach fuzz on your upper lip, for instance, that area is not a candidate for laser. Most of the reputable hair-removal facilities always ask before a laser treatment if you have recently been out in the sun, which makes your skin more sensitive to laser, as does taking antibiotics.

BEAUTIFYING THE BODY

Self-tanner

A good self-tanner not only gives the skin a golden, healthy color but produces subtle shading that camouflages imperfections like spider veins and cellulite. It can even make you look a little slimmer. There are many spas that offer professional airbrush-tanning treatments, or you can try it yourself at home. Sunless tanning products are easier to use and less messy than they used to be.

There are three types of self-tanner to choose from. The traditional formula is invisible upon application, and the color begins to show in about twenty minutes. A tinted self-tanner has bronzer in it, which adds instant color and allows you to see exactly where you are applying the product; it also minimizes the chance of ending up with streaks and missed areas. Additionally, there are gradual tanners that have a lesser amount of the tanning ingredient. These build up color over a few applications and are great for women who are fair or for those who want a mere glow to their skin.

To get uniform, streak-free color, prepare your skin first by shaving, exfoliating (very gently), and moisturizing with a light body lotion. The slippage from the moisturizer makes the tanner glide on more easily, helping to prevent streaks and allowing for even coverage, since it will not overly absorb where the skin is more dry. Nevertheless, during the self-tanner application, avoid the rough, drier areas (the tops of knees, heels and feet, elbows) and just skim over them last, using whatever product remains on your hands. Always wait a few minutes for a self-tanner to dry completely before putting on your clothes.

For the face and neck, I prefer to use a light dusting of bronzer rather than self-tanner, but many women like to have some warmth to their complexion without the appearance of makeup. In that case, be sure to choose a product that is specifically made for the face. Self-tanners that are intended for the body tend to be somewhat darker, and since the skin on the face and neck is thinner, the color should be a bit lighter. Use the same five-step self-tanning technique that is outlined for the body, but skip the oil (the last step). Moist skin not only helps with even distribution, it slightly dilutes the tanner and makes the color more subtle. Start with the nose, cheekbones, and forehead (where the sun naturally tans the face first), then smooth it on over the rest of the face and neck. Do not forget to go over the jaw, earlobes, and front and back of the neck.

PROFESSIONAL TECHNIQUE

Five steps to a perfect self-tan

1. Exfoliate
2. Moisturize
3. Apply sunblock
4. Apply self-tanner
5. Add a drop of oil on the legs and arms for a beautiful glow

Natural Remedies

The five-minute detox treatment

In traditional Chinese medicine, the skin is referred to as "the third lung" and is treated as the living, breathing organ that it is. Dry brushing of the skin has been practiced in Eastern medicine for centuries as a form of exfoliation and to increase circulation and lymph drainage as well as to assist in the elimination of toxins through the skin. On a purely aesthetic level, dry brushing once a week will also give you glowing, soft, healthier skin.

To do this quickly and efficiently, you will need two natural-bristle body brushes that can comfortably fit in the palm of each hand. Before getting into the shower, vigorously brush your skin using sweeping strokes over your entire body. Since dry brushing helps to improve circulation, your strokes should be in the direction of the heart—upward on the legs and arms and downward from the neck and chest. Your skin will start to look pink, but because of the soft natural bristles, the sloughing is gentle and feels invigorating. Brush over the skin for a few minutes, then get into the shower or bath. The steam helps your skin to eliminate the toxins that the dry brushing has brought to the surface, while the water rinses off the dead skin cells.

Lemon water

The most amazing remedy that I have found for puffy eyes (also great for the complexion in general) is to slowly sip warm lemon water every morning on an empty stomach (approximately ⅛ to ¼ of a lemon, squeezed into a cup of hot or room temperature water). This is an Asian beauty secret for flushing toxins and excess salt from the system. It also realkalinizes the body and helps to balance the pH level of the skin.

Homemade body scrub

You can make your own natural body scrub using white granulated sugar (better to put it on your body than in it!). Store the sugar in a sealed, flip-top plastic canister and add it to your favorite liquid body wash. The round granules are extremely gentle and will not scratch or irritate the skin.

Moisturizing your body with oil

You can make your regular body lotion more emollient by adding a natural oil like jojoba, coconut, or avocado to it. The combination of equal parts oil and lotion is the perfect remedy for chronically dry skin. When it feels especially dehydrated, even if it's only in specific areas, apply a thin veil of oil on the body *before* getting into the shower. The oil protects the skin from being dehydrated by the hot water, while the steam helps it penetrate the skin.

Common Mistake

Neglecting the hands

The hands are often neglected, but they broadcast a woman's real age (or even make her look older than she actually is). Compared with the face, our hands go through so much more abuse, yet receive just a fraction of the attention from an occasional layer of hand cream. Because I am a hairstylist and an avid cook, my hands get a lot of abuse. I have learned that the secret to maintaining pretty hands is always to wear rubber gloves when doing the dishes or using household cleaning products, apply hand lotion after washing your hands, and wear gloves when it is chilly or windy outside (a thin driving glove), not just in the winter months.

When using skin care products on your face, rub what remains into the tops of your hands. Whether a sunblock, a rich moisturizer, or even a retinoid cream, every little bit helps and your hands will reap the benefits of those wonderful products.

OPTICAL ILLUSION

Slimming the arms and legs with a body oil or a shimmer

The reflection of light can make the upper arms, legs, and décolletage look more defined. A few drops of body oil lend a beautiful sheen and enhance the shape and muscle tone (this is why body-builders put oil on their skin for competitions). Any body oil will do the trick, but one with shimmer added to it will give a nicer glow. If you prefer to work with a powder-shimmer product, invest in a large cosmetic body brush to apply it. A smaller powder brush made for the face tends to leave concentrated streaks on a larger area of the skin. Always keep shimmer to a minimum; just dust a touch over the clavicle bones, shoulders, sides of the upper arms, and décolletage. This is an accent, meant to provide only a hint of reflection, and should not be overdone. Apply these products after getting dressed, so that you are not sliding clothing over oily or shimmery skin.

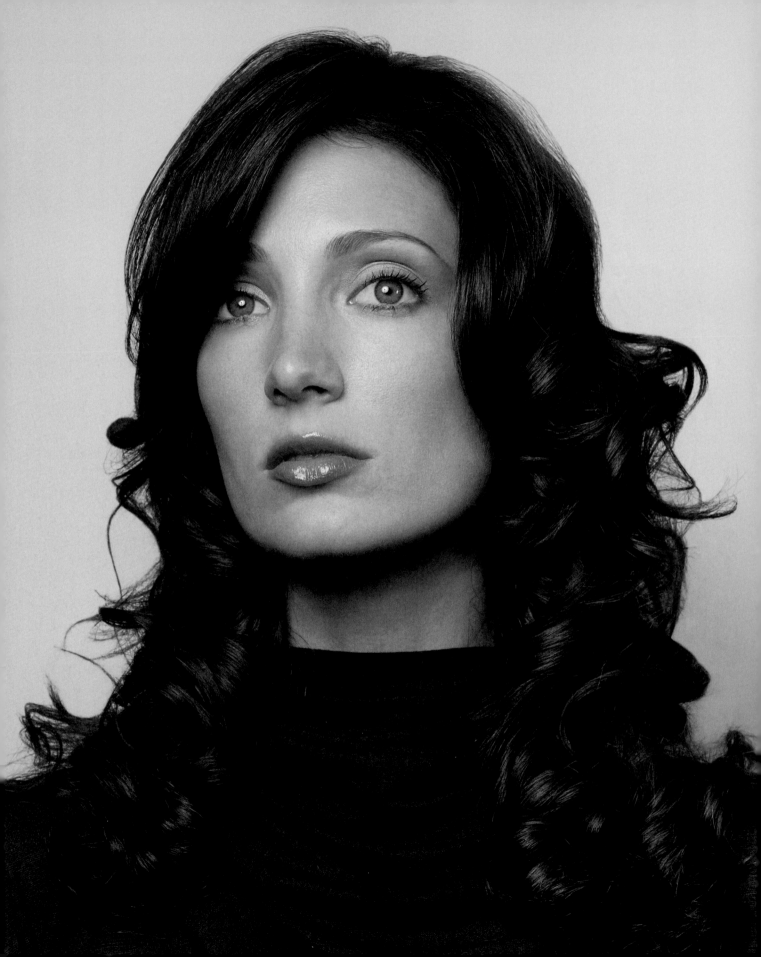

7

MASTERING MAKEUP

I became fascinated with makeup at very young age. As a little girl, I would watch my mother do her makeup, in awe of this transformative experience. She would enter the bathroom as a weary mother and housewife and emerge a glamorous and gorgeous woman. She had a renewed sense of self and a confidence in her step. Watching this amazing process taught me so much about the art and power of makeup. It can bring out the feeling a woman wants to evoke, whether feminine and pretty, confident and strong, or glamorous and daring.

My mother was the role model who inspired me to enter the beauty business. I actually became a makeup artist before I did hair professionally, perhaps because the artistic aspect of makeup came very naturally to me, having grown up around a model and observing her beauty routine. She taught me the basics, which made it easy for me to hone this art as a professional.

During her modeling career, my mother picked up a vast education from the great makeup artists and hairstylists she worked with in Hollywood. She had it down to a science and could do her face in fifteen minutes (including the application of the most natural-looking false eyelashes)! She knew how to work with her facial structure and complexion to enhance her features, which is the key to beautiful makeup and is what I aim to teach you in this chapter. You may feel unsure of your color choices and application skills, but you can learn to work with your face and make the most of what nature gave you. The tried-and-true techniques that I have used on count-less women will also give you the confidence to go beyond basic makeup and experiment with more advanced techniques such as creating a smoky eye, applying false lashes, or pulling off a more daring crimson lip color.

Most women love makeup, but learning how to work with it the right way can feel intimidating at first. I'm sure that if you ever had your makeup done by a talented makeup artist, her work seemed unattainable. Even though you wear makeup nearly every day, you may have thought, "Why can't I look this amazing all the time? What am I doing wrong?" A

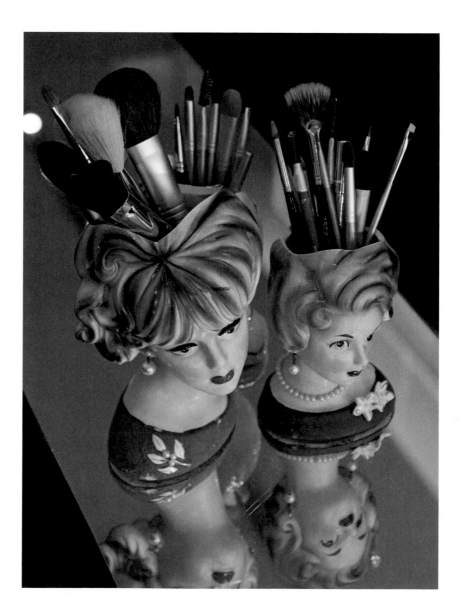

My personal makeup brushes in
vintage head vases.

better question might be, "What is the professional doing *differently?*" Because a makeup artist *does* apply makeup differently—more than you may realize. A skilled makeup artist, like a talented hairstylist, performs what appears to be magic. However, it is just the combination of a trained eye and solid techniques perfected through years of practice. I want to pass this knowledge on to you, making it simpler and less intimidating.

When it comes to makeup, subtle details make all the difference, and they are usually overlooked by most women. You can use the same makeup line that a professional works with and end up with quite inferior results because of your application and choice of colors. Lip color is a perfect example. Most women match their lip liner to their lipstick instead of their natural lip color. In addition, most do not use a brush to apply lipstick. A brush allows for better blending with the lip liner (not to mention using much less lipstick than when you apply directly from the tube). Although such details may seem inconsequential, these two simple elements completely change the finished look.

Other common makeup mistakes stem from a general misconception of what a given product is supposed to do. For instance, the majority think of foundation as "coverage" for the complexion, which results in your makeup looking too heavy. Actually, foundation is intended to even out the skin tone, while a color corrector should be used to remove redness and a concealer to cover imperfections such as blemishes and dark circles.

There are three simple yet critical rules of thumb that a professional makeup artist follows—and that most women do not. When you stick to these guiding principles of makeup application, you will be amazed by the results.

1. Apply your makeup in a systematic order.

There is a logical order to applying makeup products. If you are ever in doubt about the sequence, the basic rule is to keep the textures consistent. For example, always apply liquid, gel, or creamy makeup onto moist skin (without powder). Dry formulations in the form of eye shadow and blush should be put on dry skin that has been set with loose powder. You cannot successfully blend a cream blush over a powdered, dry surface. It will inevitably grab and stick. The same goes for applying powder blush over damp skin. The results will be streaky as opposed to blended.

2. Layer small amounts of product.

Although most women tend to use too much product at once, application of makeup should be a process of layering small amounts. For example, just one drop of foundation is perfect for the entire face and neck, if it is blended over moisturized skin. It is safer to start with the smallest amount, like the sheerest layer of blush, and build up the color gradually if you need more. Most dip a brush into makeup and apply it directly to their faces, depositing too much product, which makes it difficult to blend evenly into the skin. Makeup artists, on the other hand, tap or wipe excess makeup from their brush, puff, or sponge onto the back of their hand *before* touching the face. This simple cautionary measure is second nature to a professional.

3. Invest in the right tools and learn how to use them.

Using high-quality brushes will allow you to blend sheer layers of makeup into the skin for the most natural look. Professionals also use numerous light brushstrokes to blend makeup so that it practically becomes part of the skin. The average person uses far fewer strokes. (Count how many it takes you to dust on your blush or eye shadow—it is probably fewer than five, while I use fifteen to twenty.) This also goes for using pencils, whether on the lash line, brow, or lip. You may be using a heavy hand, drawing a line as you would with a pencil on paper. A pro uses numerous feather-light strokes to create a softer, more natural effect, lightly going over the area until the right amount of definition is created.

THE VALUE OF A PROFESSIONAL MAKEUP LESSON

Every woman should invest in one-on-one lessons with a professional makeup artist at different stages of her life. Like hairstyling, makeup is a skill and it makes perfect sense that you would need a class to learn it properly. Most of us learned to do makeup from our mothers (as I did) or from an older sister. Often, however, those well-meaning amateur teachers pass down bad habits or outdated application methods. During a private lesson, a professional will walk you through the entire makeup-application pro-

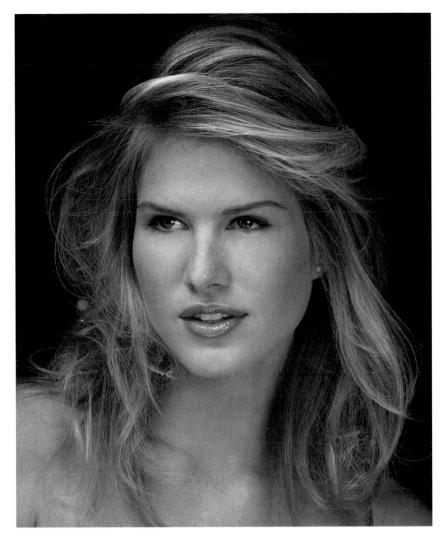

Anne Marie is wearing a sheer layer of liquid foundation blended with a concealer brush. Her pale pink eye shadow was combined with taupe as a contour shade. Rose blush and lip gloss in a shade deeper than her natural lip color completed this beautiful classic look.

cess, customizing information such as which tools, products, and colors are best for you. In the long run, taking an effective tutorial is much more cost-effective and efficient than constantly searching for the right products and buying new colors that you end up never using.

At my salon, a makeup lesson covers three components: skin care, eyebrow shaping, and makeup application. Improving the condition of your skin immediately makes your makeup look better, which is why I consider it an essential component of a lesson. I start by assessing a woman's skin type and asking about the products she uses. I then walk her through a simple and personalized skin care routine. Equally important are the eyebrows, which are an integral feature of the face; proper shaping is vital to the overall effect.

Olivia is wearing a light smoky eye using taupe eye shadow and brown pencil eyeliner. The eye shadow was extended using an angled eye shadow brush.

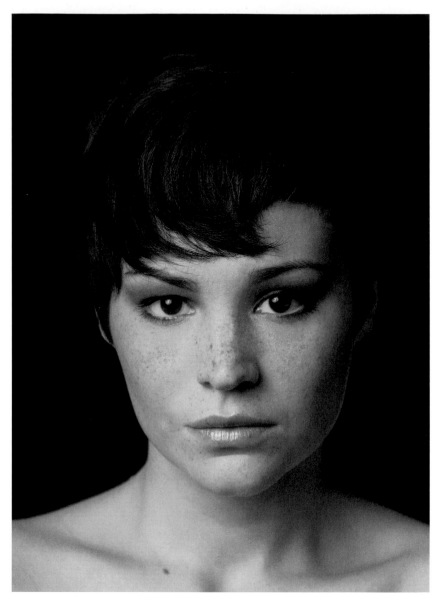

When someone books a session with me, I ask her to bring her makeup and brushes. I often see a collection of high-quality cosmetics and tools but the client simply does not know how to work with them correctly. I show her how to use the things she already has, tell her what she should get rid of, and explain what elements might be missing. I discuss her beauty routine, how and where she does her makeup, and the lighting in that room. I go over each step of basic makeup application and then move on to demonstrate some layering techniques for evening makeup. I usually have my assistant take notes about what products and colors I am using so that the client can take that information home. Essentially, as you read through this chapter, you will be having a virtual makeup lesson with me.

HOW TO FIND THE RIGHT PROFESSIONAL

A good way to find a makeup artist is to simply ask around. Perhaps someone you know used a great person for her wedding or another special event. You can also locate a talented professional at some salons and spas, or at a makeup studio or store. Many makeup artists also work on the cosmetics floors at department stores and their lessons are typically complimentary, but they are also sales driven and sometimes focused on moving certain products, so be prepared to buy something. Also, these lessons are not as extensive, because you are not paying for the service. If a makeup artist offers lessons through a salon or a makeup studio, ask to see her portfolio or just some photographs. If one has a book to show, she probably has more experience, a greater skill set, and has probably worked on weddings and photo shoots. Another way to find a local pro, especially in a smaller city, is through a popular photographer in the area. You can call the studio and ask who he or she usually hires for makeup.

CREATING YOUR BEAUTY ENVIRONMENT

Lighting

One of the biggest mistakes is made by almost everyone before the makeup process even begins—having the wrong lighting. The importance of proper lighting and an area where all your essential cosmetics and tools are at hand cannot be underestimated but is nearly always overlooked. The first thing a professional makeup artist does before beginning to work is set up the work area to make sure the lighting is right and clean brushes along with the right products are neatly organized on a table. Conversely, how many times have you attempted to put on blush, swipe on lipstick, or even apply mascara while looking in your car's rearview mirror? Or put on your makeup in a poorly lit bathroom and then surprised yourself (and your coworkers) with stripes on your cheeks? When you are not working in the right beauty environment, you start off at a disadvantage and give yourself little chance of achieving the beautiful results you want.

Everyone talks about natural light as being ideal, but it is actually more important to have an equal balance of light—and it does not necessarily have to be sunlight. In fact, if you do your makeup near a window during the day, one side of your face could be more illuminated than the other. To get even, eye-level light, install wall sconces in your bathroom on each side of the mirror. They are much more flattering and true than an overhead light that casts shadows down the face and makes you look older and tired. Also, install a dimmer switch in your bathroom so you can lower the light when preparing to go out for the evening to create an environment that is closer to the one in which your makeup will be seen. Another benefit is how a simple adjustment of lighting can make you feel. We use the bathroom numerous times throughout the day and night, and it is the one room in which we always look in the mirror. Why not feel good every time you glance at yourself? These basic lighting modifications can change your perception of and attitude toward how you look.

Comfort

In chapter 4, I recommended sitting down when blow-drying your hair, and I suggest it for putting on makeup as well. When you are comfortable, you are likely be more precise in your application. To some, creating a vanity space for makeup may sound extravagant, but it is actually very practical. Not only will you have a well-lit space with a good mirror and all your tools at hand (just like a professional), but it also inspires you to be more creative and allows you to do a better job than when you rush mindlessly through the process. A vanity area can be incorporated onto your desk or any table in a well-lit room. With a portable lighted makeup mirror, you can create a vanity for yourself almost anywhere. You will be amazed at the difference this makes in your application.

BEAUTY SUPPLIES

The right tools allow you to work with more precision. By applying concealer with a synthetic brush instead of your fingertip, you can use a smaller amount of product and blend it more easily, hiding dark circles or blemishes without making it look like cover-up. If you have never used a concealer brush, you will be shocked by the difference this one amazing tool makes: your makeup will be blended so perfectly that it appears to be part of the skin.

As we move through each step of the makeup process, I will guide you to the brush or applicator that works best with each product and explain how to work with it. If you start using the correct implements in the right way, your entire look will change, even if you use the same products. It is similar to the difference between finger painting and using the appropriate paintbrushes to create art.

SELECTING YOUR BRUSHES

The best brushes have a natural, uncut finish at the tips of the bristles. If you hold the brush up to a light, you will notice that the ends of the bristles are not all the same length. This allows the brush to hug the skin for smoother application. Brushes that are machine cut have a blunt edge, which can give a streaky and less natural-looking finish. They are typically included with cosmetics that you buy and should be tossed out.

Professionals use synthetic brushes to apply creamy or liquid foundation or concealer. The softest bristles, such as squirrel, badger, raccoon, or sable, are used for powder makeup. High-quality synthetic-fiber brushes are also available. They are beautifully crafted, soft and luxurious, and are a great alternative to brushes made from animal hair.

Storing and Cleaning Your Brushes

Makeup pros treat their brushes with the same respect that chefs give to their personal set of knives, and for the same reason: these are the tools of their trade. Once you purchase a set of brushes, take good care of them. High-quality makeup brushes can work well for years with proper maintenance and cleaning.

Do not toss your brushes into a drawer, box, or makeup bag where they will get dirty and crushed. Once the bristles become compressed and you don't have an even span, your makeup will be difficult to blend. I like to store my brushes upright in a cup or a vase—the same way that I keep my hairbrushes. It is also important to invest in a travel powder brush that comes in a case. I have done many lessons with women who open up their makeup bags to reveal old makeup and dirty brushes. They often tell me about problems with breakouts, which is no coincidence since they are using a loose makeup brush that harbors bacteria.

The bristles of a brush trap the oils from your skin, just as they do cosmetics. Just by keeping them clean you will improve the health of your skin. You should wash the synthetic brushes after each use. Just use a mild soap and rinse them under running water until it becomes clear, then lay the brushes on a towel to dry. When it comes to natural-

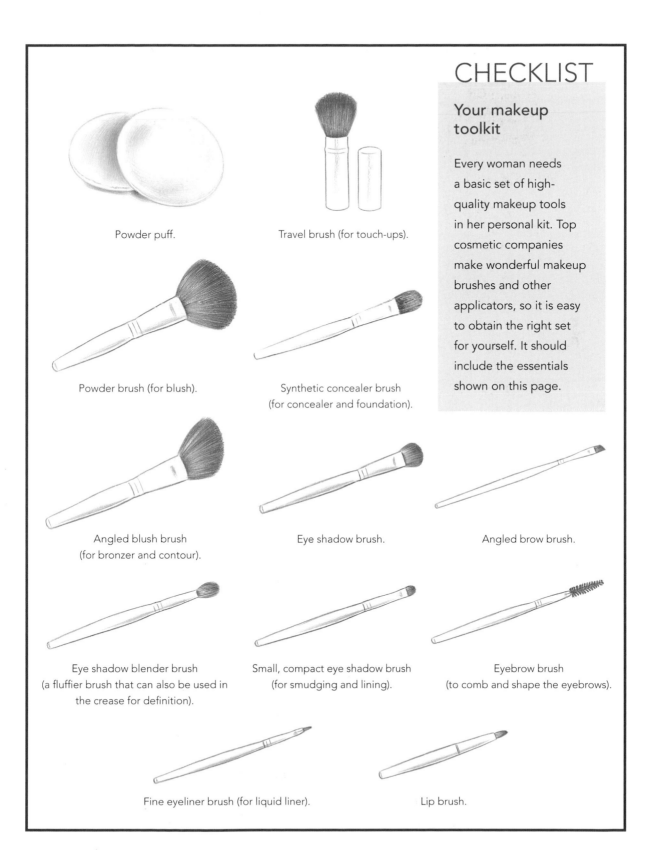

Powder puff.

Travel brush (for touch-ups).

CHECKLIST

Your makeup toolkit

Every woman needs a basic set of high-quality makeup tools in her personal kit. Top cosmetic companies make wonderful makeup brushes and other applicators, so it is easy to obtain the right set for yourself. It should include the essentials shown on this page.

Powder brush (for blush).

Synthetic concealer brush
(for concealer and foundation).

Angled blush brush
(for bronzer and contour).

Eye shadow brush.

Angled brow brush.

Eye shadow blender brush
(a fluffier brush that can also be used in
the crease for definition).

Small, compact eye shadow brush
(for smudging and lining).

Eyebrow brush
(to comb and shape the eyebrows).

Fine eyeliner brush (for liquid liner).

Lip brush.

hair brushes, cleaning them regularly will also protect their longevity. If they are not washed every couple of weeks, makeup and oil from your skin start to break down the bristles. Be especially gentle with natural bristles, making sure not to mash or manipulate them too much with your fingers. You need to maintain the original shape of the brush, whether it is pointy, flat, or fluffy. Wash your brushes in a bowl of warm soapy water (add a drop of shampoo) by swirling them in a circular motion. Do not compress the bristles at the bottom of the bowl or rough them up with your fingers. Afterward, take them out and rinse under running water in the direction of the bristles (doing it in reverse will distort their shape) until the water runs clean. Gently squeeze out the excess water, reshape them a bit with your fingers, and set them flat on a towel to air dry overnight. You should also hand-wash your powder puff once a week.

For home use, I prefer plain soap and water over a spray-on brush cleaner. Makeup artists have to use these sprays because there is no time to wash and dry their brushes between clients. But we also replace our brushes much more frequently than you should ever need to. These cleansers are loaded with alcohol and chemicals that can dry out and deteriorate the bristles. They are too harsh and unnecessary for daily use on your personal brushes.

PREPARING THE SKIN FOR MAKEUP

Makeup should never be applied to dry, thirsty skin. You have to moisturize first, and the real secret is *not* allowing the moisturizer to dry or completely absorb into the skin. Apply foundation about one minute after you moisturize, while your skin is still moist, so the makeup has plenty of slip. This ensures the most even, sheer makeup application and a radiant, glowing complexion.

When a woman tells me, "My makeup doesn't last—it totally absorbs into my skin," I know that she is not using enough moisturizer. Her cream or liquid makeup is indeed being absorbed into the dry skin, acting essentially as a moisturizer. This results in foundation that fades away quickly or looks blotchy. Right before I apply makeup to a client's face, I always

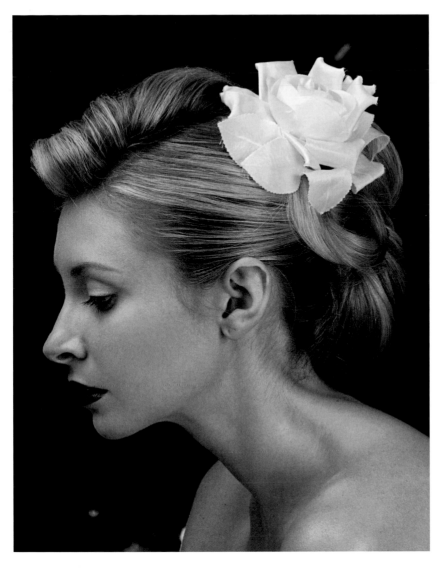

Kendra's skin was evened out with a liquid foundation with a damp sponge and concealer that is one shade lighter than her skin tone, applied with a synthetic brush. The classic red lip and upsweep were created for a bridal shoot.

mist a hydrating toner over her skin, followed by a little bit of extra moisturizer and eye cream, and only then do I start to put on foundation.

A common question is whether a makeup primer should be used. Personally, I think it is optional and may be unnecessary if you moisturize sufficiently. Primers usually contain silicone, which provides the slip that allows makeup to glide on better. However, they have become so popular precisely because most women do not moisturize and nourish their skin enough. I never use primer on myself, because I prepare my skin with the right skin care products and prefer to keep silicone off my face. (Remember the daytime skin care routine I suggested in chapter 6: toner, serum, moisturizer,

Giovanna is wearing a warm bronze foundation and a loose powder.

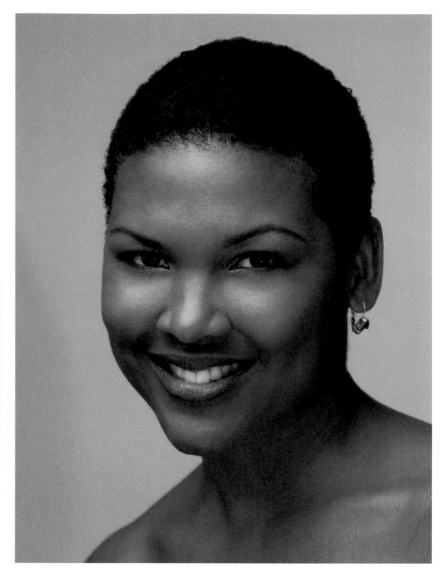

CHECKLIST

The Sequence of Applying Makeup

There is a clear, systematic order to applying makeup, which gives the best results and makes the application easier:

- Foundation
- Concealer
- Powder
- Bronzer
- Eyebrow pencil or powder
- Eye shadow
- Eyeliner
- Mascara
- Lip color
- Blush (You will learn later in this chapter why blush should be last.)

eye cream, and sunblock.) If you still find that you have a difficult time blending foundation without a primer, add a few drops of serum directly over the makeup and blend with a synthetic concealer brush.

Some people have the opposite problem: their makeup does not have staying power because their skin is too oily. In this case, an oil-absorbing product under the makeup can make the skin more matte and help keep oil at bay. It can be used just in the T-zone or applied over the entire face. This is the only exception to my rule of putting liquid foundation on moist skin.

PERFECTING THE SKIN TONE TO CREATE THE CANVAS
Foundation, Concealer, Powder, and Mineral Foundation

It is probably safe to say that the radiant, glowing complexions we see on celebrities and models are more often the result of beautifully applied makeup and airbrushing than of flawless skin. The combination of foundation, concealer, and powder can create this illusion of perfection. Most skin does not have an even tone throughout, which is why these first three steps are so important. Foundation has an undeservedly bad reputation for being heavy or cakey. This is only because it is so frequently overapplied to cover up flaws on the skin, when it is meant only to even out the skin tone. After that, you can use concealer to camouflage imperfections, and you will look ten years younger. A perfect canvas is the key to beautiful makeup.

Choosing the Right Formulation

The formulation you choose depends on the consistency you feel most comfortable wearing. Those with dry skin may prefer an emollient cream foundation. A powder or mineral-powder foundation might work well for women with oily skin. A tinted moisturizer is good for an even complexion that just needs a bit of color. Generally, a liquid foundation works beautifully on everyone. I use a liquid formula on my skin and because it is so sheer, no one ever thinks that I am wearing foundation. The goal of foundation should be an even, radiant complexion with undetectable coverage.

Choosing the Right Shade

Foundation should always match your skin. When testing one, apply it to the side of your face above the jawbone. It should disappear into your skin. Walking up to a window, under natural light, is the most accurate way to judge. Remember that if you can see the foundation, it's the wrong shade for you.

Perfect Application

I apply a liquid or cream foundation with my fingertips because the warmth from my hands helps to blend the makeup. Rub a pea-size amount between the fingers of both hands, then work it into slightly moist skin. The pads of your fingers can be the most effective makeup applicator for many cream or liquid products, but if this technique is challenging for you, then work with a synthetic concealer brush. You can also use a silicone sponge, which many cosmetics companies manufacture. (Don't bother with the cheap drugstore sponges—they are ineffective and fall apart when you try to wash and reuse them.)

Powder Foundations

Powder foundations must be applied when the face and neck are completely dry. Any moisture on the skin will soak up the powder and instantly create blotchiness. A powder formulation can end up looking too heavy when used all over the face. Instead, I prefer to use it as an accent.

My secret to a flawless, polished complexion is to follow the first three steps—foundation, concealer, loose powder—and then use a mineral or a powder foundation where you want a little more coverage, usually around the nose, the laugh lines, and the chin. A shade that is a bit lighter than your foundation (or about the same color as your concealer) will make those areas appear brighter and more luminous. You will be amazed by what the strategic application of powder makeup can do for you. It adds a touch of brightness and coverage exactly where you need it most. I use this technique on almost everyone, and it instantly makes the complexion appear smoother and more youthful.

Mineral Foundations

Mineral-powder foundations have become popular and are used by some as an alternative to traditional foundations. This, however, is not how I

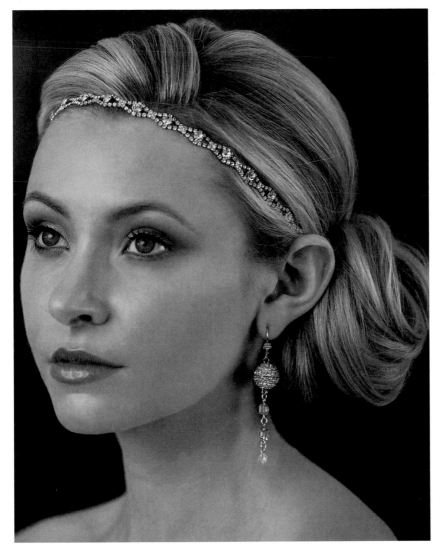

Kendra is wearing a smoky eye created with warm taupe, chocolate, and gold. The eye shadow was smudged with a compact eye shadow brush.

prefer to use them. I like to add a light dusting of mineral powder as a final step of my makeup application. Minerals reflect light and give a beautiful luminosity to the skin. Used on their own, as the sole form of coverage, mineral powders can look a bit shiny and even artificial. But they are perfect for creating a thin veil over the skin and can be a great solution for someone who has oily skin or breaks out from sunblock (the bonus of mineral powders is that they offer natural sun protection). They are also perfect for a midday touch-up, since you will give your skin some added coverage and reapply sunscreen at the same time.

CONCEALER—MY FAVORITE COSMETIC

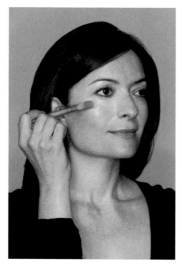

Concealer to cover and highlight.

After the complexion has been evened out with foundation, I like to apply a concealer that is one shade lighter than the foundation under the eyes to reflect light and brighten the area (applying foundation over the concealer would mask this beautiful effect). Because these areas of the face are slightly recessed, they are shadowed. Illuminating them with concealer fills these darker hollows with light and makes them appear more plump. This technique also does wonders for the corners of the nose and the laugh lines.

A liquid or cream formula works best, so look for a concealer that comes in a tube or a pot. A stick is more dry and difficult to blend and will inevitably crease. I always apply concealer with a brush. The tips of the synthetic bristles act as an eraser for broken capillaries and red or brown spots on the face. You are literally painting away imperfections. Don't forget to use the back of your hand as a palette, dabbing excess product on it before carefully patting, brushing, and blending.

Remember always to wash your concealer brush after each use with a bit of hand soap or shampoo and warm water. Especially if you are using it to cover a blemish, the brush can spread bacteria. You should never touch a dirty brush to your face, particularly if it is close your the eyes or over already irritated skin.

COMMON MISTAKE

Blending concealer with your finger

Blending concealer with your fingertips seems much faster and easier, but is a big mistake. The oils and warmth from your hands emulsify the makeup and cause it to disappear into the skin. This is what you want from your foundation, but not from your concealer, which should provide more substantial coverage. Working with a brush allows you to layer and build up that coverage with control, whereas your fingers end up rubbing the concealer right off your face. You can also maneuver the tip of the brush into the inner corners of the eyes and right up to the lash line.

PROFESSIONAL TECHNIQUES

Applying foundation for a special event

Using a sponge to press foundation into the skin allows you to build up the makeup so it is not as translucent. This is why makeup artists use a sponge to apply foundation for film and television, or if someone's complexion is particularly uneven. It works well for times when you need more opaque coverage and a more dramatic look. Dampening the sponge (squeeze out all the excess moisture) makes blending easier and produces a more flawless finish.

Red carpet tip: Creating a luminous, "high definition" complexion

High-definition makeup is becoming popular for an immaculate, radiant finish. These cosmetics were designed to create on-camera perfection for high-definition television, which magnifies every flaw, including fine lines and large pores. The foundation contains light-reflecting properties that look natural and flattering on the skin while blurring imperfections. It is the cosmetic version of a soft-focus lens. However, you can create the same luminosity with a number of products, including mineral-powder foundation or a shimmer product that comes in a liquid, cream, or powder.

A great tip is to add a drop of liquid shimmer to your foundation to make it light-reflecting. You can also apply shimmer strategically. After applying your foundation and concealer, and while your skin is still moist, rub a tiny drop of liquid shimmer between your fingertips (just as you would with foundation). Pat it lightly over the tops of your cheekbones, top of the forehead, brow bone, and chin, and just touch the bridge of the nose. These are the points of the face that naturally come forward. If you prefer to use a powder shimmer instead, graze a tiny amount over the same areas after foundation and concealer have been set with a face powder. This adds a youthful, luminescent finish to the skin while softly highlighting and defining the features.

COLOR CORRECTOR

A color corrector is used to adjust and balance the skin tone. Not everyone needs this product—for many, a foundation and concealer are sufficient. A drop of liquid or cream color corrector can be mixed with the foundation (added to the actual product before the application) to neutralize redness in the skin or to warm a sallow complexion. It can also be put directly on the skin before the concealer is applied to color-correct a small area like dark circles under the eyes (peach cancels out blue/green) or to neutralize the color of a blemish. Color correctors work under the laws of basic color theory, specifically the concept that opposites on the color wheel cancel each other out. For example, the opposite of red on the color wheel is green. Therefore, someone with rosacea, too much pink in her skin, or redness around the nose can add a drop of green color corrector to neutralize the red. If the complexion is too yellow or sallow, a touch of lavender can be added.

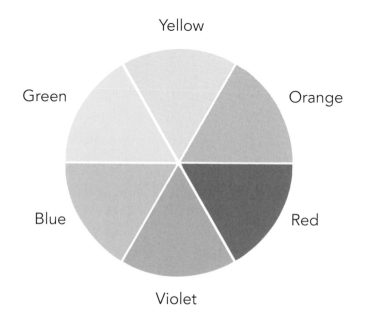

PROFESSIONAL TECHNIQUE

Covering up a blemish

Covering a blemish presents a slightly different challenge and demands a drier formulation that will stay put. This is when a stick concealer works perfectly. Use one that matches your skin tone or foundation color, and with your synthetic brush take a little bit of product at a time and tap it on with the tip. Using your finger or the stick itself just creates a big splotch around the blemish. If the spot is very red, you can dab on a tiny bit of green color corrector before applying the concealer. After covering the area, set it with a small amount of loose powder.

POWDER—TO SET

Loose powder absorbs moisture that has remained on the skin to create a dry, smooth surface upon which to apply color. Every woman needs two powders: a loose powder to set makeup and a compact powder for touch-ups and travel. Their textures are completely different, and a compact powder is too dense and heavy to set makeup. The finish from a finely milled, lightweight loose powder is much more natural. Women who have sensitive skin or acne should look for a talc-free formulation that will not clog the pores.

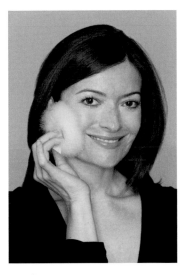

Powder—to set.

How to Choose the Right Shade

A colorless, translucent powder is always a safe bet, but you can also use a tinted powder for a subtle color correction. One that is slightly yellow will neutralize redness, and a powder with a hint of pink in it will warm and brighten a pallid complexion that has yellow or olive undertones. Tinted powders can be particularly flattering on certain skin tones. For instance, lavender is gorgeous on porcelain skin, a pure white powder can enhance a dramatic ivory complexion, while a rich bronze can warm and invigorate dark skin.

How to Apply

Almost everyone applies powder incorrectly, using a big fluffy brush to dust it all over the face. The powder ends up looking heavy and chalky and does not give good coverage. Powder should create an even, impercep-

PROFESSIONAL TECHNIQUE
Use a tinted face powder as a subtle blush

For women who don't like a lot of color on their cheeks or who blush naturally, I love to dust some pale pink face powder on the apples of the cheeks to subtly brighten, lift, and flush them. Because it adds just a hint of color, a tinted loose powder can also be used as a highlighter, applied high on the cheeks to make them pop or on very fair skin, when blush seems too bright. Darker skin looks gorgeous with a deep rose powder, which is a great way to bring a subtle, healthy glow to the complexion.

tible veil over the skin. Therefore, there is only one optimal way to apply loose powder to set makeup—with a velour or down powder puff. Dip the puff into the powder and tap it on the back of your hand. Press the puff into the face (do not rub!) and move it along until you have covered the entire face. This technique of pressing and setting the foundation and concealer is the best way to make foundation last. When you finish, your face will look way too powdery—almost like a mime. This is when you use a clean, fluffy powder brush to go over your entire face and remove the excess powder. (A powder brush should actually be called a "powder-removal brush.") This two-step powder method leaves you with the most natural and immaculate complexion.

BRONZER FOR ENHANCING BONE STRUCTURE

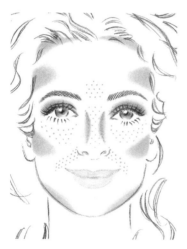

Highlighting and contouring.

—areas to highlight with concealer or a foundation two shades lighter than your skin tone.

—areas to contour with a matte bronzer or a pressed powder three to four shades darker than your skin tone.

Most people think of bronzer as something to pull out in the summertime to create a sun-kissed look on pale skin. Bronzer is actually more versatile and essential than you may think. I use a bronzer on most days, year-round, to warm and enliven my complexion and as an extraordinary contouring tool that helps enhance and define the bone structure.

It can be used in lieu of blush for women who have rosacea or who naturally have a lot of pink in their skin. The brown in bronzer can counteract some of the red tones and give the face a healthy glow without adding more pink.

Bronzers come in liquid, gel, and powder. Gels and liquids help to create a dewy, fresh look. If you prefer a classic matte finish, apply a dusting of bronzer after you have set your foundation with loose powder. It is really that simple. Always remember that once your skin has been powdered, you should not put gels, liquids, or creams on it.

HOW TO APPLY GEL, CREAM, OR STICK BRONZERS

Use the pads of your fingers to put on a liquid, stick, cream, or gel bronzer. I start on the nose (the first place where the sun naturally hits your face), then move to the cheeks, the brow bones, forehead, and hair-

OPTICAL ILLUSION

Shading the neck area

Some automatically dust a bronzer over the neck to shade and camouflage lines or sagging. However, bronzer used on the neck can sometimes end up looking a bit orange because the skin there is usually lighter than on the face. A better product to create the desired optical illusion is a pressed powder that is two to three shades darker than your skin. This is an old television technique that makeup artists used on news anchors to shade the neck and make it appear more streamlined on camera. You can also try using a darker foundation on the neck to gently shade under the jawline.

line, then around the chin and mouth, blending down the jaw area and into the neck. Your skin should still be moist, so the bronzer will be easy to blend. Another way to use liquid bronzer is to add a tiny drop directly to the foundation for an all-over golden color. Admittedly, liquid formulations can be tricky to work with, and I find that powder bronzers are much easier to control, particularly when used as a contour.

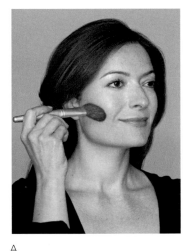

A

HOW TO APPLY POWDER BRONZER

I sometimes lightly dust bronzer all over as a final step, but more often I use it to create a contour effect under the cheekbones. This is the most amazing way to accentuate your cheekbones, or even to discover them for the first time! Slightly grin to make your cheekbones stand out and use an angled blush brush to sweep a small amount of matte (not shimmery) bronzer underneath them, in a C shape (photo A). I use this technique on almost everyone to define the cheekbones or to make a round face appear more angular. The same method can be used around the temples and hairline to make a prominent forehead look smaller (photo B), or at the jawline to make it look more defined. A darker color makes areas recede, just as a lighter shade (concealer, for instance) makes a feature stand out.

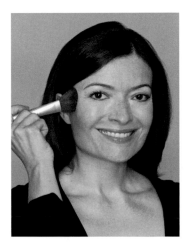

B

WHICH SHADE OF BRONZER SHOULD YOU CHOOSE?

Bronzers come in golden bronze, red-based brown, or pink-brown. Pink-browns are best for lighter skin tones, while the warmer red-orange bronzers are generally more flattering on darker skin. The best way to choose a bronzer, even if you're using it as a blush or contour (rather than to bring color to your entire face) is to match the color of your skin when it is naturally tan. For example, I do not tan very dark, so I stick with a lighter pink-brown bronzer. Those who tan easily can use a darker color like a terra-cotta brown.

EYEBROWS

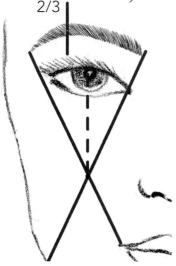

1. Draw an imaginary line from the center of your pupil to the apple of your cheek.
2. Place a ruler (or pencil) against this point and line it up with the inner corner of your eye (the bottom of the ruler will cross about an inch below the corner of your jawbone). Where the ruler ends along the brow bone is where the inner edge of your eyebrow should begin.
3. Place the ruler against the same point below the eye and angle it to the corner of your mouth. Where the ruler crosses your brow bone is where the outer edge of the eyebrow should end.
4. The arch of the eyebrow should be two-thirds of the way from the inner edge.

Eyebrows frame the eyes, enhance the eye shape, and add balance to the face, but they are often overlooked. Eyebrows are a permanent type of makeup, and when left unshaped or asymmetrical they have a profound effect on the facial structure. I define them before doing any eye makeup to clearly see the shape of the eye and have a better sense of how to contour it with makeup.

CREATING THE SHAPE: TWEEZING, WAXING, AND TRIMMING EYEBROWS

The ideal thickness and shape for your eyebrows depend on their natural form and your facial structure. You can sculpt a shape only from your original mold. So, if you are blessed with a substantial brow, you clearly have more options. The choice of brow shape also has a lot to do with your personal style. Some women may want a more natural look that requires minimal, simple grooming, while others prefer to have the sculpted, arched eyebrows that give their faces a more glamorous look.

Some eyebrows need shaping *and* coloring to get definition. I recommend having a professional create at least the initial eyebrow shape. Although I have met women who are quite adept at maintaining their own brows, there are many obstacles to doing so effectively that set almost everyone up for potential disaster. Many look into a magnifying mirror when tweezing, thinking that being able to see each hair will give them more accurate results. But this usually leads to overplucking. Up close, your eyebrows look enormous and furry, but later, when you look in a regular mirror, you may realize that you have overdone it. It is essential that you look at your face and eyebrows objectively and from a slight distance, which is also why it helps to have a professional lead the way.

Q&A

Q: *How can I keep my face from looking shiny when it's hot and humid?*

A: Rice-based powder is an absolute miracle product. It absorbs moisture better than any other kind of powder I have ever used. It is incredibly matte and keeps your face shine-free for hours. I have used it on photo shoots and in television for years. I also use it on myself, not just when I'm on television but when preparing for a dinner party and cooking in a hot kitchen. Because some of these formulations are very white and chalky, be sure to apply it sparingly. You can lightly dust it on as a final step to your makeup, or just dab some over your forehead and nose, where you tend to get the shiniest.

PROFESSIONAL TECHNIQUE

Waxing versus tweezing

Whether to wax or to tweeze is a frequently asked question when it comes to eyebrows. I prefer to create the shape using a slanted-tip tweezer because it allows for greater precision and a more individualized shape. When it comes to brows, one hair can really make a difference. Waxing is best for removing the fine, superfluous hairs under or on top of the brows. Many women ignore the blond peach fuzz that tends to form on the brow bone, thinking that it does not matter, since it's so fine. But these hairs absorb light and dull the skin. When they are removed, the smooth skin actually makes the eyes look more youthful. Even if you like a fuller, natural brow, this little bit of grooming can make a surprising difference—and it is faster to wax all those baby-fine hairs. However, when it comes to actually customizing a shape for the brows, waxing alone will not do the job. The result frequently ends up looking like a stencil, as opposed to the softer, more natural look that you get from tweezing the hairs individually.

To find a good brow expert, try to get a recommendation. When you notice a woman with especially well-shaped eyebrows, nine time out of ten she will have had them done by an expert. Ask her where she goes. Usually it will be a makeup artist or an aesthetician at a salon, a spa, or a makeup studio. (If she happens to do them herself, you will have made her day.) Some aestheticians are brilliant at shaping brows and some are not. Many makeup artists are proficient at this because the eyebrow is such a cosmetic feature. Remember, however, that just as with hair, your brow expert may have a different aesthetic than you do. Be sure to find somebody who is right for you and with whom you can easily communicate. For example, if you do not want overly arched brows, or much tweezing at all, that needs to be clearly conveyed before the work begins.

GROOMING YOUR BROWS

You can maintain your brow shape by tweezing stray hairs as they appear, but do not pluck anything that might affect the shape. However, if you feel confident enough to give do-it-yourself brow shaping a try, remember to take it one hair at a time and one row at a time, working inward from the outer ends. Do it in a systematic way, rather than tweeze hairs haphazardly here and there. Focus on the big picture and don't use a magnifying mirror, in which it is too easy to lose sight of the shape of the eyebrows in relation to your face. If you cannot see well without a magnifying mirror, you should not be doing your own eyebrows in the first place. Otherwise, be careful and take your time.

I strongly discourage women from trimming their own eyebrows. I notice that they usually overcut, making the brows look unnatural and severe. It is better to ask your hairdresser, aesthetician, or brow technician to trim them for you.

DEFINING AND FILLING IN YOUR BROWS

Some lucky women who have thicker eyebrows don't need to do anything once they have a nice shape in place, but for those with sparse or uneven brows, it is important to augment them with makeup. It is much easier to use a pencil than a powder to add more definition, a slightly stronger arch, or a bit more length. It is critical that the brow pencil is very sharp and that you work in short, feather-light strokes. The sharp point gives you complete accuracy and literally enables you to create fine, hairlike lines. Follow the natural shape of the brow, and accentuate with slight enhancements where it is clearly necessary. Be careful not to press too hard or draw a harsh line. Next, blend over the pencil strokes with a clean eyebrow brush to soften the pencil, then dust on a tiny amount of translucent powder to further take the edge off and integrate those

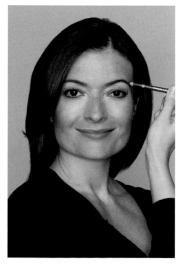

Eyebrow pencil to enhance the shape.

THE RULE

Never tweeze from the top of the brow.

THE RULE BREAKER: This is a common misconception that gets many people into trouble and is one of those myths that simply does not make practical sense. Many women start tweezing from the bottom and continue to go up until they are left with eyebrows that are too thin. Had they just tweezed one row off the top, they would have probably achieved the definition they were looking for. However, since most women simply don't know how to properly tweeze, such warnings have become the rule.

sketched lines into your brow hair. On sparse brows, I also apply an eyebrow powder after the pencil, using a stiff angled brush to better fill in and shade any empty spaces. The powder sticks to the waxy base from the pencil and produces a diffused, furrier brow. Powder alone, however, tends to appear chalky and creates too imprecise a line.

Brow pencils typically come in light, medium, and dark brown shades. It is usually safer to go a shade lighter than your natural color, since the pencil tends to appear darker once integrated into the hair. If you have cool-toned gray or dark hair, look for more of a graphite or slate shade. It will be much more natural-looking than a dark brown that tends to have more warmth to it. Redheads should use auburn or a natural, warm brown.

EYE SHADOW

Step One: Create the Canvas

When applying color to your eyelids, start with a clean canvas. This will give you a smooth surface to work on and neutralize any redness or darkness on the lid that may otherwise interfere with the eye-shadow color. I use the tiniest bit of foundation, which can be added there while you are applying it to the rest of your face. Use just the remnants from your fingertips (or sponge) to swipe over your lids. Set it with the slightest trace of powder, lightly pressing the powder puff onto the lids. This technique will also help to prevent the eye shadow from creasing.

Step Two: Perfect the Canvas

Select an eye shadow that is similar in tone and color to your skin (or slightly lighter) and dust it over the entire lid area—from the lashes to the crease of the eyelid. If you have green or yellow undertones in your skin, pale pink or peach looks beautiful. Someone with red undertones can stay with a more neutral cream or beige shade, while taupe or chocolate is flattering for darker skin. The goal is to brighten the lid without adding too much color. A dusting of one color may be all that you need for a clean, classic look.

Step Three: Add Definition

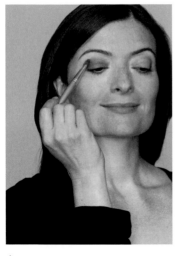

A

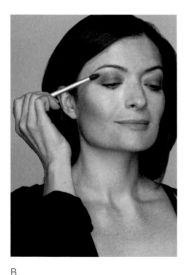

B

To create more shape and definition, you can use a second shadow that is a shade or two darker than the first one. This defining color can be a neutral tone, such as taupe, brown, gray, charcoal, or plum. Apply it with an eye-shadow brush that has a half-moon shape to hug the eyelid. First, tap the excess shadow off your brush; then, starting in the middle of the lid, work to the left and to the right with short downward strokes aimed toward the center of the lid (photo A). You can extend this color outward and beyond the lids to make the eyes appear larger (photo B). Another easy technique for definition is to use a fluffy eye-shadow brush to apply a darker shadow directly to the crease at the top of the eyelid. It is important to raise your eyebrow so that the lid is smooth and you can easily contour under the brow bone. Remember that you are using a small amount of pigment at a time. You can always layer on a bit more. Using numerous short brush strokes allows you to create a more blended look.

Q&A

Q: *Do I need an eyebrow gel to help tame or define my brows?*

A: This is an optional item that some women really love. I have found that gel can make the brow look too wet or shellacked and sometimes flakes by the end of the day. If you like using a gel, take any excess off the wand with a tissue before applying it. Generally, I find that simply brushing the brows with an eyebrow brush gives a suitably clean and polished look.

EYE LINER

Using a Pencil

FOR THE MOST NATURAL LOOK: Many women are confused about how to apply eyeliner, especially about how far to extend the line. The answer, especially for a daytime look, is simple: follow your natural lash line. It is essential to use a sharp eye pencil so you can work the point in between the roots of the lashes. You are not so much drawing a line as connecting the dots between each lash to make your lashes look more lush and accentuate the shape of your eye. If the pencil is too blunt, it will produce a thicker line that does not look as natural.

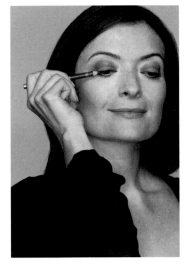

Using pencil eyeliner to frame the eye.

FOR MORE DEFINITION: Starting with a pencil that is a bit less pointy but still sharp, line above the top lash line. Begin in the very center and move the pencil point with the tiniest back-and-forth motion, as if you were sketching a miniature line between two points. Continue in this manner, connecting the points from the middle of the lash line to the outer corner and then back to the middle. Repeat this from the middle to the inner corner of the eye, just short of the tear duct, until you have an even line across your lashes. The line should be heavier at the outer than the inner corners. Starting in the middle, rather than on one end, provides you with a grounding center point to work from. It's the same idea as when you draw a heart on a piece of paper, beginning in the center and going to the right or left. Starting at either end of the eye tends to result in an uneven shape.

In terms of precision, using a lighted makeup mirror is the only way to really see what you are doing. This is especially helpful if you wear glasses and have to put them on and take them off repeatedly.

Choosing an Eyeliner Color

Eyeliner is meant to be an extension of your eyelashes, making them appear fuller near the base. Therefore, I always prefer to use a shade that matches the mascara. You cannot go wrong with dark brown or black eye pencil and liquid liner.

Using Liquid Eyeliner

If applied with a fine-hair brush, in an almost undetectable fashion, liquid liner can define the eye in a way that pencil alone cannot. As a woman ages, she begins to lose that definition around the eyes because her eyelashes are not as thick or dark as they used to be. A thin, dark line at the lashes creates depth and fullness, and always makes a woman look younger. I love to use a liquid liner day or night, in combination with a pencil, to soften the line and establish stronger definition of the eye.

Once you dip the thin eyeliner brush into your liquid liner, remove the excess from the edge of the brush back into the container. Then begin at the center of the top lash line and follow your pencil line to the outer corner of the eye, staying as close to the lashes as possible. With what remains on your brush, follow the line to the inner corner (where your lashes naturally end). The line should be barely visible at the inner corners of the eyes and more prominent at the outer corners.

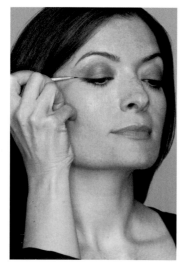

Glamorous "cat eye" created with liquid liner.

Cat Eye Liner

Crisp, clean eyeliner is glamorous, sophisticated, and timeless. This is my preferred technique for applying eye makeup, which has even become a personal signature. Some of you may think, "This look is not very daytime," but I don't care—I love it! Best of all, it is simple to execute once you get the hang of it. The pencil liner you already have on helps to establish the shape of the eye and will provide you with a clear guideline. It also softens the line if the liquid liner looks too harsh on its own.

STEP ONE: PAINT OVER THE PENCIL LINE WITH LIQUID LINER.

Use a thin eyeliner brush with brown or black liquid liner (again, swipe the excess from the sides of the brush first) to paint over the pencil line you learned how to make earlier, starting at the top center of the eye. Before you begin, tilt your chin up slightly and look down to create a flat eyelid surface. It also helps to gently raise your eyebrows to further smooth out the lid. Line from the middle to the outer corner, holding the brush at a diagonal, and extend the line ever so slightly at the end in one long stroke. Then, using the eyeliner that remains on the brush, follow the pencil line from the middle to the inner corner of the eye, stopping just short of it.

STEP TWO: ELONGATE AND WING OUT THE LINE.

Add a bit more liner to your brush, remove the excess, and make the extension at the outer corner. You are lengthening the line not straight out but slightly upward. On your right eye, aim between two and three o'clock, and on the left, aim between nine and ten o'clock. Do not pull your eye taut to do this or you will end up with an inaccurate line. I realize that trying to correctly angle the liner up and out at the corners can be frustrating when you first attempt it, but remember that practice does make perfect.

Smoky Eyes

Start with the traditional eye-makeup steps discussed earlier and intensify the look by adding a deeper shade right on top. This prevents the eye makeup from becoming too dark and messy. My aunt Jan loved big hair

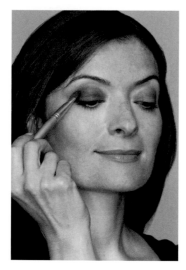

Create a smoky eye by applying dark shadow.

and lots of eye makeup. But even she was concerned about overdoing it and would always ask, "Is my eye makeup too dark, like two burned holes in a blanket?" You can avoid this by tapping the brush on the back of your hand before applying the makeup to leave only a trace of shadow on your brush. You can always add more if you need to. It is better to build the color a little bit at a time rather than all at once.

STEP ONE: ADD A RICHER EYE SHADOW.

Since you already have a nice base to work with, just add a plum, navy, charcoal, espresso, or even a soft black eye shadow over the entire lid, blending it up toward the crease. This one addition will instantly make your eyes appear more dramatic.

STEP TWO: BUILD UP THE EYELINER.

Use your eye pencil to go over the line that has already been drawn, making it a bit heavier and not so sharp. Instead of a fine, thin line at the base of the lashes, it should now be thicker and more diffused. Once the darker shadow is applied, it is easier to gauge how thick your liner should be to balance it out and keep the eye makeup in proportion. Connect the top and bottom lash lines by filling in the outer corners of the eyes. For an even more smoldering effect, you can also line the inside rim of the lower lash line. For this, I would use a brown rather than a black pencil. It is softer and easier for most women to carry off.

PROFESSIONAL TECHNIQUE

Blending eye makeup

If your eyes end up looking too dark or messy, blend the makeup with a clean, fluffy eye-shadow brush to reduce the amount of shading. If you feel that it still looks too heavy under your eyes or starts to accentuate dark circles, you might want to skip the liner on the bottom and keep all the drama on the top. If your eyes look slightly top heavy, balance them out with a more neutral eye-shadow color at the lower lash line, which helps pull it all together. To prevent eye shadow from landing under your eye or cheekbone, hold a folded tissue there as you work—it will catch any sprinkles.

STEP THREE: SMUDGE THE LINER.

Use a compact blender brush with a little bit of the dark shadow and press it right on top of your pencil line, working it into the top and bottom lash lines.

Lining Underneath the Eyes

There are a few techniques for lining the lower lash line. This is where you can get a little more creative with color. A touch of green underneath the lashes is especially gorgeous on redheads, a plum hue is flattering on brunettes, and a soft gray can look great on a blonde. Using a lighter color, like a gray or taupe, across the lower lashes is more forgiving than rimming the entire eye with dark brown or black, which can enclose the eye and make it appear smaller. In fact, a lighter shade on the bottom lash line, paired with dark brown or black on the top, can open up the eyes and make them look larger.

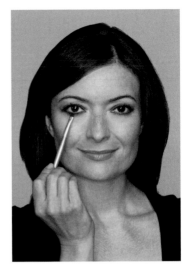

Blending the shadow to define the lower lash line.

PROFESSIONAL TECHNIQUE

Eye makeup shades to enhance your eye color

BROWN EYES: Cream, taupe, rich chocolate and espresso browns, plum, indigo, pale pinks and peaches, bronze, gold.
GREEN EYES: Taupe, light to medium browns, deep forest green, olive, bronze, plum, peach, gold.
BLUE EYES: Pale pinks, dark navy, taupe, chocolate, gray, lavender, silver.
HAZEL EYES: Cream, taupe, light to medium chocolate, olive, forest green, bronze, gold.

THE RULE
A blue pencil will enhance the color of blue eyes.

THE RULE BREAKER: This is a common belief, but nothing enhances blue eye color more than brown or taupe, because these neutral shades do not compete with it. People will notice the blue of your eyes, as opposed to your blue eyeliner.

Making your eyes appear bigger

Try using a white or peach-tone pencil on the inner lash line. It helps to visually extend the white of the eyes and make them look larger.

Some women believe that liner under their eyes is an absolute necessity, while others don't like it at all because they feel it smudges too easily and looks raccoon-like. You have to experiment and see what is right for you, but realize that lining under the eyes does not have to result in a dark, heavy look. Consider these simple options:

1. Use the same defining eye shadow that you applied on your crease and smudge it as close to the lower lashes as possible with a small eye-shadow brush.
2. Take what is left on your liquid-liner brush and trace the faintest thin line across the lower lash line. There should be almost nothing left on the brush, and you just tickle it underneath the base of the lower lashes. Then use a clean brush to soften that delicate line. A powder shadow or the tiniest bit of liquid liner will be more smudge-proof than a pencil.
3. If you're using a pencil, place a small dot in between each lash, just as you did on the top lash line. You can connect the top and bottom lines in the outer corners of the eyes for a more dramatic effect.

Making Final Adjustments

Defining the brows, lining the eyes, shading the lids, and intensifying the lashes all work to enhance the shape of your eyes. Only when completely finished with your eye makeup can you take a step back to get a clear perspective on what may need adjusting. Step one foot away from the mirror and assess your work.

MASCARA AND FALSE LASHES

The quest for the perfect mascara is universal. We either buy the latest formulation or stick to an old faithful but wish that it did more. I certainly have never found one product that could meet all my professional or personal expectations. Some mascara is better at lengthening, while another is great for thickening the lashes. After experimenting with mixing mascaras and using different brushes, what I discovered completely changed the way I apply mascara to my clients' and my own lashes.

I layer two different formulas together, one for thickening and one for lengthening. The results of this dual-mascara technique are incredible, creating fuller, darker, curled, and lifted lashes. Use the fuller wand for the first mascara (thickening) and the finer wand for the second (lengthening) to define and comb through the lashes. The use of two different brushes makes an enormous difference, as does the technique with which you use them.

How to Apply Mascara

Mascara is the one makeup item that almost every woman uses daily, but few know how to maximize its potential. Hold the fuller mascara wand horizontally at the very base of your lashes and wiggle it ever so slightly to the left and the right. Concentrate the mascara at the base, pushing and lifting the roots before beginning to brush outward and extending it to the ends. Use a thinner wand to apply a coat of the second mascara before the first coat dries. This separates the lashes and prevents clumping. You can work with mascara only when the lashes are wet and pliable, and you have to integrate the two mascaras together, not just put one on top of the other. I will take this opportunity to dispel the myth that you need to let mascara dry before putting on another coat. Applying wet mascara over dry mascara results in clumpy, spider-like lashes. So do not go from one eye to the other and back again. Keep working over the lashes of the same eye until you are happy with the results and then move on to the other eye.

PROFESSIONAL TECHNIQUES

Creating optical illusions with eye makeup

- For eyes that are close set, lighten the area at the inner corners of the upper lids to create the illusion of more space and width there. You can brush on a light eye shadow or blend a shimmery pencil or powder just below the tear duct.
- Extending the defining shadow slightly up and outward will help make the eyes appear more doe-shaped and wider set.
- If you have the opposite problem and your eyes are wide set, blend that defining shadow in the crease a bit more toward the nose. This will create some shading that brings the eyes closer together.

While the lashes are still slightly damp, gently comb through them with an eyelash comb or an eyebrow brush. This separates them and blends the mascaras even more. Whatever mascara is left on that brush can then be lightly skimmed over the bottom lashes. This is a terrific way to define the lower lash line and have it look natural.

Should You Always Wear Black?

Black mascara is usually the first choice for most woman but brown can be a wonderful alternative for many. With eye shadow, liner, and defined brows, you do not have to rely on black mascara to make your eyes stand out. Dark brown mascara can look very fresh, young, and softer for daytime. Finding the right brown is key: it should have an undertone of red in it if you are a redhead, while blondes or strawberry blondes should try an ash brown. A brunette who wants a more understated look can opt for a rich brown/black. Women who naturally have very dark hair or eyelashes look best with basic black.

Curling Your Lashes

Many makeup artists consider curling the lashes the standard, but I believe this is an optional step, which I have found to be less important when I effectively work the base of the lashes with two kinds of wands and mascaras. I stopped curling mine when I started using this technique and my lashes always look lifted and curled.

Many women are afraid to use a lash curler—perhaps because it looks like a medieval torture device or because they have used one of poor quality that pulled out their eyelashes. While it is not for everyone and is not always necessary, once in a while it's nice to curl your eyelashes,

COMMON MISTAKE

How to work with frosted eye shadow

Be cautious when using a frost, which is not the same as shimmer. A frost is heavily pigmented and more opaque. Because it is not as sheer as a shimmer, it absorbs light and can make the lines on the eyelid more pronounced. You should use less of it, keeping it just on the center of the lid or the inner corners of the eyes. If you see that it is making fine lines appear, switch to a shimmer.

particularly for a special event or a night out. Combined with the lifting and curling produced by the dual-mascara technique, it can give you the effect of natural-looking false lashes.

To curl your lashes safely and easily, open the jaw of the curler and place your lashes inside *before* applying mascara. Set the curler at the base of your lashes and depress it gently for about five to seven seconds. It helps to look down slightly as you do this; if you look straight ahead or move your eyes or lid, you may inadvertently tug on your lashes.

Applying False Lashes

Once, I found my grandma Wright smacking our kitchen counter with a flyswatter. "Spiders!" she exclaimed. When I got closer, I saw that they were actually my mother's false eyelashes! While they look creepy when detached, I love false eyelashes. To me, perfectly applied lashes are the epitome of glamour. They can even be appropriate to wear during the day if done right. The trick is not to use a full strip of lashes. Cut a strip into two or three pieces and place one on the outer edge of your lashes. If done correctly, it will not look over-the-top. Cutting a full strip into smaller sections is much easier and more manageable than attaching individual false lashes.

You will need a pair of slanted tweezers. Most use their fingers to apply them, but this can become frustrating, since your hand gets in the way while you are attaching the lashes. Put a tiny drop of hypoallergenic eyelash glue

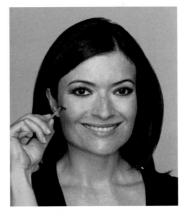

Step 1: When applying false eyelashes, start by cutting the strip in half.

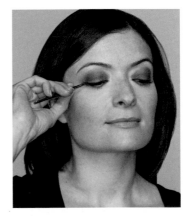

Step 2: Attach to outer corner of lash line.

Items to keep in your makeup bag

- Pressed powder
- Powder foundation (mineral powder optional)
- Travel powder brush
- Sample-size eye cream (if you feel dehydrated around the eyes)
- Cotton swabs (to clean under the eyes)
- Small bottle of spray-on toner
- Concealer
- Lip balm
- Mascara
- Bronzer
- Blush
- Lip liner/lipstick/lip brush/lip gloss

(available in most drugstores) on the back of your hand. Use the end of your tweezers or an orangewood stick to paint a thin coat of the glue onto the flat edge of the lash strip. The amount of glue should be so small that it looks as if you might not have enough. Using less glue allows it to dry faster and makes for a much cleaner application. With the tweezers, place the lash section at the outer corner and allow it to set for about ten seconds. Then, gently press it into the lash line with the tweezers to seal it. I apply a very light coat of mascara before attaching the corner lashes. You should wear less mascara with false lashes—you simply don't need as much.

HOW TO APPLY A FULL STRIP OF FALSE LASHES: When using a full strip of lashes, always add them *after* a light coat of mascara and eyeliner. Hold the lash strip with your tweezers and slightly bend it between two fingers before applying the glue. This makes the flat, straight strip easier to mold to the curvature of your lash line. With an orangewood stick, run the tiniest trace of glue along the strip and position it on your lash line with the tweezers. Make sure to tilt your chin slightly upward (you may need to reposition the mirror), so that the eyelid is smooth when you apply the strip. Aim for the center of your eye with the middle of the false eyelash, then attach each corner. Use the tweezers or orangewood stick to gently press the corners of the strip into the lash line for about ten seconds. Apply pressure where necessary, especially if the corners are flipping up. Try your best to keep the eye still and blink as little as possible so that the strip can dry. Once it is attached, you can use just a trace of liquid liner on top of the false lashes. This helps to integrate the base of the lash strip at the seam of the lash line and hides any visible adhesive. Apply any additional mascara just at the base of your lashes. Avoid brushing mascara through the false lashes. It is not necessary, and if you keep the lash strip clean, you should be able to reuse it.

Using less mascara and working it mainly at the base is how not to go overboard with this look. The lashes that you choose are also important. Generally, you don't want the lashes to be too long, but it really comes down to what you feel comfortable with. Some women can carry off lashes that take them into showgirl territory, while others would never even think of it. You can also gently trim a strip of lashes yourself by making tiny V-shaped cuts (the point-cutting method from chapter 1) into the ends with a pair of manicure scissors. (Of course, do this before the lash strip is applied.) However, it is just as easy to find shorter-length lashes—there are many beautiful options available. Finally, consider the color of the lash strip. For a softer and more natural look, I love to use false lashes that are brown in combination with dark brown mascara.

LIP COLOR

Lips are the easiest feature to enhance. A lip gloss or lipstick is undoubtedly the makeup product that most women would not leave home without. Chances are that it was the first beauty item you ever tried and is the one you buy more of than any other. It's no wonder that lipstick is such a popular impulse purchase—it has the power to make you feel better instantly.

Most women put lipstick on throughout the day, almost unconsciously and usually straight from the tube. But if you use a more thoughtful, professional approach to your application, the extra effort will be worth it.

Step One: Prepare your lips.

Lip color should be applied to a moisturized, smooth surface. Otherwise the product will overly absorb into the lips and appear dark, uneven, and too saturated with pigment. Lips have no oil glands, so we depend on lip balm to keep them hydrated. You can exfoliate and moisturize your lips as part of your nightly routine (see page 186). Before applying lipstick or gloss, put on a very thin layer of natural lip balm to create a smooth base for lip color.

COMMON MISTAKE

Neglecting your smile

Whereas certain shades of lipstick make the teeth look whiter and brighter, some women rely on this optical illusion but neglect the actual shade of their teeth. There is a reason why you see beautiful pearly-white teeth on actresses and models—it makes them look healthy, vibrant, and younger! Whether you have yours professionally whitened or use whitening strips or a custom-made tray, it does not have to entail a big investment and will make an amazing difference in your overall appearance.

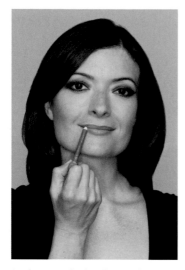

Lip liner applied with pencil to enhance shape.

Step Two: Line your lips with a pencil.

Lip liner keeps lipstick intact and increases its longevity. The real beauty of using a lip pencil, however, is that it enhances the shape of your lips, adding definition and depth to make them look fuller. This is why you need only one lip pencil in a shade that matches the natural color of your lips, extending them and accentuating their shape without that awful ring of a dark liner that tends to remain after the lipstick has partly worn off. In addition, a liner color that matches the lipstick can make the overall color look too dark and saturated once the lipstick goes over it. Most women have a pale pink, rose, plum, or natural brown tone to their lips. Beware of nude lip pencils that are too muddy or mauve—they can make your lips look deathly and unnatural.

Always work with a sharpened pencil. A blunt tip produces a thicker, blurred line. To avoid drawing a hard line, use light, sketching strokes, as opposed to the heavy-handed way you would use a pen. The pencil should be almost dancing along the lip, tickling it across the surface so as not to leave a heavy line. Holding the pencil more loosely and at a slight angle helps to achieve those light, feathery strokes. Begin at the top of the heart (or the Cupid's bow) of your lips and work from there to either end of the upper lip. Then, move to the center of the lower lip and line to the left and to the right. As when lining your eyes, starting at the center point helps to keep the shape even on both sides. Follow your natural lip line and adjust the liner where you need to even it out or to extend the line slightly so that your lips appear fuller. You can also fill in the lips, sketching lightly inside the original outline. This provides a more saturated, pigmented effect and helps the lip color, and/or lip gloss to stay on longer.

BEAUTY SECRET

How to make a nude lipstick wearable

A pale, flesh-toned lipstick can easily look pasty and flat. This is where lip gloss comes in handy. A great tip is to top a nude lip color with a sheer pink gloss. The transparency of the gloss enlivens a beige shade without altering it too much. Keep in mind that if you wear a nude lip color, you will have to compensate with color elsewhere in order not to look washed out—perhaps with stronger eye makeup and a little more blush or bronzer.

Step Three: Apply color with a brush.

Using a lip brush enables you to apply the finest, sheer layer of pigment evenly and precisely, and to blend it with the lip liner for a seamless finish. You cannot create such detail (and the details always make the look) when you spread a lipstick on from the tube (the wand of a lip gloss does give more accuracy). If you do not feel that it's realistic to reapply your lipstick with a brush throughout the day, at least do it for the initial application. My best friend, Lynn, always applies her lipstick this way and it looks so ladylike and cool! Try it—you will be amazed at the difference. This is another reason why your makeup looks so great when a pro does it—we always use a brush.

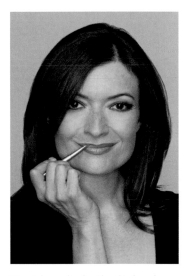

Lipstick applied with a lip brush.

Which Kind of Lip Color Formulation Is Best?

Most women have tried a myriad of different products and know the shades and textures to which they usually gravitate. There are many to choose from: tinted balms, glosses, stains, satin lipsticks, and matte formulas. As always, the choice is a matter of personal preference. One of my favorites for daytime is a transparent lipstick, which is more sheer. Its texture is that of a thinner, more natural lipstick. With a lip pencil application underneath, I have found this product to have longevity and to give a more polished and sophisticated look than a lip gloss. Matte lipsticks are even longer-lasting. Most important, remember that almost anything applied properly is going to look great.

How to Pull Off a Classic Red Lip

Red is bold, glamorous, and sexy. It always makes a statement and is easier to apply and wear than you might think, as long as you know the professional technique. First, it is important to consider the big picture when you are adding drama and color to the face. For example, doing a dark, smoky eye and a red lip may be too much. A red lip paired with a natural eye and crisp black liner is sophisticated and powerful on its own. By the same token, you should also wear a little less bronzer and blush with red lipstick. (A warm apricot or peach will be more understated and will complement red lips better than a pink blush.) Getting the right balance of drama and color is key.

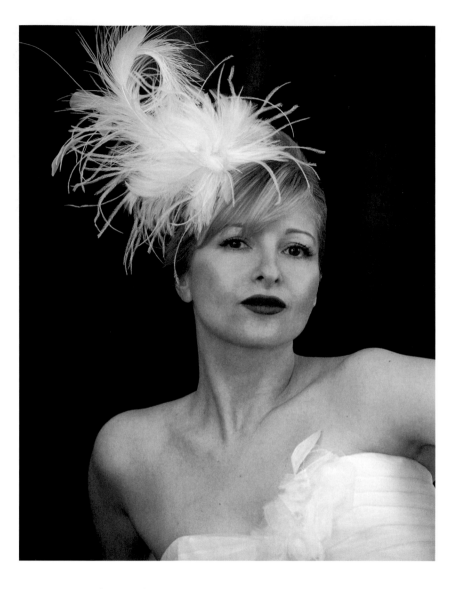

Line your lips with a natural-color lip pencil and apply a red color with a brush, blending it into the edges of the liner. To keep the color from feathering, you can use a small brush to skim the faintest amount of translucent powder around the border of the lip. Personally, I do not like to add a gloss on top, which somehow cheapens an elegant red lip.

Choosing the Right Red

Every woman wants to find the perfect red lipstick for her complexion, but almost everyone is confused by this process. It is actually very simple and depends on your skin tone.

- Porcelain, fair skin with pink undertones: blue-based red (see Lynn, opposite)
- Fair to medium complexion with a yellow undertone: brown-based red—A, or a rich true red—B
- Natural redheads: orange-based and clear-toned red—C
- Medium to dark with red undertones: brown-based red, dark cherry (not too bright)—D
- Medium to dark with yellow or olive undertones: deep Bordeaux, rich ruby—E, and darker true red

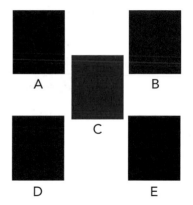

BLUSH: *The Finishing Touch*

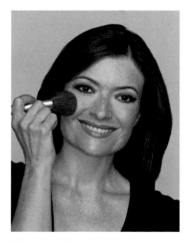

Blush to add color.

Blush is somewhat magical in the way it can instantly make you look healthier, well rested, and more youthful. Choosing the right blush formulation depends on your preference for either a dewy complexion or a more traditional matte finish. For the latter, a powder is by far the easiest to work with, especially as a last step when your face is already set with a face powder.

If you prefer a dewy complexion, do not apply any face powder to your cheeks (use it just on your T-zone). Then you can use a cream or stick blush that will be compatible with moist skin. Start with the blush on your fingertips and rub the fingers of both hands together to evenly distribute the product. Next, gently press the pads of your fingers to your cheeks, starting at the apples. Pat and blend the color up the cheekbones.

Most consider blush the primary way of bringing color to the face and typically apply it too early in the process. When putting on your blush first, it is easy to misjudge how much you need, and you can end up with too much color by the time your makeup is done. For this reason, leave blush until the end, after your eye and lip makeup has been applied. Otherwise, if you have decided to wear more eye makeup or a bright lip, it can suddenly look as if you're wearing too much. Or some natural red or pink tones in your skin are peeking through the foundation, and you realize that you don't need much blush at all. Treating blush as an accent and applying it last will help your makeup look more harmonious.

Choosing the Right Blush Color

Blush is meant to mimic the natural flush of your skin, so keep this in mind when choosing the shade. Many women look good with a pop of pink on their cheeks. Pink-rose is a universally flattering color for lighter complexions, while a deeper rose/brown looks great on darker skin. The exception is for those with too much natural red or pink in their skin, in which case a muted apricot shade, a soft brown, or a bronzer, can be a great alternative. These tones can also work well for women with a warmer hair color, such as red, chestnut brown, or honey blonde. For darker skin tones, some good options are deeper shades like cognac, berry, plum, or wine.

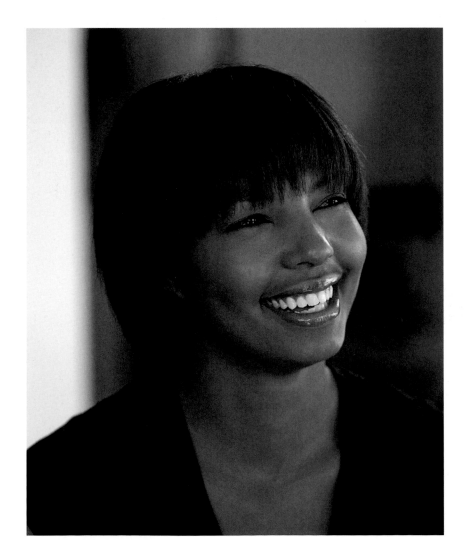

Danyelle is wearing a soft, terra-cotta blush.

Opposite: My mother, Saundra, 1963.

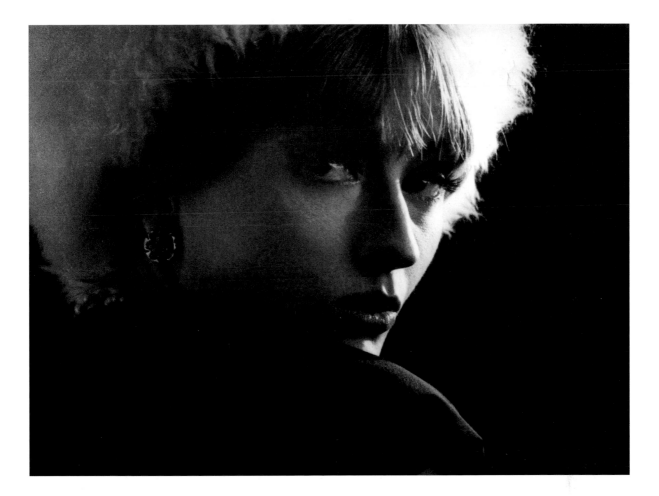

Professional Technique

Refreshing your makeup

With a few essentials stashed in your desk drawer or cosmetics bag, it is easy to touch up your makeup midday or before going out for the evening. Keep a small container of spray-on toner that you can mist over your face (you can also use water). When the skin is damp, use your fingertips to blend any areas where makeup may have settled, such as under the eyes, around the nose, and at the laugh lines. Next, reapply a tiny bit of concealer under the eyes or wherever you need it. Remember to not use a concealer on dry skin, which can look cakey. This is when a compact powder foundation or a mineral powder comes in handy. Brush it on with your travel brush, adding a bit more coverage, since some of your makeup will have worn off. A brush gives a lighter finish than a puff and allows you to use less product. If any eye makeup has smudged, use a cotton swab with a drop of concealer to clean it up. You might also want to add some color with a little bronzer, blush, or lip color.

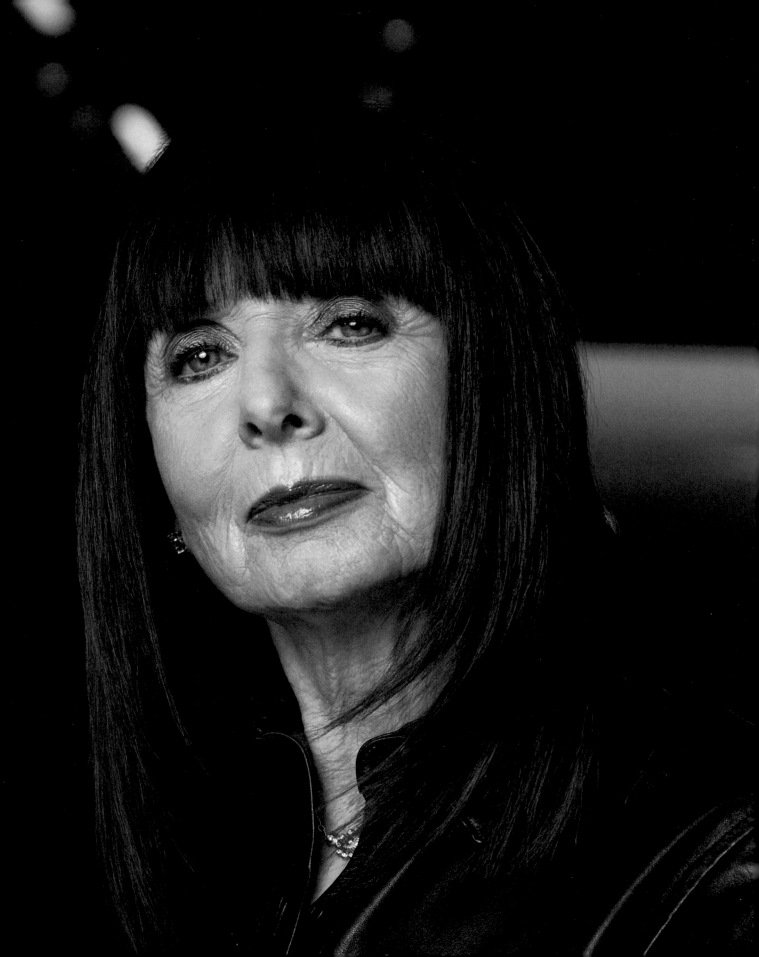

8
AGELESS MAKEOVERS
WHY CAN'T YOU?

The only real elegance is in the mind; if you've got that, the rest really comes from it.

—DIANA VREELAND

Legendary fashion icon and magazine editor Diana Vreeland penned a famous column in *Harper's Bazaar* titled, "Why Don't You?" The outlandishly chic Vreeland would suggest to readers: "Why don't you rinse your blond child's hair in champagne to keep its gold, as they do in France?" Or, "Why don't you turn your old ermine coat into a bathrobe?" I applaud her eccentrically glamorous advice and attitude, although it may have been shocking for some. Instead, I ask, "Why can't you?" Why can't a woman be stylish and a little daring after a certain age? Are we supposed to be frumpy after fifty? I definitely don't think so, and in this chapter I set out to prove that beauty is within the reach of every woman and to refute some "rules" about beauty and aging.

Sadly, age is used to narrow a woman's options in life, and too many women fall into the trap of believing that they are defined by their age, that it should slow them down or stop them from having fun, going out on a limb, or being adventurous with their life and their looks.

Maddie, age seventy.

These constraining societal attitudes serve only to pigeonhole people, often creating a self-fulfilling prophecy. If you expect to no longer be dynamic, to lose your sex appeal, or to develop health problems, then it may very well happen. *Do not buy into it*. There is no reason why you cannot be just as alluring, sexy, exciting, active, and healthy as ever, perhaps even more so!

The key to ageless beauty is a state of mind—a youthful flexibility, both physical and mental. Young people have a more malleable mind-set, but as we get older we are often gripped by the fear of change and of trying new things. The onset of this rigidity is when people start to think and act old. It is a stronger sign of the aging process than wrinkles or gray hair. New ideas, new learning experiences, and new challenges are part of the ebb and flow of life; being able to roll with it is what prevents "old age" from setting in. The best attitude to have about getting older is either to ignore it or to embrace it, but try not to be defined by a number. You are not alone—this is a universal challenge, as we are all getting older. Be more forgiving, open, and caring with yourself through each stage of life. Beauty might shift and look a bit different from what it used to be, but it never goes away. You are not the same girl you were at twenty—you are actually much better now, with all the experience and wisdom that you have gained.

So many wonderful things have come to me through the years, and time has brought much beauty into my life. With every year, I have become wiser and more compassionate, I have worked hard and become more successful, and I have learned many important life lessons. I appreciate my relationships more and have a deeper connection to others, along with a greater understanding of myself than I had when I was younger. I take even greater joy in my work, have more gratitude for my family, and get more pleasure from a big laugh with friends than ever before. I am much more appreciative of the woman I have become because the process of getting here has been so enriching.

It is in that spirit that I want to dispel paradigms about beauty that society, culture, fashion, and media impose on women—especially as they mature. This attitude pulls a woman further away from the unique person she has become. One such "rule" is that a woman should cut her hair short at a certain age. There are plenty of women I know personally who have proved this to be wrong. If you want to keep your hair long, then by all means do it! It can look beautiful on you, but the right haircut is crucial. The bottom length is actually inconsequential if you have a strong structure and shape within the haircut. This becomes even more important as the planes of the face change and the bone structure is less pronounced. With the right layers around the face and enough lift in the crown, long hair does not have to drag your face down or make you look older. Quite the opposite—it can make you sexy and more youthful.

Another myth is that as women age, they need to go much lighter with their hair color. Many women lighten their hair in an attempt to hide grays more effectively, but the shade often turns into a midrange blond-beige that washes out the complexion and makes them look tired. This drab, flat hair color, ironically, ages a woman. If being a brunette feels more like you, then you should not have to go lighter. You can still maintain a rich chocolate shade and maybe add a few highlights around the face to soften the hair color and help camouflage grays at the hairline. If the contrast between the dark hair and your complexion is too stark (which can be aging to the face), dusting a bronzer onto the skin can compensate for a lack of color. Lightening the eyebrows slightly will also brighten and soften the face. Details like these make the components of your personal brand of beauty come together and work for you.

The transformations in this chapter and the women featured break the paradigms of beauty. All of them (except Alex) are my clients. Some have been coming to me for so long that there are no "before" photos. Others have started seeing me more recently. I hope that they help to emancipate you from tired stereotypes and inspire you to escape a beauty rut that no longer serves you. Subtle changes in a woman's appearance can also affect her in ways that are more intangible and sometimes surprising, such as liberating her with a renewed sense of confidence. It is that combination of a positive attitude and self-image, along with a fresh new look, that makes a woman truly beautiful. It is never too late to feel great about how you look.

BEAUTY SECRETS

Five Golden Rules to Looking Younger

1. Have a few highlights placed around your hairline to help camouflage emerging gray hair and brighten your complexion.

2. Do not apply heavy powder under your eyes (if necessary, use a puff with just a trace of powder on it). Powder collects in the creases around the eyes and can look "crepey."

3. Apply a dual-finish makeup (a powder foundation) that is one shade lighter than your skin tone, around the corners of your nose and your laugh lines. This will help to bring light and give more coverage to the areas that naturally recede.

4. Create more height to your hair at the crown of your head. This lengthens your silhouette by an inch or two and makes for a more feminine look.

5. Stand up straighter, smile, and think about beautiful things. Others can see and feel your energy, and energy *is* beauty. Try it and everyone will notice!

Maddie (chapter opener)

Whenever Maddie comes to the salon, I am always impressed by her sense of style. Classic, yet a bit avant-garde, she wears elegant jewelry and great boots with slim jeans tucked in. The day of the shoot, she also wore a chic leather blouse. At seventy, Maddie is a mother of three, a grandmother, and has been married for more than forty years. I had always wondered about her age but had never asked until I invited her to be in this book. Maddie is a rule breaker not only in her fashion sense and personality but because her shoulder-length hair is a chestnut brown and worn with a dramatic bang. She blows out her naturally curly hair straight and polishes it with a flat iron—yet another rule breaker, since older women are taught that they should not wear their hair too straight. Maddie actually did her own makeup that day, and I thought she looked great, with her standard smoky eye shadow with blue eyeliner and a bright coral lipcolor.

Ruth

The day I met Ruth, I was so delighted to have her in my chair! She is a best-selling author, an editor, and a renowned food critic. Ruth's genuine nature showed in her warm personality, while the way she dressed and carried herself made her age a mystery. She loves her hair long and dark, which suits her feminine and somewhat bohemian style. It is cut in triangular layers and colored an espresso brown. I used a palette of soft pinks and roses to warm her complexion. At sixty-two, Ruth is passionate about her work and inspired by her life. She is the epitome of ageless beauty.

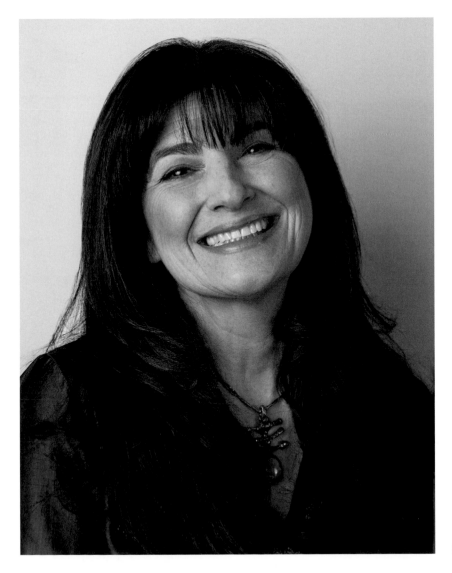

Ruth, age sixty-two.

Joy

Joy is the quintessential rock star: she's a singer, songwriter, and voice coach who has been making music for most of her life. At fifty-seven, she rides her bicycle all over Manhattan and Brooklyn, is active and energetic, and is clearly not defined by her age. Her hair is cut in concave layers, balayaged, and glazed. The makeup is neutral, using the lightest bronzer with a taupe eye shadow and a pinky-beige lipstick and gloss. Raised in England, she tells me how she loves to keep her "fringe" long. I met Joy on a shoot fifteen years ago, when I did her hair and makeup for an album cover of her band, Echo, and she has been coming to me ever since. She is just as beautiful today and continues to sing and play in her band all over the world.

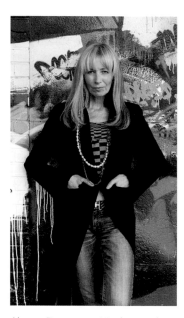

Above: Downtown Manhattan the day of the shoot.
.

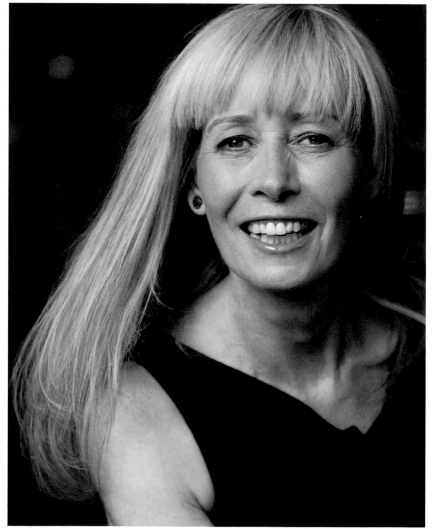

Joy, age fifty-seven.

Freddi

When I first met Freddi, she told me, "I'm in your hands." I saw her with something softer and more feminine and recommended that she grow her hair longer to give it more movement (although many women are under the misconception that gray hair should be cut short). It took some time to achieve this triangular layered cut that suits her perfectly. I also changed her makeup palette to cool tones, using a slate eye shadow and blue-pink blush and lipstick color, and shaped her eyebrows. I felt that her natural silver hair looked beautiful and could be enhanced even more with a glaze. At sixty-one, Freddi feels she is in the prime of her life! For many years she had balanced raising a family with her work as editor in chief of several national magazines. She now finally has the time to take care of herself by working out regularly and leading a healthy lifestyle, while contemplating her next business venture.

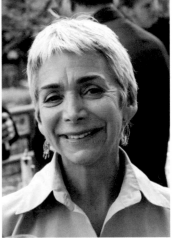

Above: Before.

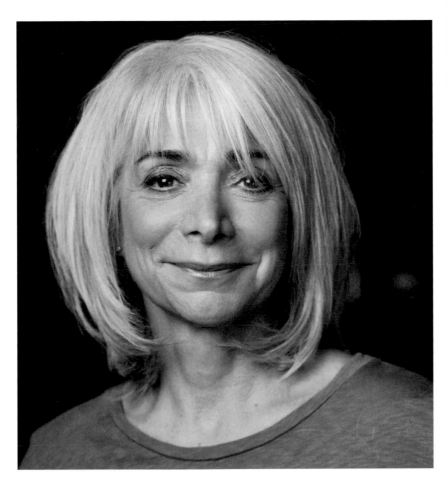

Freddi, age sixty-one.

Jyll

Jyll has been a longtime client. She prefers to wear her naturally wavy hair straight. When she first came to me, she asked for a lot of movement in her hair without sacrificing its length. Most important, she did not want the style to look boring. The cut I chose for her is my signature The UnCut, which allows her to maintain a longer length with a strong shape. The subtle golden highlights painted onto her chestnut brown color add dimension to the cut. The diamond-shaped layers were done with a razor to remove excess bulk around the bottom of the cut and add height to the crown of the head. Her makeup palette of pinks and peaches imparts warmth to her skin and balances its yellow undertone. At fifty-eight, after a long tenure as the senior vice president of advertising at *The New York Times*, Jyll is pursuing her passion for cooking and has recently graduated from a culinary institute.

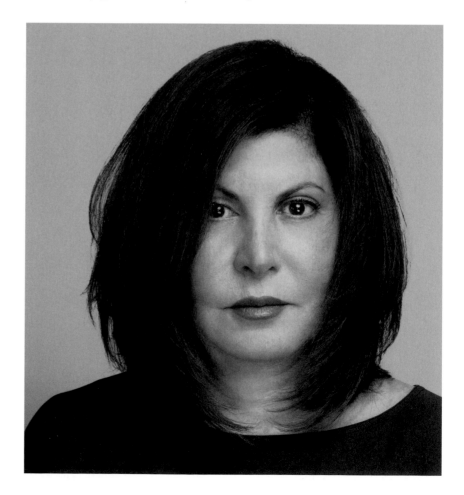

Jyll, age fifty-eight.

Joy

Having come to me as a former brunette, Joy was ready to embrace her natural gray after years of coloring her hair. However, she was afraid that the short hair that remained after having the colored ends cut off would make her look older. I explained that with a great cut a woman can look chic at any age, regardless of the hair length. When gray, the cut becomes even more important, since short hair can range from mumsy to sexy, depending on its shape. I cut her hair with a razor to make it look more modern and youthful, and reminded her that she is not gray but white, which is closer to platinum blond! Her makeup is soft and natural with pale pinks and smoky eye shadow to enhance the deep brown of her eyes. Joy loved her new hair so much that she decided to stay with the shorter length. When she comes to me for haircuts, I use a violet-based glaze to remove any yellow that naturally occurs in white hair. At sixty-two, Joy feels liberated and wishes that she had done this sooner!

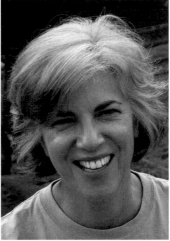

Above: Before.

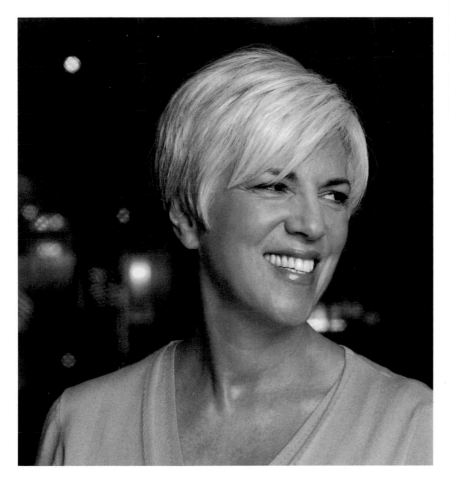

Joy, age sixty-two.

Carolyn

I have been cutting and highlighting Carolyn's hair for years and have always admired her casual downtown style. She likes to wear her hair choppy and undone. Before meeting me, she even cut it herself because she did not want it looking too "perfect." I used a razor to cut her fine, midlength layers. Her makeup palette is her signature dark eyeliner and pale pink lips. An entrepreneur and a culture aficionado, she is my go-to girl for recommendations on everything from theater to restaurants. I was inspired by her ageless style and sensuality and asked her to be in this book. Even though I had known Carolyn for years, I would never have guessed that she is seventy. Her attitude, active lifestyle, and the time she spends with her grandchildren have kept her looking and feeling young.

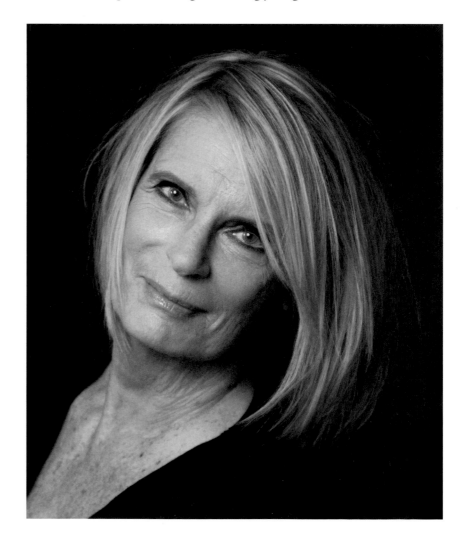

Carolyn, age seventy.

Carole

After hearing about each other for years, and with much persuasion from her daughter and my longtime client Lori, Carole and I finally met. She wanted a new look and said that her daughter had told her that if anyone could do it, it would be me. I suggested that she grow her hair out and add lowlights to the gray, to blend some "pepper back with the salt." Although it took a little time for her hair to reach the desired length, each time I saw Carole she remarked that everyone was talking about how good she looks. We finally got her typical short cut to a beautiful bob with soft, round layers. After the color, cut, and a makeup lesson, Carole said that she finally looks as good as she feels! A mother of four, she devoted her life to her children. She now enjoys traveling and spending leisure time with family and friends. The day of the shoot, we decided to also take some mother-and-daughter photographs. They had so much fun that it was hard for them to keep it together for the portraits.

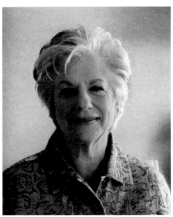

Above: Before.
Below: With her daughter, Lori.

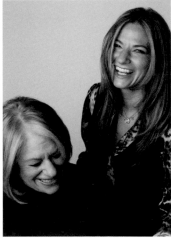

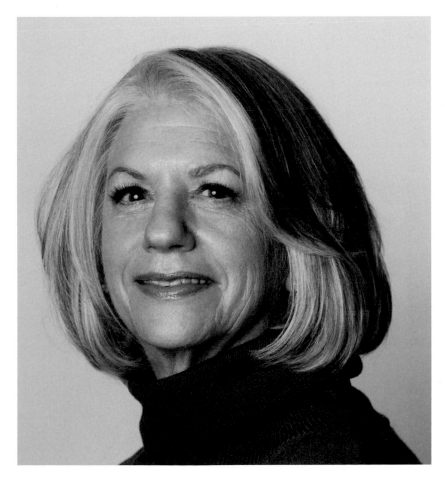

Carole, age sixty-six.

Alex

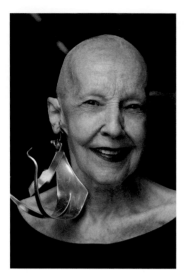

Alex, age eighty-six.
Opposite: Alex, near our salon on
Bond Street.

Alex is the ultimate rule breaker and I feel privileged to have had her as my friend for many years. At eighty-six, she not only wears shorts, high heels, and fabulous jewelry but shaves her own head by choice. Alex is an artist whose canvas is her body. She especially appreciates sculpture and considers fashion and beauty to be about "the line." Finding that her hair interrupted that line, she has shaved her head for the last twenty years. She is known for her collection of unconventional jewelry and prefers to wear her art rather than hang it on a wall. She buys only classic designer clothing, is partial to black coffee and white wine, and rarely drinks water. When I asked Alex her secret to looking great at any age, she said that it's about not doing anything in excess: "Don't eat, drink, or exercise too much. Only do what you feel comfortable with and what makes you feel happy." I also asked how others react to her avant-garde style and how she feels when they point and stare. She just shrugged and said that she pays them no mind. "I am who I am and I've always been this way." She told me how growing up in a supportive environment, with a mother who taught her to celebrate her individuality, had given Alex the confidence to express it throughout her life.

Alex still works part-time as an executive secretary to a prominent family in Manhattan. Surprisingly traditional in her views, and opinionated, she is warm, kind, and delightful to be around. She has friends of all ages and does not feel defined by her own age. Alex is a walking work of art who has been photographed by some of the most famous photographers. She serves as a reminder that the world is filled with wonderful and interesting individuals whose uniqueness is their true defining characteristic, not to be limited by societal dogmas or by their chronological ages.

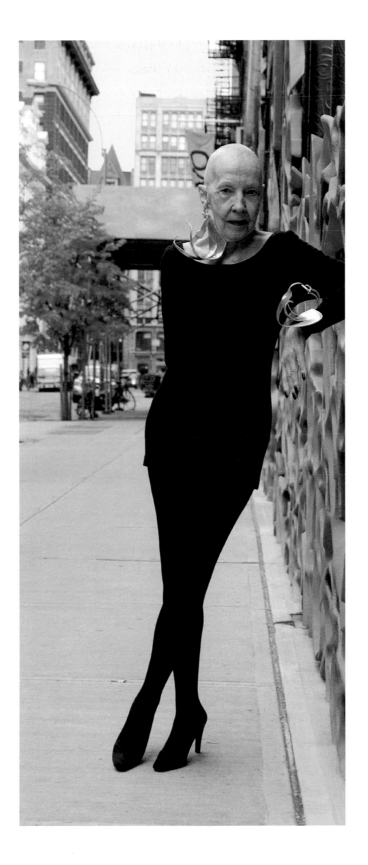

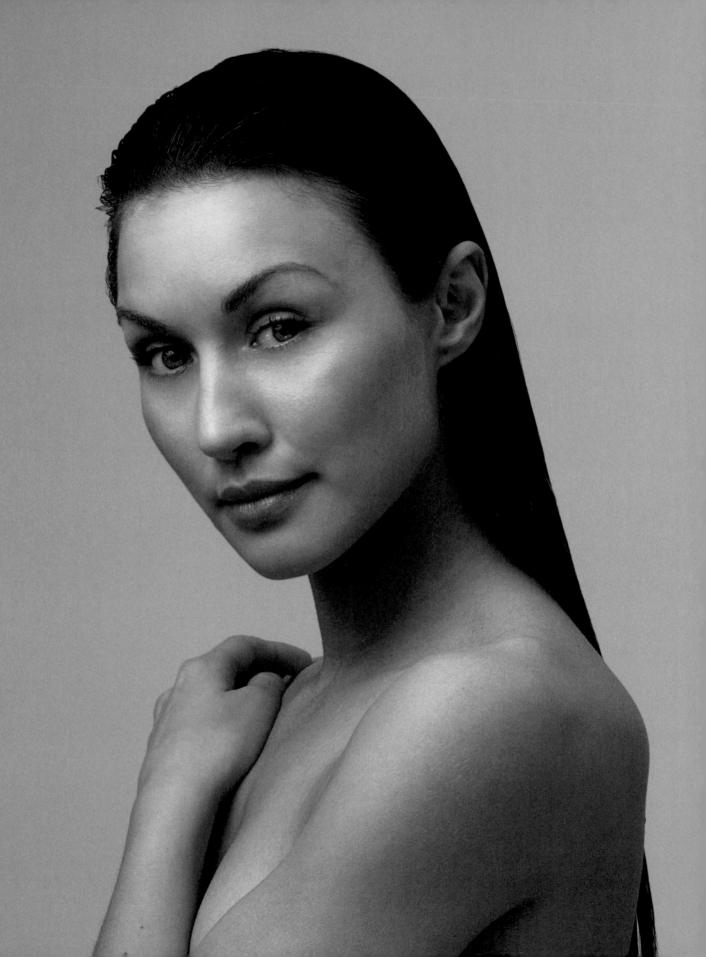

9

BEAUTY FROM THE INSIDE OUT

Everything that you have learned in this book about looking and feeling great is also influenced by what is happening *within* your body. Your job, personal relationships, and lifestyle affect your state of mind, your overall health, and ultimately your looks. Failure to take the time to care for yourself and manage how you process daily challenges and stress can manifest itself in under-eye circles, skin disorders, weight loss or gain, and a compromised immune system.

The only way to truly achieve beauty is with a holistic approach. A balance between physical and emotional health feeds an energy—a lightness of spirit—and an exuberance that are the true foundations of youth. Like anything worth having, it requires a commitment to yourself and a conscientious effort to lead a healthier and a more positive lifestyle. This entails some effort and willpower, but the payoff is nothing less than life-changing.

My fascination with wellness and nutrition started when I was fifteen years old and my father was diagnosed with adult-onset diabetes. I began studying diet and nutrition and learned that many foods have the power to heal the body. Although opinionated and sometimes stubborn, my father was open-minded enough to make the necessary changes to restore his health. As an Italian-American family in Detroit, we ate a traditional

Mediterranean diet rich in olive oil, fish, pastas, meat, and sauces, combined with some unhealthy American influences. I tossed out all processed foods and everything that contained refined sugar and simple carbohydrates. We started eating a more fresh, organic diet containing whole grains, tofu, lean protein, salads with nuts and seeds added to them, and a lot more vegetables. For diabetes, the combinations and portions were just as important as the food choices. Within only two weeks of my father's starting this rigorously healthy diet, his glucose levels went down to the normal range. He was able to regulate his diabetes through diet and lifestyle alone. He also lost ten pounds and started to feel more energetic almost immediately. It was an amazing transformation. His doctor was shocked at the change and asked what my father had been doing differently. "My daughter has me eating brown rice and kale!" he replied. "Just keep doing whatever you're doing, because it's working," said the doctor. My father maintained a healthy diet for years to come and never had to take insulin. As I watched his health improve before my eyes, I knew that I had found the answer. Since I did most of the cooking in our home, I made that a new way of life for myself and my family.

My interest in this area evolved as I got older and has continued throughout my life. It is truly a passion. Living a healthy, happy life is a conscious choice that we have the power to make. What you put into your body, how you sleep, your general health, and your personal happiness—all affect the way you look and feel. If one component is out of sync, it throws everything off-balance. I want to share the knowledge and insight that I have accumulated over many years of personal research and through experts such as doctors, acupuncturists, sleep experts, psychologists, fitness trainers, nutritionists, and body workers. It has had a profound impact on my own life and has also been passed on to my family, clients, and friends, all of whom have greatly benefited as a result. Following these principles will help put you in touch with your body, mind, and spirit, and inspire you to lead a healthier, happier, and more fulfilling life. Being open to new ideas allows us to find solutions to problems and learn to deal with life's challenges in a more positive and proactive way.

HOW TO GET STARTED
Make Yourself a Priority

Taking care of oneself is a daily practice that allows a person to stay energetic, strong, attractive, and happy. Signs of aging are grossly exacerbated by poor health and neglect. Women who make their physical and emotional health a priority look spectacular at fifty, sixty, seventy, and beyond. Unfortunately, this is often one of the first elements to get pushed aside during the juggling act of daily life. Many women actually feel guilty about spending time or money on themselves. Society instills in us that selflessness and sacrifice are virtues, but if we do not balance taking care of others with caring for ourselves, not only does our health deteriorate but we eventually become a burden to the ones we love. In this sense, neglecting your own health and happiness is actually a very selfish act.

Having seen this so many times, I am still taken aback when a woman who gives so much of herself to her work and her family feels a great deal of stress taking just one hour for herself. In her need to please and care for others, she sacrifices her own well-being, unwittingly bankrupting herself. Taking a twenty-minute walk, going to a yoga class, getting a massage, and having lunch with a friend are the most rudimentary ways of carving out some personal time, which should be part of a regular routine and seen as an investment in your health and happiness. The costs of not doing these things are much greater than the time and money spent on them. Feeling stressed, depressed, unhealthy, or unattractive carries a tremendous weight and robs you of experiencing joy in all aspects of your life. If you consider taking care of yourself a "luxury," you need to rethink your priorities. Instead, think of it as a birthright, a personal responsibility, and a sign of a healthy self-esteem.

So many people live their lives as if in a holding pattern—waiting to do the things they know they should be doing and to enjoy life's pleasures that are completely within reach. So many first-time clients have told me that they have wanted to make a big change in their hair or overall appearance for ten or even twenty years! When I ask what made them come to me now, the answer is never that they could at last afford it and rarely is it a result of some momentous occasion. The reason is simple and nearly always the same: "I have finally decided that it's time!" This attitude is prevalent in all too many aspects of our lives, whether it's our health and well-being or just the little things that make us happy. People wait to improve their diet, quit smoking, start exercising, or finally open that beautiful bottle of wine that they have wistfully glanced at for years while waiting for a "special occasion" that never seems quite special enough. Many even reserve their nice dining room for company, rarely enjoying it themselves.

In the preceding chapter, I posed the question "Why can't you?" To this I now add, "What are you waiting for?" The longer you wait to get started, the more of your precious life passes by and the longer it will take to bring yourself back to physical and emotional health. Don't be afraid to give to yourself just because it will make you feel good and to be kind to yourself in general. On an airplane, the flight attendant instructs us to put our own oxygen mask on first before helping someone else. This simple analogy is a life lesson that often takes too many years to learn. We are simply no good to anyone else unless we take care of ourselves!

You may relate to what I am saying but not know how to begin to shift your perspective and habits. Perhaps you are dealing with a troubled child or caring for an elderly parent and have neglected yourself as a result. Making a dramatic change in your lifestyle and behavior can at first seem daunting, which is probably why so many are afraid of it. Change is actually a beautiful thing—it all depends on your outlook. Being more open to new ideas and less judgmental of yourself and of others is a wonderful start. Improve the quality of your life gradually and with self-compassion. If you give to yourself only a portion of the kindness that you so freely give to others, you will be a happier and healthier person and, in turn, more positively affect those around you. It is not necessary to change your life overnight. Take it one day at a time and start moving in the right direction, whether you begin with your diet or how you cope with stressful situations. Moderate shifts to your lifestyle will soon add up to a significant change, as with each small accomplishment you build momentum and confidence. Eventually, these changes will add up to become the new you.

NUTRITIONAL SUPPORT
A Guide to More Mindful Eating

Everyone has a doctor in him; we just have to help it in its work. The natural healing force within each one of us is the greatest force in getting well. Our food should be our medicine. Our medicine should be our food. —HIPPOCRATES

We truly are what we eat. After I witnessed such a fast and dramatic improvement in my father's health as a direct result of a better diet, it became completely clear to me how food choices affect every element of our lives: our health, energy level, weight, immune system, mood, and appearance. Rather than choose foods that we crave or that are most convenient, we should base our dietary decisions on what our bodies need.

Changing your eating habits is as simple as making smart substitutions and developing a healthier palate. It does not mean a drastic diet. To me, "dieting" has a negative and even depressing connotation (the first three letters spell *die*). Dieting is more about deprivation and an unsustainable lifestyle aimed at quickly losing weight. It also distorts our relationship with food, which then becomes the "enemy" rather than a positive life force that nurtures, protects, and heals the body. A more enduring approach is to create a way of eating that you can live with—for the rest of your life. In this chapter, I will share how to make smart food choices that work for you instead of against you, are simple to implement, and will make you look and feel better. The goal of a good diet is not to get model-thin and may not even be to lose weight at all. It is simply to eat foods that nourish your body in a positive way.

Swap Processed Foods for Healthier Choices

Start by replacing processed, prepackaged foods, which are filled with sugar, preservatives, and chemicals, with foods that are grown in the ground, raised on a farm, or caught in a river or an ocean. Processing food destroys its nutrients, which manufacturers then attempt to replace by "fortifying." But it can never be as nutritious as the real thing. So, instead of snacking on unhealthy junk food, buy raw nuts (instead of the salted, roasted kind) and nibble on them with a piece of fruit. Choose nutrient-dense whole grains over refined and nutritionally deprived carbohydrates: brown rice, quinoa, millet, kasha, or spelt instead of white rice, bread, and pasta made from bleached or enriched flour. Whole grains are left in their original, unprocessed state, as opposed to being ground into flour. They are digested more slowly, which helps to maintain consistent blood sugar levels in the body and keeps you feeling full longer (thus curbing cravings for snacks and sweets). Thankfully, nature has it figured out for us: if something does not live and grow in nature, don't eat it! Anything that is chemically engineered or altered is not really food.

Eat a Wide Variety of Foods

Ideally, your diet should include a wide variety of foods, which will give you a greater chance of getting all the essential vitamins, minerals, amino acids, and fats that your body needs. Color is important when it comes to food (just as it is with hair and makeup). The easiest way to ensure that you are getting all the nutrients you need is by choosing many (natural) food colors. The contents of your plate should have an array of vibrant shades: the bright colors of fresh-cut vegetables and herbs; the deep, rich shade of a side vegetable; the beige or brown of a grain. Many protein sources such as white fish, chicken, and tofu do not necessarily have color, but the food around them should. People tend to stick with their favorite foods and end up missing out on a host of nutrients necessary for a strong, healthy body that are easy to incorporate by adding some variety to your plate.

BEAUTY SUPERFOODS

Certain vitamins and minerals are particularly beneficial for the hair and skin. I encourage you to incorporate them into your diet, preferably in the form of whole foods. In addition to a healthy diet, I also recommend daily supplements. Taking a multivitamin, for example, helps ensure that you're getting everything your body needs. However, it should be regarded as a supplement rather than a substitute for nutritious foods.

Foods for Healthy Hair

Foods that contain vitamin B are essential for healthy hair growth. Biotin (B_7) is found in eggs, milk, brewer's yeast, peanuts, and almonds. Pantothenic acid (B_5) is in whole grains, legumes, and royal jelly. B_{12}, mostly contained in animal-based proteins, such as meat, fish, and dairy products, can also be consumed by eating nutritional yeast. Folic acid (B_9) is critical for cell division and maintenance. Its naturally occurring form is folate. Prenatal vitamins are high in folate because it is essential for the production of healthy new cells, especially during the periods of rapid cell division that occur during pregnancy. Folate gets its name from the Latin word *folium,* which means "leaf." Accordingly, it is found in green leafy vegetables such as kale, spinach, and Swiss chard. Legumes and sunflower seeds are also good sources of folate. A deficiency in any of these B vitamins can be a contributing factor to hair loss. Protein is a primary building block for the body's cells and tissues. Hair and nails are actually made of it (in the form of keratin). Some of the best food sources of protein are lean meats, poultry, fish, eggs, tofu, legumes, and nuts.

Foods for Healthy Skin

Two types of nutrients primarily contribute to healthy skin: antioxidants and essential fatty acids. Antioxidants reduce and fight off oxidative stress in the body by neutralizing free radicals, which break down healthy cell function. The production of free radicals is also intensified by external factors that include sun exposure, smoking, and pollution.

Antioxidants such as vitamins C and E as well as beta-carotene (which is converted into vitamin A in the body) counteract free radical damage, strengthen the immune system, reduce inflammation, and protect the skin from environmental damage that results in loss of collagen. Vitamin C also helps repair and regenerate tissue and build collagen. Sources of vitamin C include citrus fruits such as oranges, lemons, and grapefruit, as well as goji berries, blueberries, papaya, and tomatoes. Vitamin E, which also helps to repair damaged tissue, is found in green leafy vegetables, olive oil, broccoli, avocados, sunflower seeds, and walnuts.

The minerals selenium and zinc are essential for beautiful skin. Selenium helps to maintain the skin's firmness and elasticity. It is found in foods such as Brazil nuts, button and shiitake mushrooms, tuna, beef, and garlic. (Brazil nuts are particularly high in selenium, so one or two a day is plenty.) Zinc promotes collagen synthesis (similar to vitamin C). It also regulates oil production and its anti-inflammatory properties help to heal acne. Zinc is found in oysters, beef, wheat germ, tahini (sesame butter), roasted pumpkin seeds, and dairy products.

Essential fatty acids lubricate the skin (including the scalp, resulting in more lustrous, shiny hair) and reduce inflammation. Eating fish is the easiest way to consume omega-3 fatty acid. If you do not eat fish, you can get omega-3 from fish oil supplements, walnuts, soybeans, legumes, dark leafy greens, hemp, or flaxseeds. The best way to eat flaxseeds is to grind them yourself (in a coffee bean grinder reserved just for this purpose) and to sprinkle them on top of yogurt, cereal, or salad, or blend them in a smoothie. In addition to their omega-3 content, they are a great source of fiber. Omega-6 is gamma linoleic acid (GLA), an essential fatty acid that is beneficial for dry skin and is found in plant-based oils such as borage oil, black currant seed oil, and evening primrose oil; all can be obtained in the form of supplements.

CHECKLIST

Beauty superfoods shopping list

This list will help you select nutritious beauty foods that benefit your hair, skin, and overall health. They contain essential nutrients such as omega-3, omega-6, omega-9, biotin, selenium, zinc, folate, beta-carotene, protein, minerals, and vitamins A, B, C, and E. This list is far from complete but it contains some of the more common items that can be found in many food markets and health food stores.

MEAT, POULTRY, AND EGGS: Pasture/grass-fed beef and lamb; free-range or organic chicken and turkey; chicken and duck eggs (duck eggs are especially high in nutrients).
FISH (CAUGHT IN THE WILD, NOT FARM-RAISED): Salmon, herring, rainbow trout, halibut, mackerel, sardines, tuna, cod, crab, lobster, shrimp, and oysters.
VEGETABLES: Tomatoes, red and yellow peppers, sweet potatoes, kale, Swiss chard, spinach, escarole, carrots, beets, cabbage, broccoli, cauliflower, and seaweed.
FRUITS: All berries, oranges, grapefruit, lemons, papaya, melon, mangos, goji berries, and avocados.
NUTS AND SEEDS: Brazil nuts, walnuts, almonds; sunflower seeds, pumpkin seeds, and flaxseeds.
OTHER FOODS: Green tea, red wine, and dark chocolate are all high in antioxidants; wheat germ, legumes, tofu, whole grains, milk products such as cheese and yogurt, olive oil, gingerroot, and garlic.

CONSIDER THE FOOD SOURCE

Mindful eating begins with choosing high-quality ingredients. How something is grown or raised makes an enormous difference. Fruits and vegetables that are inorganically farmed can be depleted of vital minerals due to pesticides and fertilizers, not to mention the harm that ingesting all those chemicals can do to our health. Ironically, the term *organic,* as it relates to food, was created fairly recently, as most of our food became inorganic. Until then, organic was not "special"; it was simply the way people ate, and it is how we are supposed to eat. It is basically food that is free of harmful chemicals.

It is important to select wild fish as opposed to "farm-raised," which means raised in captivity and confined in pens. These fish are generally fed protein pellets rather than the smaller fish or vegetation that they would eat in their natural habitat, while the man-made pools of water can be a breeding ground for parasites. Farm-raised salmon is often fed beta-carotene, which turns its flesh orange and makes it appear freshly caught or at least healthy. The fish also swim in their own waste matter, in which case the term *organic* (even if no chemicals are added to the fish meal) is a misnomer.

If you eat meat, make sure it is organic, pasture/grass fed, or free-range. The animal is healthier for you if it has been raised in a clean and humane environment, having been fed what it would normally eat in nature. For example, cows naturally graze on grass and plants, as opposed to being pumped full of hormones, antibiotics, and pesticide-coated, fattening corn. All those chemicals enter your body when you eat the meat or drink the milk from these cows—or eat eggs from chickens that have been fed growth hormones. Likewise, the meat and dairy products from a free-range animal pass the nutrients that the animal eats on to you. Just like humans, animals are what they eat. Learning about how most of our food is grown, raised, and slaughtered is not only astonishing and eye opening, it is heartbreaking. Eating mindfully means making agriculturally sound and ethical choices not only for your health but for the health of the environment and for the humane treatment of animals.

BEAUTY SECRET

The truth about salt and the importance of minerals

Getting enough dietary minerals such as calcium, zinc, copper, magnesium, potassium, and selenium is just as important as getting enough vitamins. Moreover, our bodies naturally crave them. Such is the case with salt. Many people crave salty foods because their bodies are deficient in essential minerals. Often this is caused by not eating the right kind of salt—that is, naturally mineralized. Instead, to satiate our mineral cravings we tend to snack on processed foods with salt that is refined and bleached of its mineral content. The best form of salt is natural sea salt, which contains the essential minerals that our bodies need for good health. Adding a small amount of it to the whole foods you cook at home will help you to achieve a balance of healthy minerals in your diet and eliminate your cravings.

HOW TO EAT MINDFULLY

Chew your drink and drink your food.　　　　　—Mahatma Gandhi

The way you eat your food is almost as important as what you eat. Too often, we grab something and eat it on the run, in the car, or on autopilot in front of the television. We sometimes do not even remember what we ate. The answer to overeating is not dieting but simply slowing down, paying attention to what we are eating, and truly savoring it.

Practice Portion Control

Most people in Western culture consume way too much food in one sitting, usually from eating so fast that they do not realize they are full until they have overdone it. Your brain takes about twenty minutes to receive signals from your stomach as it gets filled. Therefore, if you must eat quickly, keep in mind that you may not know that you are full until it is too late. The other extreme has dieters measuring out their portions in tablespoons and ounces. A better way to gauge (and remember) the appropriate portion size is to hold out your hands, palms up in an open prayer position. The right amount of food for one meal should be no more than what would fill your hands.

The way to practice such self-control is not to wait until you are ravenously hungry. At that point, you will inevitably make bad choices, such as attacking a basket of bread at a restaurant, grabbing a high-fat muffin, or digging into a block of cheese without a thought. Plan ahead for yourself, just as moms do for their kids. Have healthy snacks handy so that you don't end up feeling vulnerable and famished.

Eat More Slowly

One of the most challenging but important things to do consistently is to slow down and chew your food properly. Like most people, I am guilty of eating too fast. Being a hairdresser often means wolfing down lunch in five to ten minutes between clients, so there is rarely time to sit down and enjoy a meal. If I have to eat in a rush during busy days at work, I try to practice more mindful eating at breakfast and dinner. The simple act of properly chewing your food well makes an enormous difference in how it is digested and how you feel as a result. Gandhi's quote about chewing your drink and drinking your food is a wonderful reminder that the digestion process actually begins in the mouth, with digestive enzymes from the salivary glands. "Chewing your drink" refers to how the act of chewing activates those glands to signal the stomach that something is coming. "Drinking your food" means that if chewed sufficiently, it becomes almost liquefied before being swallowed, which allows the body to assimilate the nutrients more efficiently. Many digestive problems can be helped or even eliminated by following this simple wisdom.

Make Smart Food Selections

The right foods go a long way toward helping you naturally control your appetite and portions. The glycemic food index is a measure of the effects of carbohydrates on blood sugar levels. Foods that are low on the glycemic index, such as lean proteins, vegetables, and whole grains, will keep you feeling full longer, since the body digests them more slowly. They also prevent your blood sugar from rising and falling like a roller coaster. Proteins such as chicken, fish, turkey, and tofu work on the same principle, as do healthy monounsaturated fats found in avocados, nuts, and olives. Conversely, foods that measure high on the glycemic index (high in sugar) increase blood sugar and insulin production, slowing the metabolism and storing most of these empty calories in the body as fat. If you have tried losing weight to no avail, check your food choices against a glycemic index that can be found on the Internet.

Even with the best intentions, it is still challenging to regularly eat healthy, whole foods. Remember that good habits form gradually. Many of us eat out frequently or get take-out. Due to my crazy schedule, I often eat at restaurants or order lunch from them. Nevertheless, I have found many ways to make healthier choices, such as ordering fish or chicken baked or broiled with sauces on the side, and vegetables and salad to replace fries. Simply requesting that your meal be prepared with light oil and salt will reduce calories and bloating.

Prepare More Meals at Home

Cooking at home, something I love to do, gives you complete control over your food so you can make the most healthful choices. If you want to start making positive changes in your and your family's diet, begin by taking small, practical steps that will set you up for success. Maybe you cannot eat all the right things daily and at every meal, but integrating better choices into your diet at home is going to make a big impact on your health, energy level, and looks. Make a decision to cook something with fresh ingredients just twice a week—perhaps on the weekend, when you have more time. Meals could be as simple as a vegetable soup or a stew; brown rice with a salad of diced tomatoes, cucumbers, and herbs; or sautéed greens with tofu. Many dishes can be stored in the refrigerator or frozen so that they last more than one meal. Planning ahead and doing the prep work makes it simpler. For example, if you wash and cut salad greens and vegetables and refrigerate them in airtight containers, it is faster and easier to assemble a salad or whip up a simple dinner when you come home from work. People say that they don't have the time to make something healthful, but it still takes time and effort to place an order or sit in a restaurant. You will make wiser choices (and actually know what is in your food) when you make the meal yourself. Think of the rewards and benefits of looking and feeling better, and the satisfaction of using fresh ingredients.

Remember that this is a lifestyle, not a diet, so there needs to be a period of adjustment to get comfortable with the changes you are making. Try not to be too hard on yourself. Certain foods that bring you pleasure do not have to be eliminated. You can enjoy a chocolate chip cookie, a little ice cream, or your favorite comfort food now and then. These are wonderful pleasures, and as long as they do not become daily indulgences, there is no reason to feel guilty. Food should be a positive experience that brings you enjoyment, as long as you treat yourself and everything you eat with respect.

THE HEALING POWER OF NUTRIENTS
Raw Foods and Juicing

When your body is in a weakened state due to illness, injury, or emotional trauma, replenishing it with additional nutrients is essential to help yourself heal, recover, and rebuild your immune system so that you can return to your old self again. I look to nutritional support when I feel especially run-down, stressed, or exhausted, or when I am on the verge of (or recovering from) a cold or flu. You will be amazed at how reparative and restorative these natural remedies can be.

Eat More Raw Foods

Raw, as opposed to cooked, foods have a highly concentrated vitamin, mineral, and enzyme content. Heating food above 118°F destroys natural enzymes that aid in the digestion and absorption of nutrients. Incorporating raw or "live" foods into your diet is actually easier and tastier than you might think, and you do not have to be fanatical about it. You can integrate raw foods effortlessly by adding fresh fruits and vegetables to salads and snacking on raw seeds and nuts or sprinkling them on cereals and grains.

. . . Or Just Drink Them

For many of us, a busy lifestyle that includes work and travel, or just cooking meals for finicky eaters at home, makes it hard to eat enough fruits and vegetables. This is when drinking them is an easy alternative. Juicing gives you the freshest, most concentrated quantity of vitamins, antioxidants, minerals, and enzymes from raw food, and since those nutrients

BEAUTY SECRET

Supplements to boost your nutrient intake

Getting your daily nutritional requirements from natural food sources is optimal, but it is not always possible. Dietary supplements can be a great insurance policy or just give an added boost of specific nutrients. Generally, a good multivitamin taken once a day covers most bases.

are in liquid form, they are easily and more quickly absorbed into your system. You are essentially drinking a bushel of fruits and vegetables in one glass. This should not be confused with processed, packaged juices that are available in supermarkets. The goal is to extract the nutrient-rich juice without adding any sugar or preservatives.

Years ago, I started drinking a vegetable juice every afternoon, around that four-o'clock lull when most people reach for a sugar or caffeine fix. Not only has this energized me and strengthened my immune system, but it improved my complexion. If you do not have a juice bar nearby, I encourage you to invest in a good juicer. Juicers are easier to use and to clean than they used to be. Fresh juice is most nutritious when you drink it immediately, but it can be stored in a tightly sealed glass container in the refrigerator for up to two days.

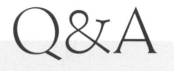

Q: *Is the help of a nutritionist worthwhile?*

A: If you are unsure which foods to stay away from and which to eat more of, it is absolutely a good idea to consult a nutritionist. Many people who have tried dieting to no avail eventually find lasting success once they have the support of a professional. He or she can provide invaluable insights on your eating habits and educate you about food combinations and portion control to create a sustainable diet plan that is customized just for you. This can be truly life-changing.

COMMON MISTAKE

The myth of the salad bar

You may feel that opting for the salad bar over a cheeseburger is a smart choice, but this seemingly good idea can be deceptive. When you break down the ingredients that most people pile high on their salad plates, they might as well order burgers with all the fixings. Leave it to Americans to turn a salad into a cheeseburger by adding meat, cheese, bacon bits, croutons, and creamy dressings. Even the vegetables (such as beets and corn) can be deceptively high in sugar and starch. If a typical salad bar is your answer to healthful eating, you may just be fooling yourself.

MY PERSONAL ROUTINE

FIRST THING IN THE MORNING: I start with half a glass of apple juice mixed with water (equal parts) with a scoop of daily greens (a powdered supplement found at the health food store). I use this drink to wash down three or four capsules of omega-3 fish oil. Next, I make a cup of yerba maté, a South American tea that is loaded with powerful antioxidants (and caffeine) or a cup of fresh ginger tea or lemon water, depending on how I feel. If I am going to work out that morning, I will also eat one piece of fruit, whatever is in season.

BREAKFAST: I am not a big breakfast person, but I do try to eat something, especially since my workday is so physical. I usually have a small portion of one of the following: oatmeal, muesli, or kasha (buckwheat groats); fresh fruit with yogurt; a piece of wheat-free toast with one slice of cheese or a little peanut butter; one egg (usually poached or scrambled) with a piece of dry toast.

I also take my vitamins: a multivitamin, borage oil, and vitamin C, plus whatever I feel my body needs that day. For example, if I feel run-down or a cold is coming on, I may also take lysine, a protein amino acid that boosts the immune system, before eating anything (I like the kind with echinacea and garlic). Most vitamins are assimilated in the body with protein, so they should be taken with a meal. Fish oil is a protein carrier and can be taken on an empty stomach.

I usually have organic French-pressed coffee with breakfast. I rarely drink coffee on an empty stomach, because it is so acidic. If you find that stomach problems consistently accompany your caffeine fix, try combining it with food (if cutting it out completely is not an option).

LUNCH: I typically have a salad with some type of protein (tofu, hummus, a grain/veggie burger, or sometimes a piece of fish or meat). I also add a whole grain such as brown rice, millet, or quinoa. The protein and the grains keep me full through the day. Nuts, seeds, and raisins are also delicious and easy to sprinkle onto your salad to make it more filling.

MIDAFTERNOON SNACK: A glass of fresh vegetable juice (a delicious mix is kale, spinach, carrot, beet, apple, lemon, and ginger) is my favorite healthful pick-me-up. I might have an apple with some almond butter, or a cup of soup (one with vegetables and legumes for more energy). I like to have raw walnuts or almonds handy to snack on.

DINNER: I choose to eat vegetarian meals most of the time, but occasionally I have sushi or a lean piece of organic meat. I try to have a variety of foods each day: one dinner might be a salad with a small portion of pasta and another may consist of some fresh fish with sautéed vegetables. I love Indian, Middle Eastern, and Asian cuisines that include lots of vegetables and meat-free protein sources such as tofu, beans, and grains. I nearly always have a glass of red wine with dinner. It is rich in antioxidants and makes all food taste better.

I rarely eat dessert. The more sugar you have, the more you want, and those are empty calories. I feel that the best way to satiate a craving for sugar is to eat more protein-rich foods. Try it and you will begin to notice that your sweet tooth diminishes. And if that doesn't work, imagine that what you are eating is going straight to your hips; perhaps even visualize slathering the food directly onto a specific body part to be absorbed without bothering to eat it (this one usually works for me!). Another good reminder: nothing tastes as good as healthy feels!

BEAUTY SECRET

Balancing alkaline and acid foods

The body's pH—its measure of alkalinity and acidity levels—is a delicate chemical balance that affects your overall health. You can keep your pH in check with the foods you choose. There are even at-home pH testing kits to check your acid/alkaline levels. The pH balance of the body influences the amount of inflammation that occurs within it. An acidic pH can trigger skin conditions such as rosacea, acne, and eczema. It can make you feel fatigued and compromise your immune system. Eating too many acid-producing foods such as beef, dairy, and wheat contributes to this problem. Alkaline foods such as dark leafy greens, tofu, miso soup, celery, and cucumber reduce inflammation and keep the body's pH in a healthy balance. Ideally, you should eat both alkaline and acid foods to feel your best. Alkaline/acid food charts are readily available on the Internet.

KEEPING FIT

The benefits of regular exercise are extraordinary. It is the key to maintaining your ideal weight or losing weight and keeping it off. It boosts your metabolism, increases your energy level, helps you sleep better, strengthens your immune system, reduces stress, and builds strength, endurance, and flexibility. By increasing circulation, it also naturally helps the body cleanse through perspiration. Regular physical activity has even been found to slow the aging process.

The psychological benefits of regular, vigorous activity are just as great. It improves your mood and emotional well-being by releasing endorphins and elevating serotonin levels in the body that help to alleviate depression and anxiety and to decrease the "stress hormone," cortisol. It also makes an immediate and powerful improvement in your body image and self-confidence. Think of exercise as something you do for your mental health and getting in better shape as the added benefit. Consider it to be a privilege and a true blessing. Think about the millions of people who are physically unable to run, stretch, play, or even be mobile, and would love to use their bodies as you do. You will quickly forget your excuses. I admit that I am not a big lover of working out, but I like to be active because I feel so much better mentally and physically afterward. I have three easy ways of keeping my workouts fresh and interesting.

BEAUTY SECRET

Improving your digestion for better skin

An imbalance in the digestive tract can lead to all sorts of health problems as well as common discomforts such as bloating, constipation, and indigestion. It can also affect your immune system, decrease your energy level, and cause skin problems, since inadequate elimination of toxins and waste affects the health of the skin. It helps to eat more fiber-rich foods in the form of raw fruits and vegetables, raw juices, and whole grains. Increase your intake of water throughout the day and consider supplementing with plant-based food enzymes (in capsule form) that can be taken with each meal. Since the enzymes in food are significantly reduced when heated, supplements help to replenish the stomach's natural enzymatic balance. Probiotics and acidophilus also promote better digestion and regularity by adding healthy bacteria to the digestive tract.

1. Make Your Workout Fun

The secret to sticking to a consistant exercise plan is to find one or two physical activities that you actually enjoy. One reason why most children are naturally fit is that they run and play every day for fun. As adults, we tend to compartmentalize exercise as a chore to accomplish a few times a week. If you create a positive experience around a daily workout, it can actually become the part of your day that you look forward to most. But be honest with yourself: if you hate going to the gym, don't go. Instead, take a brisk walk or go for a run, go to a yoga or Pilates class, join a softball team, learn to play tennis, or take dance lessons. Exercise does not have to be a typical workout—it can be a fun bike ride, a weekend hike, walking the dog, or playing with your kids.

2. Vary Your Exercise Routine

The best exercise formula is to combine an aerobic activity that raises your heart rate with some type of weight-resistance exercise. Mix up your activities: a walk one day, a bike ride another, a yoga class twice a week; and ideally rotate your strength-training exercises to work different muscle groups. Otherwise, your body adjusts to doing the same thing all the time, and eventually you will see diminished results. Variety also ensures that you will not get bored. My weekly routine usually includes working out at the gym, walking, swimming, and yoga. I have recently taken up cross-country skiing, which is an amazing workout!

3. Incorporate Daily Physical Activity

Generally, we are not as active as we should be, which can be blamed partly on conveniences such as cars, escalators, and elevators. In New York City, we use our feet as our main method of transportation. We walk everywhere and go up and down stairs in subway stations (and many apartments). I have a client who does not like to work out at a gym, but lives on the twelfth floor (of an elevator building) and walks up the stairs to her apartment. For her, it's like one big StairMaster. Whether you park your car farther away from your destination, take the stairs instead of the escalator or elevator, or run errands on foot instead of in a car, simply using your body the way it was intended to be used will make a big difference in how you look and feel.

BEAUTY SECRET

Your posture affects your energy

Standing and sitting up straight instantly creates a more flattering silhouette, making you look stronger, leaner, taller, more confident, and years younger. When you enter a room with your shoulders slouched, people probably take little notice of you, but if you walk in with your shoulders back and your head held high, looking people in the eye, the reaction is completely different and much more positive. When I am aware of my posture and stand up straighter is when my husband tells me how beautiful I look (regardless of what I'm wearing). This energy and air of confidence is what people can actually see and feel, and is what attracts them to us. Become more aware of your alignment and tap in to your personal beauty energy: stand up straight, pull your shoulders back, and tuck your tailbone and pelvis slightly. Even though it may feel unnatural at first, once you are in perfect alignment, everyone will take notice (and your back will feel better).

Legend has it that Marilyn Monroe could go completely unnoticed in public when she covered her famous platinum blond hair with a scarf and wore sunglasses and no makeup. While in this incognito mode, she once asked a friend if she wanted to see what happens when she turned on "the Marilyn." Off came the scarf, and she flipped her hair back and walked that famous walk. Using only her energy and without a stitch of makeup, she transformed herself into the most beautiful woman on the planet. Cars screeched to a halt, people began to flock to her . . . The truth is that some of this allure and sex appeal is inside all of us. We just have to tap into it, believe it, and present it to the world. Self-assurance is captivating. Your energy and individuality attract people, and physical perfection has little to do with it.

Q&A

Q: *Is a juice fast a good way to detoxify the body and to lose weight?*
A: A juice detox typically entails drinking lots of fresh, organic juice throughout the day in place of meals and usually lasts three to five days. This can be a wonderful practice that gives the liver a rest and can make you feel more energetic, lighter, and less bloated. However, when you incorporate healthful, nutrient-dense, fiber-rich whole foods into your daily life, your body will naturally detoxify itself. If you want to try a juice cleanse, I recommend working with a nutritionist or an integrative doctor who can suggest an appropriate plan for you.

BEAUTY SLEEP

Without adequate sleep, the body does not have an opportunity to restore and repair itself, or recover from illness or stress. Exhaustion contributes to a compromised immune system, which affects the body in a myriad of adverse ways. Lack of sleep also results in a dull, pallid complexion, which accentuates dark circles under the eyes. It has even been found to contribute to weight gain by activating production of the hormone ghrelin, which stimulates the appetite.

Unfortunately, for many, restful sleep is an elusive pleasure, which may be due to numerous factors. You may have young children or too much stimulation before bedtime from watching television, working on the computer, or talking on the phone. Consuming caffeine, sugar, or alcohol in the evening can also interfere with sleep. And we all know that stress and daily worries can keep us awake. I have certainly had my struggles with sleepless nights, and have therefore collected a wealth of knowledge from numerous therapists and sleep experts about how to facilitate restful sleep. The self-tested advice that follows will help you get to sleep easier and stay asleep through the night. Your body and state of mind will be healthier for it.

Five Ways to Get a Better Night's Sleep

1. REDUCE MENTAL STIMULATION.

Too much mental activity and technological stimulation close to bedtime can make it difficult to fall asleep. Watching television (especially something scary or violent) or working on the computer can make you agitated and alert. Move the TV and the computer out of the bedroom, and turn them both off at least thirty minutes before going to bed. This will give your mind a chance to slow down and relax. Consider moving the telephone to another room as well, and if you have a digital alarm clock, put it on the floor (or cover it) so that its glow is not at eye level.

2. PREPARE TO RELAX.

Getting into a mode of relaxation before bed means switching from mentally stimulating activities to more relaxing ones so that your mind and body can unwind. For example, I like to take a hot bath and read a bit afterward. It also helps to create a relaxing atmosphere in your bedroom with dimmer lighting and comfortable, high-quality bed linens and pillows. Investing in a good mattress will be worth every dollar you spend.

3. WATCH WHAT YOU EAT AND DRINK.

Abstain from caffeine after about 4:00 p.m., including coffee, tea, and soda. Also, stay away from sugar, which can boost insulin in the body and temporarily increase your energy level. Try not to drink liquids an hour before bedtime to avoid having to get up in the middle of the night to go to the bathroom. And make a conscious effort not to overeat at dinner. When your body is actively digesting food, it is more difficult to sleep. Overindulgence in alcohol is another thing to avoid. Although it may initially put you to sleep, alcohol turns into sugar and ends up stimulating and possibly waking you up in the middle of the night.

4. IDENTIFY AND CONFRONT ISSUES THAT DISRUPT YOUR PEACE OF MIND.

There is a strong psychological aspect to sleep. Stress and anxiety can literally keep you up at night, as your troubles seep into your subconscious. Often, when racing thoughts disrupt our sleep, we are trying to produce a different outcome by obsessively going over particular situations with regrettable real-life results. It may be something that happened at work or in your relationship over which you are in denial and/or feel that you have little control. Keeping some paper and a pen by your bed can really help. When you are awakened by these disturbing thoughts, try to write them down to target the problem and get it out of your system, and then deal with it on a conscious level during the day, when you can actually do something about it.

5. LOOK TO NATURAL SLEEP REMEDIES.

Herbal supplements such as passionflower and valerian root are natural sedatives and make a good combination. Kava is another herbal remedy that has long been used for insomnia and anxiety. Melatonin is helpful for many people as well, and is often recommended by physicians as an antidote for jet lag. You have to experiment to see what works best for you.

STRESS MANAGEMENT

It ain't about how hard you hit, it's about how hard you can get hit and keep moving forward. That's how winning is done.

—ROCKY BALBOA IN THE MOVIE *ROCKY BALBOA* (2006)

Stress affects your sleep, eating habits, and happiness, and is clearly linked to depression and anxiety disorders. It can lead to gastrointestinal problems, headaches, muscle tension, and grinding of the teeth. Stress can cause weight gain because it increases appetite, slows the metabolism, and affects insulin regulation. It can even alter where fat is stored in the body (usually, the abdomen). It lowers the immune system and elevates inflammation and blood sugar, making you more susceptible to illnesses such as diabetes, heart disease, and cancer.

If stress can make you sick and even kill you, it can certainly destroy precious beauty cells. Not only does stress exacerbate inflammatory skin conditions, but the resulting elevated cortisol levels can deplete collagen and cause the body's cells to age more rapidly. Stress, worry, and sadness put a negative film over everything in your life.

Since we generally cannot prevent stress from entering our lives, we have to focus on how we deal with it. A dear friend and client, as well as a fellow woman entrepreneur, once said something very wise to me when we were discussing the trials and tribulations of running a business: "Bad things happen to everyone; what separates people is how they recover from them." We then went on to talk about how some people are devastated and depressed for months (or even longer) over something fairly insignificant, while others suffer truly horrific events but find the strength to go on to lead happy and productive lives. My friend epitomizes this positive attitude and emotional endurance. Having recently gone through an extremely difficult time and loss in her business, she has always appeared upbeat and smiling, and when discussing her challenges she has focused on the brighter future rather than dwelled on what went wrong. She has also shared other inspirational stories about building her business as a single mother.

Although some people are innately more positive and emotionally stronger, anyone can make a conscious choice to deal with a problem by moving through it or wallowing in it. You can beat yourself up for your mistakes and costly decisions, or accept that they are a part of life and learning. Forgive yourself and focus on the choices you can make from this day forward, since you cannot change the past. You can allow yourself to feel like a victim when something bad happens or someone hurts you, or you can have the confidence to know that circumstances and other people do not have to control your life—only you have that power. The way we deal with stress and difficult situations determines how they affect us physically and emotionally, and the extent to which they set us back.

I have understood this well over the years, hearing so much on the subject from others and having gone through some very difficult times myself. Not long ago, I had to care for my father after he had multiple strokes in his old age, losing his vision and ability to walk. At the time, he lived in Michigan and the doctors gave him only three months to live.

I wanted to be near him during his last days and found him a nursing home in New York. I hired a physical therapist who helped him walk again and a private nurse's aide to take him out to the park, read to him, bring him good food, and be by his side while my sister and I were at work. My father lived for another three years. Although I was glad to be with him during that time, the experience of caring for a sick parent took a profound emotional and physical toll on me. I actually saw my face change, as it started to reflect the sadness and anxiety I felt from constantly seeing my father in such a terrible state, and even guilt from not being able to do more for him. I had to change my lifestyle to protect my health from deteriorating as a result. Since that time I have learned a great deal about coping with stress and staying physically and emotionally healthy during particularly trying times. These practices have continued to help me cope with the everyday challenges of running a business and managing professional and personal relationships.

COPING TECHNIQUES FOR STRESS, ANXIETY, AND LIFE IN GENERAL

Along with your general outlook on life and how you process difficult situations, regular exercise has been scientifically proven to combat stress. Nutritional support also becomes even more vital. For instance, B vitamins supply energy and fuel cell function and growth. As a result, these vitamins are the first to be depleted by stress. Replenish them with foods high in B's. I have also found the herb holy basil incredible for reducing anxiety. Native to India, it is often used in ayurvedic medicine to treat a variety of conditions and to calm the nerves.

As opposed to taking better care of ourselves during times of stress, our instinct is actually the opposite and we end up making matters worse. The following are practices that will help immensely. Even if some of them sound strange at first, try to have an open mind. Perhaps not all of them are for you, and that's okay. The good news is that if you lead a healthy lifestyle and take good care of yourself during such times, the routines will probably become a way of life, keeping you more flexible and resilient.

The Body-Mind Connection: The Value of Integrative Medicine

In Western culture we tend to separate the mind and emotions from the physical body, compartmentalizing stress and anxiety as something different from physical illness. Integrative medicine, on the other hand, adopts a holistic approach and combines Eastern healing practices with conventional Western medicine. It embraces the interconnection between the physical and the emotional and mental aspects of health.

An integrative physician looks at all aspects of a patient's lifestyle to detect the underlying cause of the symptoms, whether a vitamin deficiency or chronic stress. Once the root of the problem is identified, the doctor can prescribe a medication, vitamin supplement, and/or a healing therapy to relieve the symptoms. Since integrative medicine literally integrates traditional and alternative therapies and philosophies, you get the benefits of both. I believe that this approach is the best way to achieve good health. Wellness is more than mainstream medical treatment and prescriptions.

The Healing Practices of Yoga, Breathing, and Meditation

In addition to being an amazing form of physical exercise, yoga connects you to a deeper part of yourself through breathing. On a physical level, it stretches the muscles, makes you stronger, helps lengthen the spine (alleviating many back problems), and improves blood circulation, sleep, and digestion. There are many types of yoga to choose from. I recommend trying different classes and teachers to find the style that you feel most comfortable practicing.

Equally important to the more physical aspects of yoga are the deep-breathing techniques. In times of stress, we tend to take very shallow breaths. The act of elongating and slowing down the breath while pushing our bodies physically teaches us to use our breath effectively in everyday life during strenuous situations. Breathing in the face of adversity will help you to cope more effectively by lowering your blood pressure and calming your anxiety.

Yoga meditation is a powerful way to clear the mind, similar to how exercise cleans and detoxifies the body. An ayurvedic healer once explained to me that the Western version of meditation is to become ill in order to stare at four walls in a state of silence. Sickness is our no-excuse opportunity to be in restorative solitude, while in Eastern cultures it is meditation. This healer described the mind by drawing an analogy with an old-fashioned switchboard. When the wires and messages become chaotic with racing thoughts and mental chatter, signals get crossed and short-circuit. It is not until you can clear your mind that you can see situations and people for what and who they really are, and interpret things with more clarity.

NATURAL REMEDY

Beginning a meditation practice

It may sound easy enough to sit quietly and empty your mind, but if you have never tried it, you will find that it is actually quite challenging. Begin by sitting comfortably in a quiet space, with your legs crossed in front of you, Indian style. Sit on a folded towel so that you are slightly tilted forward. Rest your hands on your knees with your palms open and facing upward. Close your eyes, observe your breath, and allow yourself to drift into this empty space in your mind. When a thought enters, imagine it drifting away, as if it were a cloud, and focus back on the empty space in the center of your mind's eye, the third eye. You can welcome thoughts and outward sounds, but then let them go. Start with any amount of meditation time you can manage, even if just sixty seconds, and you will gradually be able to build on it.

BODY AND ENERGY WORK

Life takes us out of alignment in so many ways, and bodywork helps to rebalance the body and mind. For example, we hold so much stress in our neck and back that sometimes it literally feels as though the weight of the world is on our shoulders. Several forms of physical therapy, such as massage, acupuncture, acupressure, and reflexology, put us back in touch with this body that we live in. They not only relieve tension, aches, and pains, but make us aware that all parts of the body are interconnected. Working out muscle tension through massage or a practice like yoga can be healing on more than just the physical level.

Massage

Massage works hand in hand with exercise to release muscle tension, reduce stress, and increase circulation. Regular massages should be integrated into your budget and lifestyle, whether once a month, every three months, or however frequently you can afford them. Many people consider massage a luxury, but in numerous cultures it is part of the lifestyle.

Acupuncture

Acupuncture involves the insertion and manipulation of delicate needles into specific points on the body to help heal one's physical and emotional state, as well as relieve pain. This practice has been around for thousands of years. It focuses on moving qi (pronounced "chee"), which is the body's energy. According to traditional Chinese medicine, once this flow of energy stagnates or becomes stuck, it can cause illness and/or pain. Releasing qi opens the meridians, or lines of the body through which energy flows to nourish its different parts. Acupuncture treats a host of problems, but it is especially beneficial for relieving back pain, anxiety, sleep disorders, infertility, and menopause symptoms such at hot flashes and insomnia. Like many other "alternative" healing therapies, acupuncture is becoming more mainstream, so you should be able to find skilled practitioners in every major city. It is also starting to be more accepted by conventional medicine and is now used in many pain-management facilities and hospitals.

Reflexology

Reflexology is another ancient practice that is acknowledged by integrative doctors not only as a method of healing but as a diagnostic tool. It is based on the principle that nerve endings on the feet and hands correspond to other parts of the body. By applying pressure to one of these points, a reflexologist can stimulate a response in another area. A particularly sore spot on your foot, for instance, can give you information about, and relief from, a more significant problem elsewhere in your body. The toes and fingers, for example, mirror the head and neck, and the ball of the foot is the reflex point for the chest, heart, and lungs.

Reiki

Reiki is a form of energy work based on the idea that the gentle placement of hands on the body can help unblock trapped qi to maintain the flow of energy. This is a spiritual as well as a physical practice, since it is believed that traumatic past experiences, memories, and tension deposit in the body and can be cleared. Craniosacral therapy is another such technique, which involves aligning the body and releasing restricted energy channels in the head and neck.

PROFESSIONAL TECHNIQUE
Chiropractic care

Chiropractic medicine can realign the spine, unlike any form of exercise or bodywork. A chiropractor diagnoses problems of the body's musculoskeletal and nervous systems and uses a hands-on approach to adjust and manipulate joints or tissue, to alleviate discomfort, and to restore mobility, which in turn improves your overall health. As with everything else, it's the expertise of the professional that makes the difference. Many chiropractors are amazing healers, so it is important to get a referral and find the right one. Today, even traditional medicine has begun to appreciate and refer patients for chiropractic care.

THE HAPPINESS QUOTIENT

There is no cosmetic for beauty like happiness.

—Lady Marguerite Blessington, nineteenth-century Irish novelist

The most vital aspect of beauty is perhaps the most elusive and the least obvious. The way a woman feels about herself and her life, as well as the energy that she emanates, can often be the one element that throws everything off. Unhappiness, insecurity, and anxiety chip away at beauty. The eyes really are a mirror of the soul, and your appearance is a reflection of your inner world—not just your physical health, but your self-image and perspective on life. Additionally, this psychological component often determines how you take care of yourself, creating very real physical consequences. No matter how physically perfect a woman may be, if she does not feel that beauty within herself, it will not come across. Beauty emanates from confidence and emotional health. Finding these things within you can take time and dedication. We often forget that we, not others, hold the key to our own happiness.

Happiness *is* beauty—a smile creates warmth and brings a glint to the eye that cannot be captured with the most skillfully applied makeup. Cultivating a sense of joy, self-acceptance, and gratitude is much easier said than done, but it is a commitment that we have to make to ourselves. There are many avenues of insight in this area, whether through counseling, therapy, support groups, spiritual practices, or meditation. At certain times in our lives we all need to deal with the feelings, past traumas, and patterns of behavior that might be holding us back. Perhaps you are unhappy in your relationship, feel devalued by others, or have always struggled with insecurity. This inner dialogue that you battle with could be due to the messages you received as a child or to defining relationships in your adolescence, but if these feelings are faced openly and constructively, you can let them go and be set free. If you are not ready to commit either emotionally or financially to traditional therapy, there are support groups held at community centers and churches. Many universities offer counseling with graduate students for a small fraction of the price of a licensed therapist. Do some research and, when you're ready, take advantage of the resources available to you.

Learning more about the healing practices that I have touched on here will nourish your life in ways that should never be discounted. The greatest beauty secret of all is to create more balance between the internal and external aspects of your life. The most appealing and outwardly beautiful woman is one who is healthy and happy with herself and her life.

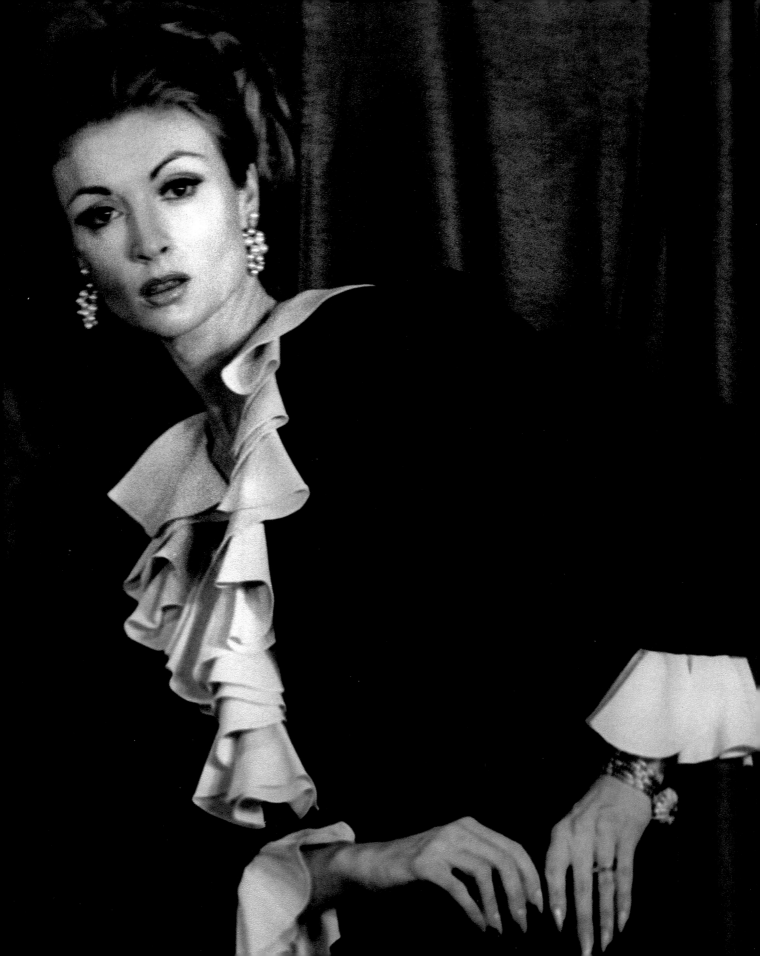

10

FASHION AND STYLE
THE FINISHING TOUCH

Fashion is architecture: it is a matter of proportions.　　　　—COCO CHANEL

Pulling your entire look together with clothes and accessories is just as important as designing your perfect haircut and hair color. Fashion defines how you present yourself to the world, how others perceive you, and, ultimately, how you see yourself. The fit, silhouette, colors, and quality of the clothing you wear speak volumes. Yet fashion can be a difficult language to learn. Becoming fluent enough to have fun with your look involves knowing a few basic rules, understanding which styles suit you, and having the confidence to find your own creative interpretation within those parameters.

Your clothing works hand in hand with your hair and makeup to project an image. It is all linked by the concepts of design, proportion, and color. When a woman knows how to pull all these elements together, she turns heads. In my line of work, I am always onstage. My credibility as a

Left: Mom, 1965.

beauty expert comes in part from the way I put together my whole look. The way I present myself is a big responsibility in a business that is all about the visual. I never just "throw something on" when getting ready for work—my outfits are always thoughtfully planned. Each day the look is a bit different, and I try to get everything—my hair, makeup, and clothing—to work together. I hope that sharing my personal philosophies about fashion and the guiding principles that I have followed over the years will make it easier for you to pull together your look. I also aim to help you get organized with all the right pieces, so that getting ready becomes less of a chore and something you actually enjoy doing.

Having my fashion-model mother with her exquisite taste as a mentor turned fashion into my second love. What I did not learn from my mother, I later picked up from my best friend, Lynn. We have known each other since beauty school (she is a fabulous hairstylist) and were inseparable until I moved from Michigan, remaining lifelong friends. In addition to doing hair and makeup, Lynn is a painter, designs jewelry, and has always had a knack for putting together stunning ensembles from random pieces in her closet. She helped me hone the skill of mixing, matching, and accessorizing clothing, which came in handy when we could not afford to buy designer labels.

My mother's wardrobe, on the other hand, was truly incredible—like that of a movie star. In the 1970s she wore tight suede knee-high boots that she owned in every color. She was also known for her jumpsuits, while her best friend, my aunt Jan, was the queen of those long, knit maxi dresses (they made her look so sexy that she once caused a car accident started by a man who was trying to flirt with her while driving as she walked on the sidewalk!). They wore fabulous wigs and falls, big sunglasses, and gorgeous fur coats (when fur was socially acceptable to wear)—Aunt Jan's was a silver fox that matched her platinum hair and my mother's red fox coat matched her strawberry-blond mane. They were impossibly chic, sexy, and glamorous women. My mother was my father's muse—he was her biggest fan.

With the trained eye of a designer and the passion of a southern Italian, my father could look at a woman and immediately see how she could improve her makeup or dress in a more flattering way. He had a true affinity for women, loved to connect with them, and found them fascinating and much more interesting to be around than men. He loved working with them and being in their company at home (he was completely surrounded; even our cats were females!). It is from my father that I inherited a genuine appreciation for working with women and helping them become their most beautiful.

My father was incredibly artistic by nature and skilled with his hands. He was a jack of many trades and had mastered most of them. He could design and decorate interiors, make clothes and jewelry, do makeup and hair, paint, fix anything that was broken, and was even a skilled mechanic who could take apart an entire car and put it back together. (I actually loved to help him when he made car repairs in our garage. I often compare being a hairdresser to being a mechanic because both professions are technical and require one to think strategically and be a problem-solver.) My dad loved to take me and my sister shopping, and afterward he personally hemmed and tailored our purchases. He would also try to re-create what we had seen in a store and perhaps could not afford. Or he would just come home, inspired to create a stylish belt made from scraps of leather that he pulled out of his sample books. His profession, interior-decoration, was clearly displayed throughout our house, with textiles and fabric swatches scattered everywhere; his designs and layouts of home interiors were piled high. Growing up around all this helped me to absorb an intuitive understanding of color, fabric, texture, and design.

The art of putting together an outfit and the laws of proportion and design are actually simpler to grasp and apply than you might think. This chapter will help you understand fashion in a straightforward and uncomplicated way. Once you learn to see clothing as basic lines silhouetting your frame, distinguishing what shapes look best on you will become easier.

I will help you assemble a classic wardrobe and combine different pieces to create a complete look. Even if you are a no-frills, jeans and T-shirt kind of girl, you will acquire valuable tips about working with accessories, gauging proportion to get the right fit from your clothing, and successfully transitioning your casual daytime ensemble to an evening look without a complete costume change. (A sharp blazer, a pair of heels, the right jewelry, and a great blowout can take jeans and a T-shirt right out to dinner!)

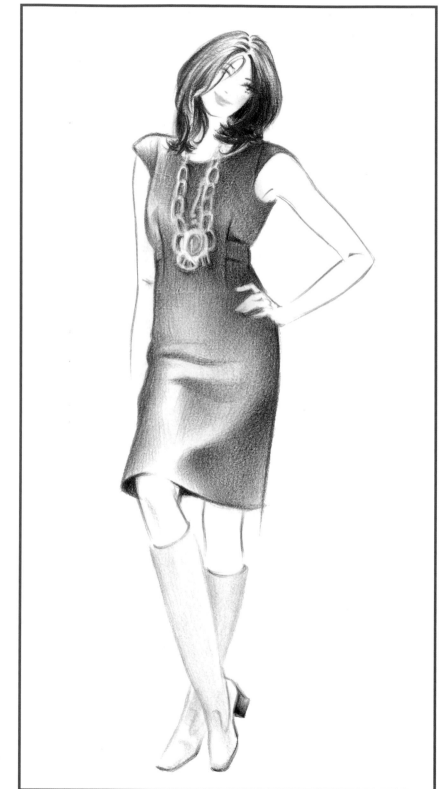

Simple blue cotton dress worn with
neutral leather boots and vintage
jewelry.

As with hair and makeup, once you learn the basics you can begin to push the envelope to develop your own distinctive style. We often see well-executed fashion-rule breakers, whether on women in the public eye or just women with great taste. Their creativity and individuality are inspiring and remind us that people create their personal styles by taking risks. After all, the most profound fashion trends began with experimentation.

PULLING YOUR LOOK TOGETHER WITH CLOTHES, HAIR, AND MAKEUP

Your wardrobe is the icing on the cake. Obviously, the tones and colors of your clothes must be flattering, but the secret to getting this right starts with your hair! A great haircut and color are permanent fashion accessories and your greatest assets. They bring you more than halfway there. (Perhaps you have noticed that after you leave the salon with fresh color and a great cut, even your casual clothes look more chic!) With these grounding elements in place, a world of opportunities with color and style will open up to you.

You can probably tell immediately whether a certain fabric color is right for you. If it washes you out, it is obviously not the right choice. If it brightens your face and really pops against your skin tone, then voilà! However, once your hair color and makeup are in balance, your clothing color palette expands, leaving you with fewer rules to follow. For example, a woman with yellow undertones in her skin tends to look sallow unless she wears warmer or brighter clothing colors that enliven her complexion. Typically, cool hues, such as silver and charcoal, may wash her out, but hair color with a warm undertone will bring warmth to her skin tone, allowing her to wear both warm and cool colors. Someone with pink or red undertones in her skin would instinctually shy away from wearing bright blue-based colors, instead gravitating toward neutral tones that help balance the red in her skin. However, hair color with a cooler tone will create the same balance, so that brighter shades of clothing will not seem to intensify her ruddy complexion.

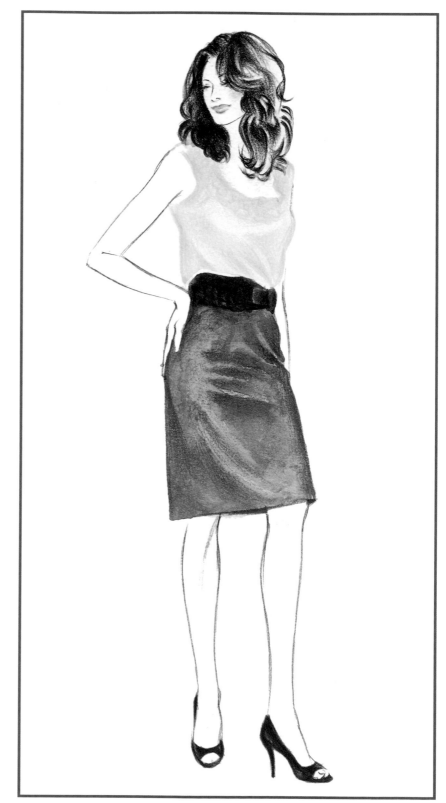

Pencil skirt, paired with a wool tank and a wide leather belt, and worn with a peep-toe pump.

TEN FASHION RULES TO LIVE BY

1. Buy Quality

You get what you pay for. Beautifully made apparel that fits well will last for years, even a lifetime, and a classic piece may never go out of style. Look for clothing made from fine fabrics that are well constructed and stitched and that display an overall attention to detail. It is these timeless pieces that are the go-to items in my closet—the staples I put on time and again because they always look great. They even include pieces that my mother used to wear, which still look beautiful and are more valuable today than ever.

Many people cannot stop themselves from overbuying needless things simply because these items are on sale. This obsession not to pass up a deal ultimately results in spending too much on too many impulsive purchases that do not fit, last, or look good on you. Unless throwaway clothing is your specific intent, it is always better to purchase fewer higher-priced but well-made pieces than many cheaply manufactured ones. Add up the money spent on all the sale items you have amassed that you never wear because they look too trendy and dated, have lost their shape, or never fit well in the first place. Instead, you could probably have purchased the one full-price piece that you really wanted and out of which you would have gotten much more use and pleasure. If you buy less and pay more, you will look much better and may actually save money in the long run.

2. Own Classic Pieces on Which You Can Rely

A wardrobe of well-made, well-fitting key pieces is indispensable. These timeless staples always make you look and feel good and can easily be mixed and matched with other, trendier odds and ends in your closet. These essentials will serve as the foundation for your wardrobe.

- **A BEAUTIFUL SUIT:** Tailored trousers or a well-fitting skirt with a fitted blazer, to wear together or separately.
- **A FEW BASIC SKIRTS:** Perhaps an A-line shape or a pencil skirt, depending on what is more flattering for your frame.

- **THE PERFECT LITTLE BLACK DRESS:** Whether it is vintage or new, this is not only a classic staple for the evening but a dress you can throw on when you are running late and need to look pulled together.
- **A FEW PAIRS OF FLATTERING TROUSERS:** Black, brown, or other neutral colors.
- **A SHEATH DRESS:** Simple, straight cut, and not too form-fitting. It is versatile enough to pair with a blazer and/or wear belted. Looks great with boots, heels, or flats.
- **A PAIR OF JEANS** that fit you perfectly. (Refer to rule 9 on page 313.)
- **A FEW SWEATERS:** Simple pullover styles and a cardigan or two that can be thrown over a sleeveless blouse or dress to make it feel more professional. Make sure that the cardigans are more form-fitting, so that they do not look sloppy or make you look heavy. You can also put a slim belt around a cardigan to better define your waistline.
- **TOPS AND BLOUSES:** From classic to sexy, a variety to choose from to be paired with skirts and pants.
- **A CLASSIC PUMP:** This basic shoe instantly makes a skirt or pants (even a pair of jeans) look stylish. Select a few neutral shades such as black, brown, and nude.
- **A FABRIC SHOE:** This is a dressier shoe for the evening or more formal attire (a leather pump can look too corporate when paired with a delicate cocktail dress). Invest in a pair of silk or satin shoes that can be a pump, peep-toe, sling-back, or strappy high heel.
- **OUTERWEAR:** Every woman needs the following: a great trench or raincoat, a thin wool coat that ends at the knee for spring and fall, a casual jacket to wear with jeans, a warm winter coat, and a dressier cocktail coat (in a fabric like suede or velvet) that feels more appropriate for the evening. You do not want to put on a puffy down coat over a pretty cocktail dress.

3. Get the Right Fit—Size Matters

It is sometimes hard to admit, especially to yourself, that you are a size larger than you want to be. Unfortunately, purchasing one size smaller does not make you that size, but actually makes you look even heavier because your clothing is too tight. So be honest with yourself and get the right fit. Every-

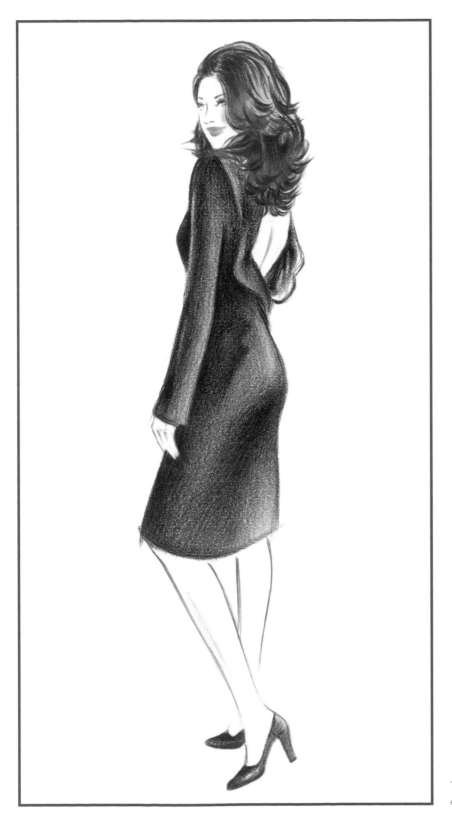

The black dress. Simple, yet
elegant.

one looks and feels thinner in clothing that comfortably drapes the body, as opposed to feeling like you have been stuffed into it, with the waistline uncomfortably digging into you and the fabric pulling across your backside, or pants that feel too short-waisted. You also run the risk of sporting the dreaded "camel toe," which is a look to be avoided at all costs. It is generally a good idea to try on garments before buying them, unless you regularly get clothing from a particular designer and know your size in that line.

4. Be Aware of Proportion

In the same way as a great haircut is designed in proportion to a woman's facial structure, the length of her neck, and her overall height and frame, a flattering article of clothing follows the same laws of balance.

Think about your height and body shape in conjunction with the silhouette of an article of clothing. Do you have long or short legs? Are you tall and thin, voluptuous, or petite? What features of your figure do you love and which ones would you like to play down? What length skirt looks best on you? Does a wide-legged trouser make you look short, whereas a slimmer leg gives the illusion of more length and height? Be discerning and listen to your instincts—if you feel that something makes you look heavier or shorter, it is probably not the right proportion for you.

Proportion is about geometric lines. In chapter 1, I explained how the perimeter line is the outline or silhouette of the haircut. The same is true with the lines of your clothing. If you can visualize the overall outline of the clothes on your body it will help you gauge how something looks on your figure. For example, a wider trouser and a boxy jacket create an overall square shape, so by wearing something more form-fitting on top (or below) you can minimize what could otherwise be an unflattering silhouette. This is similar to the optical illusions that can be created with the layers, length, and lines of a haircut to make the face look slimmer or the neck longer.

USE A FULL-LENGTH MIRROR

You need a full-length mirror for a head-to-toe view of yourself. You also need to look at the lines of your clothing from a few angles, which is why many stores have three-way mirrors in the dressing rooms. Evaluate the balance of your clothes, including your shoes, with your entire silhouette.

Is the height of your heels in proportion to the length and shape of your pants, skirt, or dress? Is the length of your boots flattering to your legs? For example, boots that hit at midcalf visually cut the lower legs in half, so they usually look best on taller women. Women of petite or average height will find that they look taller and slimmer wearing a longer boot that hits just below the knee to elongate the line of the lower leg.

PROPORTION IS ALSO IMPORTANT FOR OUTERWEAR

Take one last glance in a full-length mirror right before you leave the house, so that you can see your overall look when everything is on. Do not neglect to check the length of your coat against the hemline of your skirt, or consider whether a shorter jacket might be a better choice with your pants or jeans. Generally, shorter coats and jackets look best with pants, while longer coats that hit above or just below the knee work well with most skirts and dresses.

CHECK YOUR OUTFIT IN THE LIGHT TO AVOID ANY SURPRISES

Look in a full-length mirror in *good lighting* so that you can see panty lines or if your skirt or dress is too sheer. If the fabric is a bit transparent, you can throw on a slip or another type of nude-color undergarment in order to obscure the silhouette of your legs. Taking a last look is important to make sure that your dress does not become see-through in bright daylight.

STYLE GUIDE

How to look taller and slimmer

The proportion of your clothes, the color or print of the fabric, and even the shade of hosiery or an accessory such as a belt can create the illusion of height and a leaner figure. For example, wearing a dark shoe or bootie with matching dark hosiery extends the line of the foot and leg, making them look longer. Sheer nude panty hose with a neutral-tone shoe works the same magic and looks fantastic with a little black dress in springtime. If you want to look taller, avoid the disjointed effect of a dark shoe and a dark skirt or dress with light hose, or a light shirt with a dark skirt or pants. The stark contrast in colors makes you look shorter because the eye does not continue to travel along the length of your frame. You become essentially "color-blocked." Conversely, wearing colors in the same family from top to bottom elongates the body and gives you a taller and slimmer figure.

Neutral shades:
Beyond black

When shopping, keep
in mind that black is
not the only basic color.
Consider other neutral
hues that are universally
flattering, such as gray
(from dove to charcoal),
rich browns, navy, olive
green, and plum.

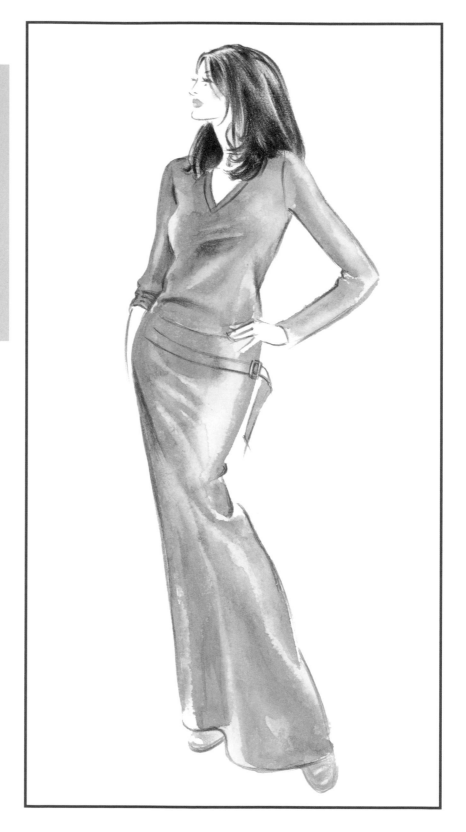

Long gray skirt with matching
V-neck sweater, belted at the hip.

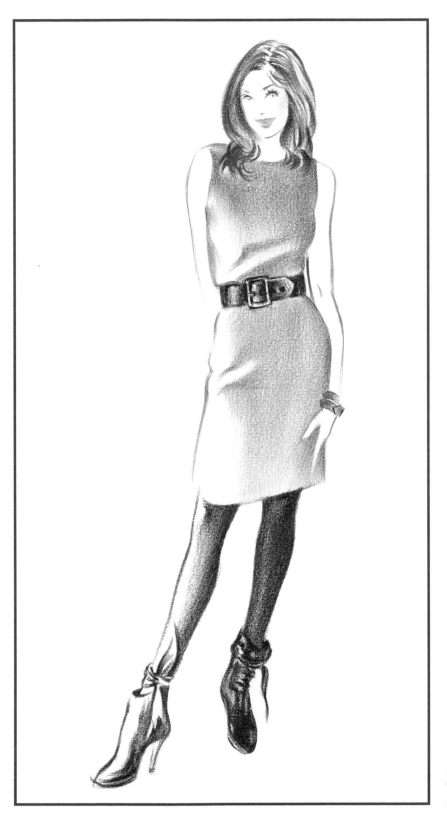

Simple sheath dress, belted. Worn
with dark hose to match leather
booties.

Q&A

Q: *Are lower-priced lines from top designers a great deal or too good to be true?*

A: Many well-known designers sell collections at popular discount retail chains. The prices are shockingly low, but are they really a good buy? If you're just looking for the fun trend of the season, the answer is, absolutely. Just know that this apparel is nowhere near the quality of the designer's higher-end line. The inspiration may be there, but the construction and the fabric are not. It is impossible to construct a piece of high-quality clothing at such a low price. Although a designer piece at a fraction of the cost is appealing, you get what you pay for.

HOW TO WEAR A DRESS THAT IS TOO SHORT

We all have dresses that are too short to wear at work or that we simply no longer feel comfortable wearing. A great way of incorporating them into your attire is to slip on a tight-fitting skirt underneath. Choose one in a complementary color that is a few inches longer than the dress, to elongate your ensemble.

CHOOSING THE RIGHT BELT FOR YOUR FIGURE

Belts can work wonders for the figure and your entire look. They are a versatile and flattering accessory when chosen correctly, serving as instant tailoring to give your body more shape and your clothing more appeal. Here are a few basic belt guidelines for different body types.

SHORT-WAISTED (OR HIGH-WAISTED): A thinner belt or one worn slightly lower on the hip helps to visually elongate the midsection. Wearing a belt that is too wide and hits too high on the body can make that area appear even shorter.

LONG-WAISTED: With a long midsection, a wider belt worn directly at the waistline (not low on the hip) directs the eye higher on the body, making the legs appear longer and the entire frame more balanced.

HOURGLASS FIGURE: A wider belt or one worn directly at the waistline accentuates the smaller waist and natural curves.

PETITE FRAME: A belt in a color or tone that blends with the rest of the outfit does not "cut" the body in half.

HOW BEST TO WEAR PRINTS AND PATTERNS

Prints and patterns worn head-to-toe can make you look heavier. With a print dress, a belt will add more shape to the body and ground the ensemble with a solid color. Another good option is to combine a print top with a skirt or pants in a solid color to slim the silhouette from the waist down.

HOW YOUR HAIRSTYLE CAN COMPLEMENT THE SILHOUETTE OF YOUR CLOTHING

Ideally, the scale and shape of your hairstyle should work with the lines of your clothing. There is actually a method to keeping them in balance. If the silhouette of your outfit is soft and flowing, your hair can follow those lines by being worn loose and wavy or curly. With something more structural and tailored, the hair looks best smoothed or straightened. This is why a blowout with a suit is such a great combination. A chic ponytail with a suit can be stunning as well. With a higher neckline, a turtleneck, or a ruffle detail near the neck, wearing the hair up and off the face visually lengthens the neck that is partially covered with fabric. For a lower neckline, I find that wearing the hair down is more flattering and can softly conceal the neck and chest (depending on the length of your hair) if you feel self-conscious about baring so much. Wearing several chain necklaces together can also help to camouflage cleavage.

PROFESSIONAL TECHNIQUE

A good tailor for alterations

It is important to find a skilled tailor who can hem a pair of pants or take something in. This is not to say that you should buy things that don't fit and have them altered for your body. If you have to re-construct an item of clothing to make it fit, you are not buying the right one. The exception is vintage clothing, whether passed down in your family or purchased. If it's a one-of-a-kind piece, expert altera-tion can certainly be worth the investment. Otherwise, start with a basic, good fit, then use a tailor for more minor and precise adjustments.

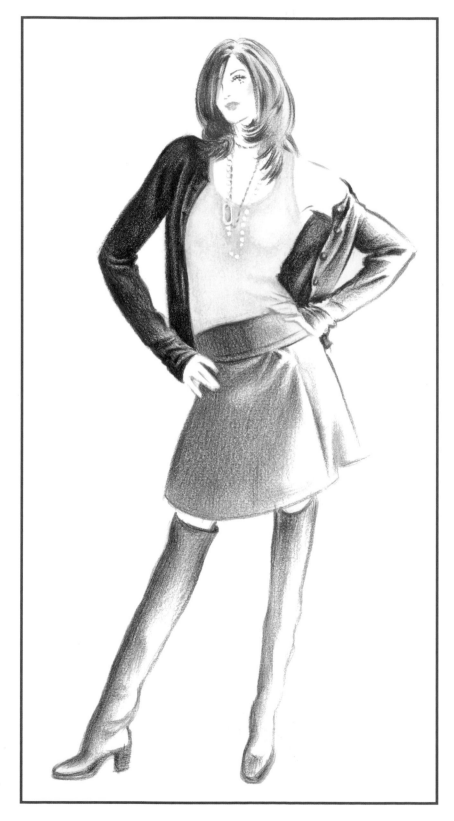

A-line skirt and tank top with cardigan. Worn with over-the-knee boots.

5. Purchase Only Pieces That You Absolutely Love

If something does not make you feel and look good, it has negative value. This is a good rule of thumb to follow when shopping or cleaning out your closets. Most of us have too many choices in our wardrobe, although only a small percentage of them are actually flattering. If you edit your clothing down to those items, there will be much less room for error when choosing an outfit. We all have a few garments that feel too tight or too loose, but that we cannot bear to part with. Store these in a separate area and pull them out if you lose or gain a few pounds, but don't keep them in the front of your closet as a reminder that you used to be thinner or heavier. Your clothes should never make you feel bad about yourself. On the contrary, your wardrobe should make you feel attractive and confident.

6. Make Sure You Are Comfortable

You should be able to move around freely in your clothes. When trying on a possible new purchase, think about all the different movements you make during the course of a day: lifting your kids, getting into and out of a car, rushing to the subway, sitting down, bending over or reaching overhead for something. Bend forward and backward, raise your arms, crouch down, and determine if the garment is too tight or if too much skin gets exposed. I probably look like a gymnast when in a dressing room. It is quite hilarious! But because of my job, these movements help me to simulate my daily environment when trying on clothes to see if I will be comfortable wearing them. Be careful not to hurt yourself, however. One time, my aunt Jan fell through the curtain of the dressing room, right out on the shopping floor, as she lost her balance when her leg got stuck in a pair of jeans that she was trying on!

PROFESSIONAL TECHNIQUE

The best way to clean leather

You can clean leather (even a leather sofa) with one drop of natural liquid soap. My father taught me this secret years ago, and it is the most gentle way to clean leather goods. Dampen a sponge in a bowl of warm water with a drop of liquid soap. Go over the leather, wiping it a second time with a sponge containing only clean water. Dry it immediately and completely with a soft cloth.

7. Dress Appropriately for the Occasion

First impressions really do matter, and wearing the right thing at the right time is the key to looking fabulous whether you are going to work, to a recreational event, or to a cocktail party. The best-dressed people dress appropriately for the occasion. They do not have to be wearing the most expensive clothing, but can stylishly differentiate between casual, business, and evening apparel within their wardrobe. In a business setting, dressing professionally can make or break a job interview or an important deal. People size you up in less than thirty seconds, and your clothes have a lot to do with how others perceive you. Dressing for success truly makes a difference and helps to create opportunities.

LEGGINGS ARE NOT PANTS

Leggings are designed to be worn under skirts, tunics, and short dresses, where too much skin would be exposed with bare legs or panty hose. They are not meant to be worn as pants unless you are exercising. Think of them as a more substantial version of tights. Even if you are in the best shape of your life, it is still not appropriate to wear tights around town or at work.

HOW TO WEAR EVENING WEAR DURING THE DAY

Most of us do not get enough opportunities to wear a cocktail dress or other evening clothes. A great way to enjoy those beautiful pieces is to dress them down by casually surrounding the fancy dress or blouse with more relaxed accoutrements. For example, try pairing a cocktail dress with leggings and boots, or throw a cardigan on top to make it more casual. You could even wear such an outfit to work with flats or a low-heeled shoe and a blazer. In a more conservative work environment, you can get away with wearing a shimmery blouse or shell underneath a fitted blazer as well as a beaded scarf with a classic suit.

8. Do Not Overlook the Undergarments

The shape and silhouette of your body are dramatically influenced by what you wear under your clothing. The right foundations allow clothes to drape and fit on the body in a much more flattering way. Wearing a bra *that actually fits you* will make an extraordinary difference in how any garment looks on your body.

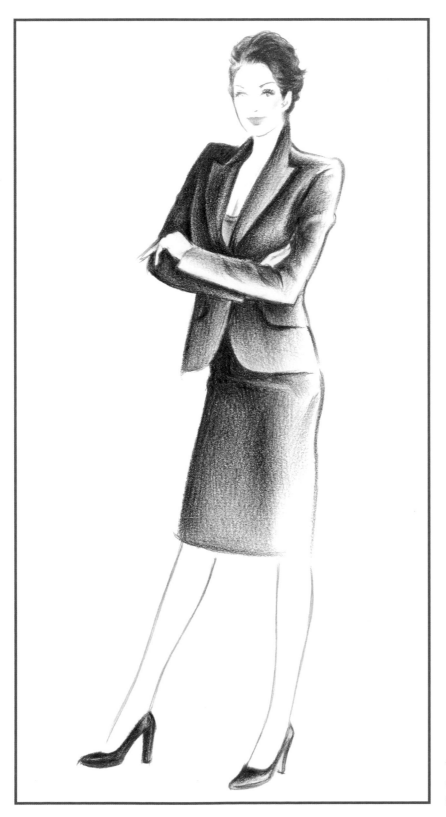

The classic suit. Fitted blazer and a straight skirt worn with leather pumps.

Every woman should be measured and fitted for a bra by an expert at a lingerie or department store (you may be surprised by your actual measurement). Also, take note of the bra's fabric: under a thinner material such as cotton or silk, you need a smooth bra with no seams or embellishments. For larger busts, lace provides the best support. And pay attention to the color of your lingerie. My personal rule is to buy only black and nude underwear—everything else, including white, can show through clothing.

As for your lower half, the goal is to shape and smooth your behind under skirts and pants, and to avoid panty lines—or worse—a double butt (also referred to as "double stuff," when your butt is horizontally split in two by your panties). Under a pair of pants I recommend wearing a thong, rather than full panties. The very reason thongs became so popular is that they solve the panty-line problem. Panty hose are an easy way to smooth and slim the legs and butt under your pants. A pair of hose (skip the control tops, which are too uncomfortable) creates the smoothest, sheerest, and most unnoticeable lining. A wonderful option under form-fitting skirts and dresses (and also during warmer months when panty hose are not an option) is a pair of body-slimming spandex boy shorts. They smartly smooth the line of your behind and hips under a snug or clingy skirt or dress. I prefer to wear them with skirts rather than with slim trousers to avoid a noticeable line on the upper thigh. I also consider them to be mandatory when I am walking around on a windy day while wearing a loose-fitting skirt. If the wind happens to blow up your skirt, you will not be caught in an em-bare-ass-ing situation.

HOW TO LAUNDER UNDERGARMENTS

Most women do not wash their bras frequently enough. A bra should be hand washed after having been worn once or twice, not necessarily because it is dirty but because the elastic gets stretched out. Gentle laundering allows the bra to snap back into shape and ensures that the delicate undergarment lasts longer. The best way to launder bras, hosiery, and bathing suits is by hand-washing them in warm or cool water with a drop of mild shampoo and letting them air dry. Since shampoo is gentle enough to use on your hair, it is better for fine fabrics with elastic or spandex than a detergent made for wool.

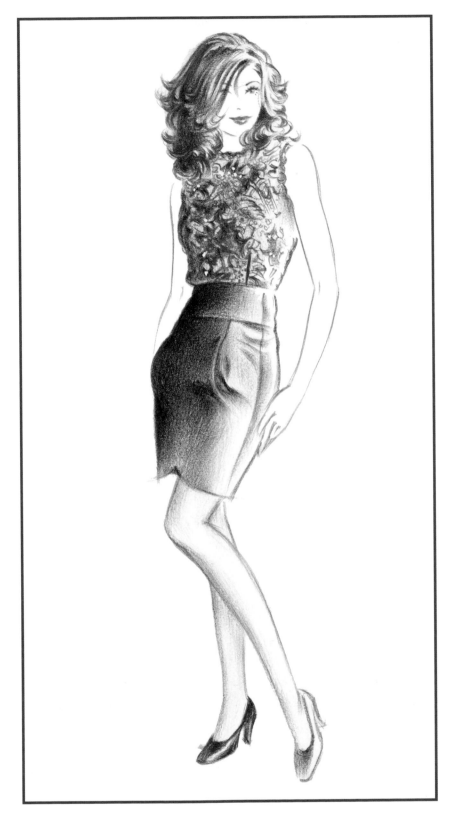

Vintage, beaded top and fitted
skirt worn with a silk pump.

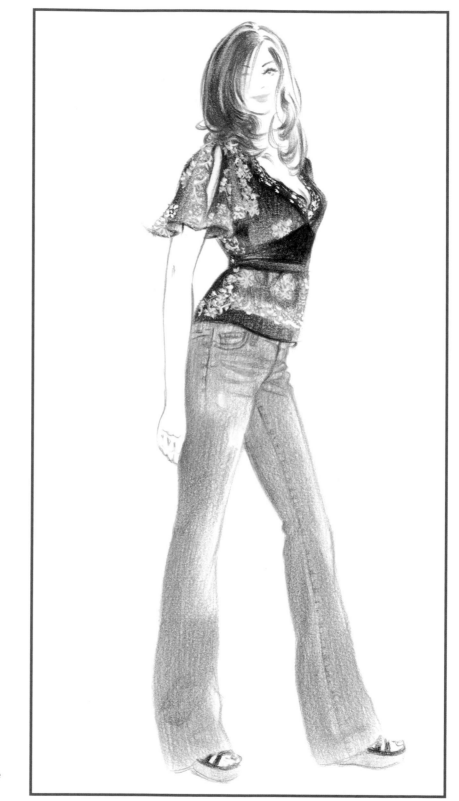

Boot-cut jeans paired with a cute
top and wedges.

At the risk of sounding like Helen Gurley Brown circa 1965, here is some good advice: if you want to have a happy, healthy love life with your husband/lover/partner, do not wear ugly things to bed unless you have the flu. It is generally wise to refrain from wearing something around the house that you would not be caught dead in outside. People have a tendency to get too comfortable and start to wear unflattering clothing when relaxing at home with the one they love. There are plenty of comfy lounging clothes that are flattering and that match.

9. Choose the Right Cut of Jeans

Wearing the wrong cut, size, and style of jeans may be the most common and egregious fashion faux pas. In my opinion, jeans are simply not as comfortable or easy to wear as they seem to be. I have found that for the majority of women, a straight-leg style is the most flattering. For those who are more curvaceous, a slightly wider boot cut will balance out the hips and create a long, lean, attractive line.

Unless you have a perfectly flat stomach, do not attempt to wear low-rise jeans. Squeezing into this style, if you have even a trace of a tummy, creates an unattractive "muffin top." Jeans that hit a bit higher on the hip (slightly below the waist) are much more becoming on most women. And remember: *skinny jeans are only for skinny people*. They do not make you look skinny—quite the opposite if you are not rail thin. Not every fashion trend works for every person. It is better to be honest with yourself and wear a cut of jeans that actually flatters your shape and that you feel comfortable in.

10. Invest in Accessories

Well-selected pieces of jewelry and beautiful scarves will never go out of style. These items add versatility to your wardrobe and can work with everything in your closet. Accessorizing properly and creatively with a few important, stylish pieces instantly transforms an outfit, making it more pulled together and chic. The most fashionable women in the world have understood the importance of the right accessories.

Jacqueline Onassis made a simple pair of capri pants and a blouse into an iconic fashion statement by adding big sunglasses, along with a silk scarf over her hair. Her combinations of simple but high-quality clothing with one or two bold accents work just as beautifully today as they did in the sixties. Fashion designer Coco Chanel, who set the precedent for layering costume jewelry in the 1930s, famously adorned herself with ropes of faux pearls. An icon and an iconoclast, Chanel would drape striking costume jewelry over a daytime ensemble and often wore no jewelry at all with evening clothes—proving that fashion rules are meant to be broken, as long as it is done with good taste.

The layering of numerous necklaces can be a beautiful classic or alternative look, depending on the style of jewelry. If you feel that a necklace on its own looks a bit boring, combining it with others and mixing different lengths instantly makes the ensemble more interesting. The key to not looking over the top is to pick your focus—wear several necklaces (or just one that makes a statement), or big earrings, but not both. If your clothes have a lot going on—a printed fabric, a scarf, or lots of detailing such as ruffles or lace—a simple pair of earrings might be enough. Accessories and jewelry become more important with clean lines and solid colors in clothing. I have always preferred this style, since busy prints can sometimes "wear you," as people notice the clothing before seeing you.

ARE YOUR ACCESSORIES IN BALANCE WITH YOUR OUTFIT?

The wrong accessory can undermine a great outfit. Carrying a purse that is too large for your frame while wearing a delicate dress can look out of balance. Like your clothing, accessories should be complementary to your overall silhouette. I always "try on" a handbag in the store before I buy it, finding a full-length mirror so I can strike a pose to make sure that it's not too big for my frame. I have actually owned purses since age three (at that time I just carried around an empty one), and they have grown up with my body.

ACCESSORIES CAN TRANSITION YOUR LOOK FROM DAY TO EVENING

Hair, makeup, shoes, and jewelry are the key components that can completely change your look. You can wear exactly the same outfit you had on at work, and with a few adjustments be ready for a dinner or an evening

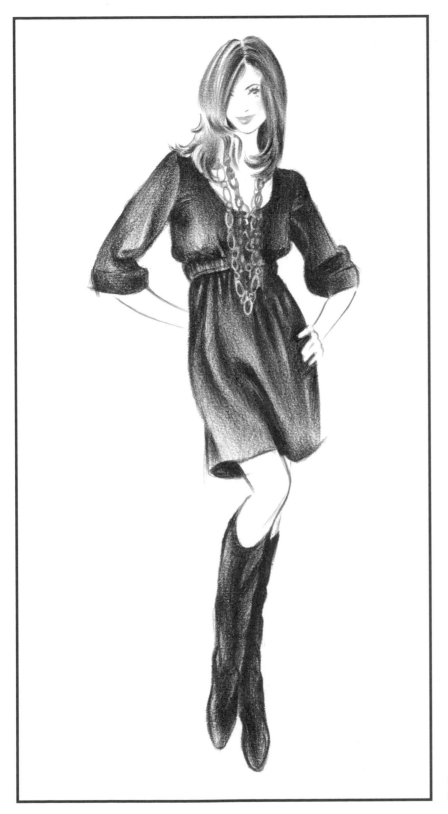

Short dress paired with a relaxed
boot and layered necklaces.

STYLE GUIDE

How to wear skinny jeans

The most flattering way to wear skinny jeans is to pair them with boots. Adding some "weight" around the calves will balance out the hips and make your thighs look slimmer.

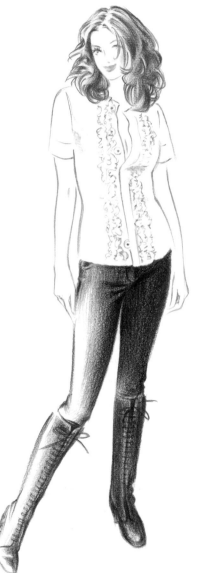

Skinny black jeans worn with fitted ruffled shirt and black boots.

out. For example, simply switch your shoes to a higher heel, add one piece of great jewelry, and use some of the makeup and hair techniques you have learned in this book. When you know that you will be making this kind of quick change at work, bring along a smaller purse. A slim clutch is perfect to hold your lipstick, money, credit cards, and phone, and you can always leave your larger daytime handbag locked in your desk at work or at the coat check of the restaurant.

HOW TO COVER YOUR ARMS WHEN WEARING A SLEEVELESS TOP

If you do not feel comfortable exposing your upper arms but have sleeveless pieces of clothing that you love, a simple and chic solution is to add a shrug. This is basically a sweater for your arms that looks great over a dress or top. Another way to cover your arms, especially in the evening, is by draping a silk or beaded scarf over your shoulders.

CARING FOR LEATHER SHOES AND HANDBAGS

Even the most gorgeous and expensive pair of shoes looks awful with scuffs and worn-down heels. Make no mistake—these are the details that people notice. I have shoes that I bought more than ten years ago that still look good because I have maintained them with regular repairs. Utilizing the services of a good cobbler will keep your footwear looking beautiful for years. Along with an excellent tailor, this person should be an integral part of your fashion support team. Take your favorite shoes and boots in for annual heel replacements and have rubber half-soles put on the bottoms of all brand-new shoes to safeguard them from wear and tear. Well-made shoes and boots cost a fortune, and simple maintenance protects your investment.

TRAVEL TIPS

Look your best for photographs

Unlike photographs taken at events such as weddings or reunions, pictures from a vacation usually do not capture us looking our best. Yet we show them off for years to come. If you know you will be photographed at a special destination or a picturesque spot, make sure that your clothing does not clash with the backdrop. During my trip to India, on the day I visited the Taj Mahal I wore a cream-colored top and scarf that I knew would look great in the photo with the surroundings. This may sound like compulsive planning, but being photographed at one of the wonders of the world is a once-in-a-lifetime experience. I knew that I was going to have those photos forever. You will be thankful for years to come by making sure that at times like these you are wearing something flattering and your hair and makeup look good.

Smart packing tip 1: How to select clothing for travel

Plan ahead and lay out your wardrobe on the bed to begin the "editing" process. I place my shoes on the floor near my potential outfits so that I can mix and match and see how everything works together. Omit items that you can do without to avoid overpacking. Think about ways to maximize what you have by pairing things and layering them, which should allow you to pack even less. For instance, bring a cardigan that can work with a skirt, pants, and a dress. Select a blouse that is versatile enough to go with the pants and the skirts you are bringing. And choose a pair of shoes that look good with all your outfits. Always pack flats for walking and heels for going out to dinner.

Smart packing tip 2: The space-saving, wrinkle-free packing solution

Because I often travel for work, I have gotten packing down to a science. Here is the most effective way to fit more items into carry-on luggage and ensure that they will not be wrinkled upon arrival. Instead of folding each garment, lay them out on top of each other and roll them into one large, compact parcel. Start with one article of clothing and smooth it out on a flat surface. Be sure to smooth away any wrinkles with your hands, since creases will lock into the fabric once it is packed. Place another piece of clothing on top of that one and smooth it out, and so on, stacking them like pancakes until you have assembled a nice flat stack. Fold in the sleeves on top of the pile and carefully roll the entire stack inward, as if it were a yoga mat, into one big roll. Your shoes (tucked in shoe bags) should be placed around the perimeter of your suitcase, with the roll of clothes in the middle. Compress it with your hands before closing the bag. Upon arrival, you will be surprised at how smooth your clothes have remained.

CONCLUSION

Although written over the course of two years, this book has been many years in the making. In effect, you could say that I have been preparing it my whole life. I am honored to have had this opportunity to share twenty-plus years of tried-and-true professional techniques, research, and personal philosophies about beauty and life in general. When it comes to your looks, health, and attitude, my greatest hope is that I was able to inspire you to reach for more, to believe that you can have it, and provide you with the insight and the skills to achieve it. Rather than a conclusion, I like to think of this as a new beginning to an ever-evolving process of learning.

The time spent writing this book has given me so much. In order to articulate a visual craft, I had to break it down into its most rudimentary elements and reconstruct it. This made me even better at what I do, provoking many questions and inspiring me both personally and professionally. I thank you for that and for allowing me to connect with you in this meaningful way.

It has also served as a reminder that the greatest teachers truly honor their profession and thus never stop learning. They have boundless curiosity and a lifelong commitment to education—expanding their own repertoire while inspiring others. Likewise, I still consider myself very much a student. This quest for knowledge motivates me each and every day and allows me to continue sharing all that beauty has to offer.

I hope that I have shown you that creating beauty is not magic and is not about "tricks." It's a combination of having the right professionals in your life and learning a set of skills that you can continue to practice until these routines become a part of your everyday life and, eventually, of who you are. You can then share what you have learned with your friends, your sister, or your daughter. Beauty is a legacy that women pass down to one another, just as some of the lessons that have been handed down by my mentors and role models, as well as the years I spent studying, practicing, and teaching the craft, have laid the groundwork for me to share my experience with you.

I started this book by making a promise to empower you with the knowledge to improve your looks and your health. I now believe more than ever that beauty is not just physical, but a state of mind that shapes your attitude and feeds the energy you exude. This energy influences how you move through the world and how others perceive you. It makes you stand up straighter, smile more, make eye contact, and carry yourself with poise and confidence, opening doors in your life that may have been closed before, or that you did not even know were there. It all begins with a small shift of consciousness that leads to a beautiful transformation.

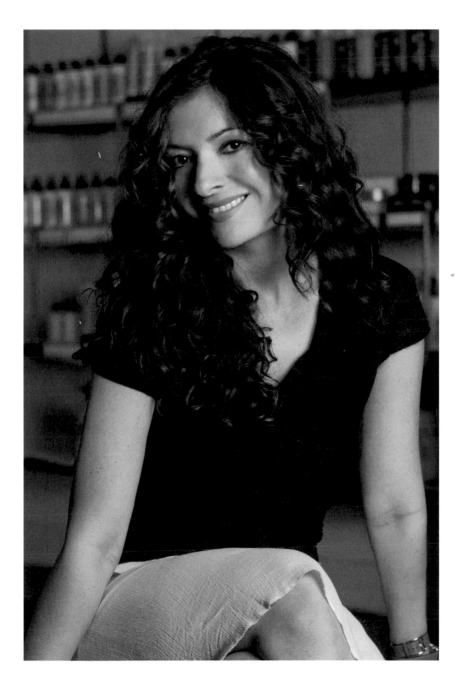

ACKNOWLEDGMENTS

My husband, Arik Efros, for your writing talent, business acumen, and your unparalleled belief in me. Your love, patience, and guidance have brought me to where I am today.

My publisher, Judith Curr, for recognizing that I had this book inside of me. Your belief in my philosophies and artistic vision have given me the latitude to openly express them and share them with others.

My editor, Greer Hendricks, whose exuberance, patience, and faith in my professional judgment have supported me as a first-time author. Thank you for trusting me and teaching me this process. And her assistant editor, Sarah Cantin, for helping to organize this enormous project.

My agent, Robin Straus, for your watchful eye and support.

Kerstin Picht, whose editing skill, made us aware of every nuance.

Martha Stewart, always the visionary, for being the first to put beauty education on the radio.

Irene Azar, for your friendship and insight. You gave me an education that I never dreamt of.

My brother-in-law, Vladimir Efros, for your frequent advice and unwavering belief in my business.

Lynn Blanchard, my best friend and soul sister. For everything we laughed and cried about, and for patiently listening to my stories. Our friendship has been like medicine and our false eyelashes like penicillin!

My sister, Vinnetta, for your support, creativity, and sense of humor. For helping me to build this business and for everything we are to each other today.

Mom, Dad, and Aunt Jan, for always believing in me and supporting the notion that my path in life would be different.

All the stylists and aestheticians who have been a part of my salon. You have pushed me in ways I could not have imagined and made me stronger. I am grateful to have been a mentor to so many who have in turn taught me so much about myself and life in general.

Last, but certainly not least, to all my clients—past and present. Without you none of this would have been possible.

INDEX

Cameron, *5*

Carole, 257, *257*

Carolyn, 256, *256*

catagen phase, 109

"cat eye" liner, 230

chamomile tea, 91, 186, 187

Chanel, Coco, 314

"chemical cut," 62

chemicals, 47, 269

chiropractic care, 288

Christine, *20*

circles, dark, 185

clarifying shampoo, 96, 107

clay mask, 182, 188

climate:

    adjusting haircut for, 36

    and frizz, 105

clips, 119–20, 143

clothes, *see* fashion and style

collagen, 177, 191

color corrector, 219–20

color wheel, 220

combs, 119

comfort, 307

concealer, 218

concealer brush, *211,* 218

conditioning, 97–101

    deep treatments, 97–98

    how much to use, 97

    leave-in, 98, 128

    rinsing out, 99

    salon vs. home treatments, 98–99

    for treated hair, 90–91

    two-in-one shampoo and, 103

cortisol, 277

cortisone shot, 185

cradle cap, 106

cream, styling, 127

cream bronzers, 222

crimping iron, 122–23

crow's feet, 191

cucumber slices, 186, 187

curl cream, 127

curling iron, 122, 123

cuticle (hair), 4

D

dandruff, 107, 108–9

Danyelle, *244*

dermatitis, 108

detox, juice fast, 279

Devin, *74,* 87

diffuser, 141

digestion, and skin, 277

dinner, 276

Donna, *40, 41*

dry cutting, 37–38

dry hair, 104

dry shampoo, 108, 126

duckbill clips, 119, 143

E

Efros, Arik, *viii,* xi–xii

elastics, 120

emollients, 177

Ena, *24*

exercise, 277–78

exfoliation, 177, 186, 193

extensions, 111

eyebrow brushes, *211,* 228